Sugar in the Social Life of Medieval Islam

Islamic Area Studies

VOLUME 1

The titles published in this series are listed at *brill.com/isas*

Sugar in the Social Life of Medieval Islam

By

Tsugitaka Sato

BRILL

LEIDEN | BOSTON

Cover illustration: The *ublūj* at the ʿAjlūn Castle Museum, Jordan (photo taken by the author).

Library of Congress Cataloging-in-Publication Data

Sato, Tsugitaka, 1942-2011
Sugar in the social life of medieval islam / by Tsugitaka Sato.
pages cm. -- (Islamic area studies ; v. 1)
Includes bibliographical references and index.
ISBN 978-90-04-27752-6 (hardback : alk. paper) -- ISBN 978-90-04-28156-1 (e-book) 1. Sugar--Social aspects--Islamic empire. 2. Islamic empire--Social life and customs. I. Title.
GT2869.S28 2015
641.3'36--dc23
2014032287

This publication has been typeset in the multilingual "Brill" typeface. With over 5,100 characters covering Latin, IPA, Greek, and Cyrillic, this typeface is especially suitable for use in the humanities. For more information, please see brill.com/brill-typeface.

ISSN 2214-6555
ISBN 978-90-04-27752-6 (hardback)
ISBN 978-90-04-28156-1 (e-book)

This book is printed on acid-free paper.

Contents

Series Editor's Acknowledgements

This is the second Brill publication written by Professor Tsugitaka Sato, following his previous work, *State and Rural Society in Medieval Islam: Sultans, Muqta's and Fallahun* in 1997. Professor Sato was a prominent scholar of Islamic history, having published a great many articles and books in both Japanese and English since 1967. He was a luminary of Islamic and Middle Eastern studies in Japan, serving as head of the research department at the Toyo Bunko (The Oriental Library) for twenty years, and marshaling two joint-research programs for Islamic Area Studies, one based at the University of Tokyo (1997–2002) and another based at Waseda University (2006–). He planned for the publication of a series of books that explore the dynamics in Islamic areas and beyond. He completed the manuscript for this, the inaugural volume of the series, shortly before his sudden death in April 2011.

Professor Sato was born in Yokohama on August 27, 1942. His parents were farmers, and he himself said that helping out on the family farm naturally fostered his interest in rural society. The first topic that captured his interest was the *iqṭāʿ* system of land management. His research showed that, from the tenth century on, this system moreover served as the core of relations between state and rural societies. His second research interest was the Mamluks, who were given *iqṭāʿ* lands to manage as a source of tax revenue. In 1991, he published a Japanese book titled *Mamlūks: Muslim Rulers from the non-Islamic World*. As the subtitle hints, he was captivated by how the *mamlūk*s, purchased as slaves, rose to become an elite group with political power, which shows intriguing aspects of how Islamic societies accepted and employed "the other". His third interest was local societies, as the intersection of rural, agricultural, and urban networks. He published a history of *The Syrian Coastal Town of Jabala* (1988) in English, and a monograph in Japanese on the legend of wandering saint Sultan Ibrahim, who was buried in Jabala. In 1995, he edited a unique Japanese book focusing on the outlaws of the Islamic world, including a paper of his own about the *ʿayyārūn* in medieval Baghdad.

His fourth interest was the connections between lifestyles and material objects. This culminated in his final publication, *Sugar in the Social Life of Medieval Islam* in Japanese in 2008 (Iwanami Shoten, Tokyo). The book you are reading is the English revised edition. Bringing together a wide variety of historical sources, this work shed light on the production and use of sugar in the Middle East, previously a lacuna in the world history of sugar. His interest in sugar originated with research he did on sugar production and taxation in the

Fayyūm region, a rural Egyptian society. For more than forty years, he gathered information from medical and pharmaceutical texts, cookery books, literary works, and other historical sources, and hand-wrote it onto index cards, a practice he maintained even after the advent of personal computers. This book is a testament to both his inquisitive mind and his patience in hunting down source materials to "draw a single picture" from fragmentary facts, as he was fond of saying. A bibliography of Professor Sato's works is included in my paper "Professor Sato Tsugitaka and His Achievements", in *Memoirs of the Research Department of the Toyo Bunko*, vol.69 (2011).

I would like to express our gratitude to Professor Kentaro Sato at Hokkaido University for his diligent efforts in checking over the entire manuscript the author left behind, and proofreading it in cooperation with Jeff Gedert. This book could not have been published without their careful work. With the consent of Setsuko Sato, the author's wife and pillar of support for nearly forty years, we have changed the order of family name and given name, from Sato Tsugitaka in his previous book, to Tsugitaka Sato in this book. Professor Sato firmly embraced the long-standing tradition in Japan and other East Asian countries that authors put their family names first, even when writing for publication in English. However, this can lead to confusion among scholars and librarians unfamiliar with the convention when referring to the family and given names of Japanese scholars. In the pursuit of clarity and consistency, the editorial committee has decided to adopt a uniform *family name comes last* arrangement for all names, including Japanese, European, and Middle Eastern names.

Sato, the Japanese word for sugar, is homophonic with author's family name, though their meanings are different. Professor Sato often joked that he was writing Sato's book on *sato*. He must be pleased with this publication, drinking a toast to it in paradise, which according to Buddhist traditions is located in the west.

Toru Miura
Series Editor
Ochanomizu University, Tokyo, 15 May, 2014

Preface

On 16 June 2006, just after the Second World Congress for Middle Eastern Studies (WOCMES2) in Amman had concluded, my Japanese colleagues and I made a short trip to the old city of ʿAjlūn in North Jordan. Syrian geographer al-Dimashqī (654–727/1256–1327) once described ʿAjlūn as having a robust fortress (*ḥiṣn*) and numerous fruits trees irrigated by a river that runs through the city (*Nukhbat al-Dahr*, Petersburg, 1866; repr. Osnabrück, 1982, 200). Ibn Baṭṭūṭa (d. 770/1368–9 or 779/1377) also described ʿAjlūn as a beautiful city with many markets and a strong citadel (*qalʿa*) (*Tuḥfat al-Nuẓẓār*, Paris, 1854; repr. 1969, I, 129).

As we walked through the castle museum there, I found myself transfixed in front of a case displaying an *ublūj*, a cone-shaped piece of unglazed earthenware pottery. The *ublūj* (pl. *abālīj*) was about 30 centimeters in height and maximum diameter, and had three small holes at the bottom. It was designed to separate out sugar from molasses. This was a rare and precious experience to see an *ublūj* in person. When I described my experience in ʿAjlūn to Doctor Mutsuo Kawatoko (Director, Institute of Islamic Archaeology in Tokyo), he explained that he had found a similar type of *ublūj* in his excavations in al-Fusṭāṭ, and kindly made pristine photocopies for me. According to Professor Christian Daniels, a specialist in the history of sugar production in China, this type of earthenware separating device has as yet never been found in any part of China.

I first gave a presentation about the spread of sugar production through the Islamic world back in 1985 at the Institute for the Study of Languages and Cultures of Asia and Africa, a division of the Tokyo University of Foreign Studies. It took me quite a while to compile the book you are reading, partly because my attention was diverted by the history of the Mamluks, the sufi legend of Sultan Ibrāhīm b. Adham, and the states and kingship of medieval Islam. But the main reason for the delay seems to have been that details about the history of sugar resided in a daunting variety of sources, including Arabic language chronicles, urban histories, geographies, travel accounts, biographies, medical books, and pharmacological sources. It is no light task to locate within these voluminous primary sources and then extract the few accounts of sugarcane cultivation, sugar production, sugar trade, and sugar as medicine.

This book mainly covers from the time sugarcane cultivation expanded from India to Iran and Iraq in the seventh century to the decline of sugar production in Egypt and Syria in the fifteenth century. It attempts to show what Muslim societies were like in the medieval ages, focusing on sugarcane cultivation, sugar production technologies, and sugar as a commodity, a medicine, and a festival treat. The primary sources used for this study were Arabic and Persian books, as well as Arabic manuscripts. The details of these sources are thoroughly discussed in the Prologue. The research on the Arabic manuscripts was done in the years 1969–70, 1974, 1984, 1986–87, 1988, 1992, 1993–94, 1996, 1999, 2001, 2003, 2005, 2006, 2007, and 2010 under funding from the University of Tokyo, the Japanese Ministry of Education, Science, Culture, and Technology, the Japan Foundation, the Toyo Bunko (Oriental Library), and Waseda University.

My thanks go out to the staff of Dār al-Kutub al-Miṣrīya in Cairo, Maktabat al-Ẓāhirīya & Maktabat al-Asad in Damascus, Süleymaniye Kütüphanesi in Istanbul, the Bibliothèque Nationale in Paris, the British Library in London, and the Institute of Oriental Studies in St. Petersburg for their kind help and advice in the course of my study of the Arabic manuscripts. I would also like to acknowledge my debt to Professor Muḥammad Aafif (Muḥammad V University), Professor Abdul-Karim Rafeq (The College of William and Mary), Dr. Mutsuo Kawatoko (The Institute of Islamic Archaeology), Mr. Ḥāfiẓ Fatḥī (Cairo branch of the Institute of Islamic Archaeology), Professor Yuzo Shitomi (The University of Tokyo), Associate Professor Kentaro Sato (Organization for Islamic Area Studies, Waseda University), Professor Christian Daniels (Institute for the Study of Languages and Cultures of Asia and Africa, Tokyo University of Foreign Studies), and Associate Professor Kikuko Suzuki (National Defence Academy of Japan), all of whom served as sources of invaluable information on the history of sugar.

I also express my sincere gratitude to Professor Bruce D. Craig, for inviting me to the University of Chicago to give a lecture entitled "Sugar in the Economic Life of Mamluk Egypt" in May of 2003. This encouraged me to complete my study of the history of sugar in the Islamic world and finish writing this book, which was initially released in Japanese under the title *Sato no Isuramu seikatsushi* (*Sugar in the Social Life of Medieval Islam*) in December 2008. With the goal of a revised and enlarged edition, I then started to translate it into English with the help of Jeff Gedert, to whom I am much obliged for his careful proofreading of the manuscript. Last but not least, I could never have written this book without the warm encouragement and understanding of my colleagues at Waseda University's Organization for Islamic Area Studies.

Tsugitaka Sato
Waseda University, 15 October, 2010

List of Abbreviations

Annales: ESC	*Annales: Économies, Sociétés, Civilisations*
AI	*Annales Islamologiques*
BEO	*Bulletin d'Études Orientales de l'Institut Français de Damas*
BGA	*Bibliotheca Geographorum Arabicorum, 8 vols., Leiden, 1870–94; repr., Leiden, 1967.*
BSOAS	*Bulletin of the School of Oriental and African Studies*
BSRGE	*Bulletin de la Société Royale de Géographie d'Égypte*
EI^2	*The Encyclopaedia of Islam, new edition, Leiden, 1954–2004.*
IC	*Islamic Culture*
IJMES	*International Journal of Middle East Studies*
JAOS	*Journal of the American Oriental Society*
JESHO	*Journal of the Economic and Social History of the Orient*
REI	*Revue des Études Islamiques*
SI	*Studia Islamica*

Transliteration of Arabic and Persian

The following list shows the Roman equivalents of the Arabic and Persian letters used in the text.

ʾ, b, p, t, th, j, ch, ḥ, kh, d, dh, r, z, zh, s, sh, ṣ, ḍ, ṭ, ẓ,
ʿ, gh, f, q, k, g, l, m, n, w, h, y, ā, ī, ū, aw, ay, īy

The Arabic definite article and the Persian ezāfe are always represented by al- and -i respectively. Words commonly cited in English (e.g. Damascus, Jerusalem, Mecca, sultan, amir, qadi) are generally not transliterated except to denote official posts such as Ṣāḥib Dimashq and Nāʾib al-Quds.

List of Figures and Map

Figures

Map

Prologue

Islamic Social History through Sugar

From the time of its invention, refined sugar has been a part of our day-to-day life. Sugar was first produced from sugarcane plants in northern India sometime after the first century. Over the centuries, sugar spread both eastward and westward. Eastward, sugarcane cultivation travelled slowly, passing through southeast China in the Ming and Qing periods, and finally arriving in Okinawa Japan in the early seventeenth century.

But westward, it leaped from country to country. It is believed that by the mid-seventh century sugarcane was already being grown in both Iran and Iraq at the end of the Sasanian period (224–651). Abū ʿUthmān ʿAmr al-Jāḥiẓ (d. 255/868–9), an ʿAbbasid writer from al-Baṣra, relates that the district of Ahwāz, being irrigated by the Dujayl River in western Iran, was particularly well known as a major producer of sugar (*sukkar*), silk brocade (*al-dībāj al-khazz*), as well as various kinds of dates (*tamr*), condensed juice (*dibs*),[1] and raw sugar (*qand*).[2] According to Andrew M. Watson, sugar production spread from western Iran to southern Iraq, further to the Jordan valley, and up the coast of Syria, arriving in Bāniyās around the tenth century.[3]

The first reference to sugarcane as a crop in Egypt comes from a papyrus from the mid-eighth century.[4] According to D. Müller-Wodarg, sugarcane cultivation expanded further in ninth century Egypt.[5] However, the main sugarcane-producing districts noted in the Arabic sources up to the end of the eleventh century were mostly limited to the outskirts of al-Fusṭāṭ and the villages of Lower Egypt. So, it wasn't until the eleventh-twelfth centuries that sugarcane plantations on a large scale spread to Upper Egypt, as well as the Mediterranean islands, Maghrib, and Andalusia. The Iberian Christians brought the sugar production techniques they had learned from the Muslims to the New World. They established numerous large sugarcane plantations in the Caribbean islands and Brazil in the sixteenth century, employing a large number of black slaves from Africa.

1 For *dibs* as sweetener, see Chapter Three (1. The Prosperity of al-Karkh in Baghdad).

2 Al-Jāḥiẓ, *Kitāb al-Tabaṣṣur bil-Tijāra*, ed. H.A. al-Tūnisī, Cairo, 1935, 32–33.

3 A.M. Watson, *Agricultural Innovation in the Early Islamic World*, Cambridge, 1983, p. 26.

4 Watson, *Agricultural Innovation*, p. 28.

5 D. Müller-Wodarg, "Die Landwirtschaft Ägyptens in der frühen ʿAbbasidenzeit," *Der Islam*, 32 (1956), pp. 47–48.

 | DOI 10.1163/9789004281561_002

The Arabic word for sugar is *sukkar*. This is adapted from the Persian word *shakar*, which in turn comes from *sharkarā* in Sanskrit. The Crusaders, who first tasted the distinctive sweetness of sugar in Syria and Egypt, brought it back to Europe with them in the twelfth-thirteenth centuries. It is widely known that the terms *sugar* in English, *sucre* in French, and *Zucker* in German, all adapted from *sukkar*, became commonplace among upper class Europeans in the medieval period. In the Ayyubid and Mamluk eras, Egyptian sugar was sold in large quantities, alongside spices and crops, to Italian merchants arriving at Alexandria. Thus, sugar became a staple commodity traded between Europe and the Islamic world in the twelfth century.

What can we learn about Muslim societies by studying sugar in Islamic history? Growing sugarcane required advanced farming techniques. The technologies to refine raw sugar (*qand*) improved. Refined sugar was used as a medicine and as a treat during certain festivals, and was a valuable trading commodity. So, examing the multiple facets of sugar, we can see the realities of everyday life in Muslim societies, such as the technological innovations needed for sugar production, the conduct of sugar merchants, and the medical effects of sugar to prevent and treat diseases. We can also see some other interesting sides of sugar, how it was given as gifts by caliphs and sultans during Ramaḍān and for pilgrimages to Mecca, and how it was sold as candy at annual festivals during the sacred months.

Sugar in Arabic Literature: Favorite Sweets

Compared to honey and the traditional thick syrup made from ripe fruits, the newly appearing sugar was a sweetener of a much higher purity. Let me first cite a passage by an Arab scholar in the early Islamic period. Abū Ḥanīfa al-Dīnawarī (d. 282/895) gives the following account of sugarcane and sugar in his *Botanical Dictionary* (*Kitāb al-Nabāt*).

> Sugarcane (*qaṣab al-sukkar*) is classified by color into three varieties: white, yellow, and black. Of these, the black variety is not pressed, due to its thin and barren nature, unsuitable even for a shroud (*kaffān*). The pressed juice from the white and yellow canes is called the "honey of the cane" (*ʿaṣal al-qaṣab*), the best of which comes from cane from Zanj (East Africa), producing a lemon yellow colored juice. The pressed juice is solidified to produce raw sugar (*qand*), and then, refined sugar (*sukkar*).[6]

6 Al-Dīnawarī, *Kitāb al-Nabāt*, II, ed. Muḥammad Ḥamīdullāh, Cairo, 1973, 211–212. See also al-Badrī, *Nuzhat al-Anām fī Maḥāsin al-Shām*, Beirut, 1980, 210; M. Ouerfelli, *Le sucre: production,*

As I will explain later, raw sugar, which is brown in color, is generally made by separating out the black molasses from boiled sugarcane juice, and refined sugar is made by boiling liquified raw sugar twice. In the passage above, sugar made from *qand* seems to indicate this kind of refined sugar.

In *The Thousand and One Nights* we find the following questions and answers in an exchange between Ibrāhīm al-Naẓẓām (d. ca. 845), a poet of the ʿAbbasid court, and Tawaddud, a female slave accomplished in the Islamic arts and sciences.

> Next, tell me what it is that a poet describes as follows:
> Its legs are slender, and its taste is quite sweet.
> It is shaped like a spear, but has no head.
> Everyone loves it.
> We often chew on it after sunset during Ramaḍān."
> She answered, "It is *qaṣab al-sukkar*."[7]

This story seems to have originated in Iraq around the ninth or tenth century,[8] and refers, interestingly enough, to the close association of *qaṣab al-sukkar* with the month of Ramaḍān. We will revisit this topic later on.

In 567/1171, as a rift between Nūr al-Dīn in Damascus and Ṣalāḥ al-Dīn in Egypt deepend, Najm al-Dīn Ayyūb, Ṣalāḥ al-Dīn's father, spoke to his son as follows.

> By God, if Nūr al-Dīn wanted a piece of sugarcane (*qaṣab al-sukkar*) [from Egypt], I myself would fight until death to stop him.[9]

Although Najm al-Dīn had sought a reconciliation between Ṣalāḥ al-Dīn and Nūr al-Dīn, this passage reveals he himself was prepared to fight Nūr al-Dīn if necessary. Next, I will cite a poem by Ibn al-ʿAdīm (588–660/1192–1262) that refers to sugar.

---

commercialisation et usages dans la Méditerranée médiévale, Leiden and Boston, 2008, p. 143.

7 Anon., *Alf Layla wa-Layla*, 2 vols., Bulaq, 1252H., I, 634 (The Four Hundred and Sixtieth Night). The story is not included in the Arabic text edited by M. Mahdi (*Kitāb Alf Layla wa-Layla*, Leiden, 1984).

8 Some scholars regard this story as being of tenth-century Iraqi origin, while the others think it originated in Egypt in the Ayyubid period (the thirteenth century) (U. Marzolph and R. van Leeuwen, *The Arabian Nights Encyclopedia*, 2 vols., Santa Barbara, 2004, I, pp. 408–410).

9 Ibn al-Athīr, *al-Kāmil fī al-Taʾrīkh*, ed. C.J. Tornberg, 12 vols., Leiden, 1853; repr. Beirut, 1965–66, XI, 373.

You see, I aged fifty years or more,
as mistaking bdellium (*muql*) for hazel-nut (*bunduq*)
or salt (*milḥ*) for sugar (*sukkar*).[10]

Reflecting back on his more than fifty years, Ibn al-ʿAdīm, a qadi in Aleppo, seems to have thought his life as much a chance as mistaking salt for sugar. In 658/1260, he fled to Cairo during the Mongol invasion of Aleppo. When he returned home to Aleppo the following year, he found it in ruins, slaughtered and pillaged by the Mongol armies.[11] Having witnessed such tragedy, he felt the need to include the above poem in his book on Arabic cuisine *al-Wuṣla ilā al-Ḥabīb.*

And lastly, Najm al-Dīn Hāshim al-Baʿlabakkī (d. 733/1331), a jurist (*faqīh*) in Damascus, composed the following poem about sugar.

I heard from you an account of sugar,
which you must make repeatedly.
I suppose that sugar is sweet and tasty,
but I've never tasted it personally.[12]

The second line "you must make repeatedly" might mean that one should produce fine sugar through repeated refining. The examples cited above show that sugar, specifically white sugar, was as a symbol of personal excellence. We will revisit the appearances of sugar in *Alf Layla wa-Layla* again in Chapter Seven.

Historical Overview and Perspectives

Since it was first produced in around the first century of the common era, the sweet taste of sugar has garnered a great deal of attention. There have been a good number of studies done on the history of sugar in ancient and medieval times. Since it is impossible for me to cover all these studies, I will only cite the works required to understand the aims of this book.

---

10 Ibn al-ʿAdīm, *al-Wuṣla ilā al-Ḥabīb fī Waṣf al-Ṭayyibāt wal-Ṭayyib*, ed. S. Maḥbūb and D. al-Khaṭīb, 2 vols., Aleppo, 1986–88, I, 315.

11 *EI*², s.v. Ibn al-ʿAdīm (B. Lewis); Ibn Shākir al-Kutubī, *Fawāt al-Wafayāt*, ed. I. ʿAbbās, 5 vols., Beirut, 1973–74, III, 126–129.

12 Ibn al-Jazarī, *Taʾrīkh Ḥawādith al-Zamān wa-Anbāʾih*, ed. U.A. Tadmurī, 3 vols., Beirut, 1998, II, 494.

First, I will look at Edmund O. von Lippmann's pioneering work *Geschichte des Zuckers*,[13] which uses the source materials known to nineteenth century Europeans (including Arabic and Persian texts translated into European languages) to trace the history of sugar production across the globe. The book often refers to sugar production in the Islamic world. However, one drawback to this elaborate work is that when he finds a single account of sugarcane cultivation in a given district, he writes as if sugar refining was wide-spread there. *The History of Sugar* by Noel Deerr[14] is a voluminous work that delineates the spread of sugarcane and sugar production through medieval Islamic countries and the early modern New World. It also refers to the appearance of beet sugar in Europe at the end of the eighteenth century. He states that sugar production spread to other countries immediately following the Arab conquests, but this argument flies in the face of descriptions found in contemporary Arabic sources. Helmut Blume's *Geography of Sugar Cane* is a geographic study of sugarcane. However, regarding the spread of sugarcane throughout the world, he relies on the above-mentioned inaccurate description by von Lippmann. Moreover, he mistakenly states that this kind of agricultural work only truly developed in the medieval Levant after it was captured by the Crusaders.[15]

Sweetness and Power by Sidney W. Mintz is quite useful for understanding the history of sugar production, the increase in sugar consumption in modern Europe, and the relationship between "sweetness and power", as he puts it.[16] However, he is obviously mistaken in assuming that slavery played an important role in sugar production in the medieval Islamic world.[17] Minoru Kawakita, who translated *Sweetness and Power* into Japanese,[18] also asserts a close relationship between sugar and slavery in Muslim societies,[19] a view I will later refute based on contemporary Arabic sources.

While these studies represent the main works on sugar production and consumption in Europe from the sixteenth century on, we also find several important studies on sugar's journey eastward to China. *The Evolution of Sugar*

---

13 E.O. von Lippmann, *Geschichte des Zuckers*, Leipzig, 1890.

14 N. Deerr, *The History of Sugar*, 2 vols., London, 1949–50.

15 H. Blume, *Geography of Sugar Cane*, Berlin, 1985, p. 164. As I mention in Chapter Three, sugar production in the Islamic world developed mostly in Egypt during the eleventh-fourteenth centuries, not in the Levant after the conquest of the Crusaders.

16 S.W. Mintz, *Sweetness and Power: The Place of Sugar in Modern History*, New York, 1985.

17 Mintz, *Sweetness and Power*, p. 27.

18 *Amasa to kenryoku: Sato ga kataru kindaishi* (in Japanese), tr. by M. Kawakita and K. Wada, Tokyo, 1988.

19 M. Kawakita, *A World History of Sugar* (*Sato no sekaishi*, in Japanese), Tokyo, 1996, p. 16.

Production in China by Kokuki Tai[20] is a work that taught me the importance of research on the production of sugar. It shows, based on original Chinese sources, the origins of sugarcane as a crop, the expansion of sugarcane since the Song dynasty, and further developments in sugar production technologies during the Ming and Qing dynasties. Christian Daniels's *Agro-Industries: Sugarcane Technology*, his contribution to the massive work *Science and Civilization in China*, is a monumental historical study of sugar in China, fastidiously detailing the evolution of sugarcane and sugar technologies, and culled from a vast array of original sources.[21] It provides a treasure trove of data for comparative studies with sugar technologies in the Islamic world. Elsewhere, Sucheta Mazumdar describes, in her also voluminous work *Sugar and Society in China: Peasants, Technology, and the World Market*,[22] how the relationship between landlords and peasants in China was transformed by the integration of sugar as a global commodity in the Ming and Qing periods.

Regarding Japanese sugar production in the Amami Islands and Okinawa, *Wind and Earthenware: An Account of Sugar* by Toyotoshi Matsuura[23] provides detailed information based on his personal experiences with sugar production in Okinawa. He gives a deliberate explanation of how white sugar was produced from boiled sugar juice in pre-modern China and Japan. As I will explain later, in the Islamic world, white sugar was made using a cone-shaped piece of earthenware pottery, for which Matsuura notes a lack of information. The recent work *A Cultural History of Sugar*, edited by Hiroshi Ito,[24] is an anthology recounting the assorted roles of sugar in Japan since the early modern period.

What is the current state of research on sugar in the Islamic world? We can cite *Le sucre en Égypte* by Jean Mazuel[25] among a small number of historical works on sugar in the Islamic world from Iran to Andalusia. Although he does give an historical overview of manual sugar production in Egypt, his main focus is on the mechanized sugar production of the ninteenth and twentieth centuries. Another work, *Les anciennes sucreries du Maroc et leur réseaux*

20 K. Tai, *The Evolution of Sugar Production in China* (*Chūgoku Kansho-togyo no tenkai*, in Japanese), Tokyo, 1967.

21 C. Daniels, *Science and Civilization in China* (Joseph Needham). Vol. 6, Biology and Biological Technology, part III, *Agro-Industries: Sugarcane Technology*, Cambridge, 1996.

22 S. Mazumdar, *Sugar and Society in China: Peasants, Technology, and the World Market*, Cambridge, Mass., 1998.

23 T. Matsuura, *Wind and Earthenware: An Account of Sugar* (*Kaze to Kame: Sato no Hanashi*, in Japanese), Fukuoka, 1987.

24 H. Ito ed., *A Cultural History of Sugar: Japanese and Sugar* (*Sato no bunkashi: Nihonjin to sato*, in Japanese), Tokyo, 2008.

25 J. Mazuel, *Le sucre en Égypte: étude de géographie historique et économique*, Cairo, 1937.

hydrauliques by Paul Berthier,[26] is based on documentary and archeological evidence, and suits our purposes in examining the history of sugar in Islamic countries beyond Morocco. The source materials cited here, however, are limited to Arabic books translated into French or English.

Agricultural Innovation in the Early Islamic World by Andrew M. Watson[27] is an indispensable work. Based on contemporary Arabic source materials, it describes the expansion of new crops such as rice, cotton, sugarcane, eggplants, watermelons, bananas, oranges, and lemons. However, only seven pages including plates are spared to discuss sugarcane plantations and sugar production, not enough to fully elucidate sugar as a commodity, a medicine, and a festival offering. In *Handelsgeschichte Ägyptens im Spätmittelalter*, Subhi Y. Labib provides us with valuable accounts of the sugar trade in Ayyubid and Mamluk Egypt,[28] while Eliyahu Ashtor reveals the technological decline of the Levantine sugar industry in the late middle ages.[29] In my own article "Sugar in the Economic Life of Mamluk Egypt,"[30] a preliminary study for the present work, I discuss the origins and expansion of sugar production, the development of the related technologies, and the significance of sugar as a commodity, a medicine, and a festival offering in Mamluk Egypt. We also find works in Arabic that mention sugarcane and sugar in medieval Egypt and Syria. Unfortunately, most of these works offer only a few pages of passing descriptions without delving fully into the original Arabic sources.[31]

More recently, a wonderful work by Mohamed Ouerfelli entitled *Le sucre: Production, commercialisation et usages dans la Méditerranée médiévale* was

---

26 P. Berthier, *Les anciennes sucreries du Maroc et leur réseaux hydrauliques*, 2 vols., Rabat, 1966.

27 Watson, *Agricultural Innovation*.

28 S.Y. Labib, *Handelsgeschichte Ägyptens im Spätmittelalter* (1171–1517), Wiesbaden, 1965.

29 E. Ashtor, "Levantine Sugar Industry in the Late Middle Ages: A Case of Technological Decline," A.L. Udovitch ed., *The Islamic Middle East, 700–1900*, Princeton, 1981, pp. 91–132.

30 T. Sato, "Sugar in the Economic Life of Mamluk Egypt," *Mamlūk Studies Review*, 8–2 (2004), pp. 87–107. For sugar production under the *iqṭāʿ* system, see also T. Sato, *State and Rural Society in Medieval Islam: Sultans, Muqtaʿs and Fallahun*, Leiden, 1997, pp. 210–220.

31 M.J. Surūr, *Dawlat Banī Qalāwūn fī Miṣr: al-Ḥālat al-Siyāsīya wal-Iqtiṣādīya fī ʿAhdihā bi-Wajh Khāṣṣ*, Cairo, 1947, pp. 319–320; S.A. ʿĀshūr, *al-Mujtamaʿ al-Miṣrī fī ʿAṣr Salāṭīn al-Mamālīk*, Cairo, 1962, pp. 178, 184, 187, 189; A.M. ʿAbd al-Raḥmān, *Marākiz al-Ṣināʿa fī Miṣr al-Islāmīya*, Cairo, 1989, pp. 24–25, 70–71; S.T.S. Abū Sadīra, *al-Ḥiraf wal-Ṣināʿāt fī Miṣr al-Islāmīya*, Cairo, 1991, pp. 354–363; S.A.M. ʿAbd Allāh, *Mudun Miṣr al-Ṣināʿīya fī al-ʿAṣr al-Islāmī*, Cairo, 2000, pp. 185–192; Sh.I.I. al-Juʿaydī, *al-Azamāt wal-Awbiʾa fī Miṣr fī ʿAṣr al-Mamālīk al-Jarākisa*, Alexandria, 2002, pp. 111–113, 198–199; A.N.M. Nāṣir, *al-Ḥayāt al-Iqtiṣādīya fī Miṣr fī al-ʿAṣr al-Mamlūkī*, Amman, 2003, pp. 257–261; Y.H. Ghawānima, *Dimashq fī ʿAṣr Dawlat al-Mamālīk al-Thāniya*, Beirut, 2005, p. 121.

published.[32] It is the first examination of the entire history of sugar, focusing on sugar production technologies, domestic and international sugar trade, and sugar consumption in the medieval Mediterranean world. Nevertheless, we can still identify points for further careful examination: (1) Although ample information is provided on sugar in the Mediterranean world, the situations in Iran and Iraq are not necessarily discussed in full. Also, the thorough account of Egyptian sugar production provided by al-Nuwayrī requires a more detailed analysis. (2) The *ublūj* (a cone-shaped earthenware device) had a crucial role in the refining of sugar, but the author does not give a concrete explanation about how it was used. (3) The *Dār al-Qand* (the storehouse for raw sugar) in al-Fusṭāṭ, which played an important role in the tax revenue levied upon raw sugar carried in from various districts, is not examined in detail. Also, the personal name "al-Nashw" of a Coptic bureaucrat is mistaken for a managerial position title. (4) The contemporary Arabic sources can give us a better understanding of the relationship between "sugar and power," showing examples of sugar as offerings at festivals, sugar given as gifts from caliphs and sultans during Ramaḍān, and sugar used in various banquets held by sultans in the Ayyubid and Mamluk periods.

Summing up these studies to date, we find the topics of sugar plantations in the New World from the sixteenth century on, and the refining, trade, and consumption of sugar in Europe have been thoroughly examined using contemporary source materials, as have sugarcane cultivation and sugar production in medieval and early modern China. But for the Islamic areas that fall between Europe, East Asia, and the Mediterranean Sea, we lack a sufficient study of the origins and expansion of sugarcane, the development of sugar-making technologies, the sugar trade, and the relationship between the "sweetness and power" of sugar. So, based on primary sources in Arabic and Persian, I intend to delineate aspects of social life in medieval Islam by examining sugarcane as a crop, sugar production technologies, and also sugar as a commodity, a medicine, and a festival offering. Taken together, these findings should facilitate a comprehensive understanding of the interactions of East Asia, Islam, the Mediterranean Sea, Europe, and even the New World.

Primary Sources in Arabic and Persian

The primary sources used for this study were printed books in Arabic and Persian, and hand-written manuscripts in Arabic. These sources, listed in the

32 Ouerfelli, *Le sucre*.

bibliography, include geographies, topographies, travel books, encyclopedias, biographies, literary works, agricultural, pharmacological, and cooking references, as well as chronicles, and urban and regional histories. The content and nature of the main Arabic and Persian sources are examined in the pages that follow.

First, regarding the situations in Iran and Iraq in the early Islamic period, there are Arabic books on geography that give us some details about the production and consumption of sugar. For example, Shams al-Dīn Muḥammad al-Muqaddasī (fourth/tenth century), an Arabic geographer from Jerusalem, provides us with ample and reliable information on sugar production in the Islamic world (*Aqālīm al-Islām*) in the second half of the tenth century.[33] Abū al-Qāsim Ibn Ḥawqal al-Naṣībī (fourth/tenth century), a geographer from North Iraq and contemporary of al-Muqaddasī, compiled a unique geographical book entitled *Kitāb Ṣūrat al-Arḍ* based on his travels as a merchant through Egypt, Maghrib, and Andalusia.[34] His account includes useful information about sugarcane cultivation and sugar production in the early Islamic period. Both he and al-Muqaddasī collected their data personally. Abū ʿAbd Allāh Muḥammad al-Sharīf al-Idrīsī (493–560/1100–65), born in Ceuta and raised in Córdoba, wrote a descriptive geography entitled *Kitāb Nuzhat al-Mushtāq fī Ikhtirāq al-Āfāq*. It was dedicated to Roger II, the Norman king of Sicily.[35] The book, which was completed in 548/1154, presents ample information on sugar production in Egypt, Syria, and other regions around the Mediterranean Sea, but curiously enough, omits sugar in Sicily, where al-Idrīsī lived for many years until his death in 560/1165.

In Egypt after the Arab conquest in the second half of the seventh century, there appeared a tradition of compiling topographies (*khiṭaṭ*) to record the histories of the settled districts of Lower and Upper Egypt.[36] Ibrāhīm Ibn Duqmāq al-ʿAlāʾī (d. 809/1406), for example, wrote a book entitled *Kitāb al-Intiṣār li-Wāsiṭat ʿIqd al-Amṣār*, which gives us invaluable information on the owners and managers of sugar refineries (*maṭbakh al-sukkar*), mainly those located in al-Fusṭāṭ[37] One of his disciples, Taqī al-Dīn Aḥmad al-Maqrīzī (ca.766–845/

33 Al-Muqaddasī, *Aḥsan al-Taqāsīm fī Maʿrifat al-Aqālīm*, BGA. III, ed. M.J. de Goeje, Leiden, 1906; English tr. by B. Collins, *The Best Divisions for Knowledge of the Regions*, Reading, 2001.

34 Ibn Ḥawqal, *Kitāb Ṣūrat al-Arḍ*, BGA, II, ed. J.H. Krammers, 3rd ed., Leiden, 1967; French tr. by J.H. Krammers and G. Wiet, *Configuration de la terre*, 2 vols., Paris, 1964.

35 Al-Idrīsī, *Kitāb Nuzhat al-Mushtāq fī Ikhtirāq al-Āfāq*, 9 vols., Napoli-Roma, 1970–84.

36 M.A. ʿInān, *Miṣr al-Islāmīya wa-Taʾrīkh al-Khiṭaṭ al-Miṣrīya*, Cairo, 1969; B. Lewis and P.M. Holt ed., *Historians of the Middle East*, London, 1962, pp. 412–413.

37 Ibn Duqmāq, *Kitāb al-Intiṣār li-Wāsiṭat ʿIqd al-Amṣār*, ed. K. Vollers, 2 vols., Cairo, 1893.

ca.1364–1442) born in Cairo, compiled the voluminous work *Kitāb al-Mawāʿiẓ wal-Iʿtibār bi-Dhikr al-Khiṭaṭ wal-Āthār* by gathering together previous records of Egyptian topographies.[38] The book provides us with detailed and vivid accounts of sugarcane pressing factories (*maʿṣara li-qaṣab al-sukkar*), sugar refineries, sugar exports to Italian merchants, and sugar candies (*ḥalawī*) for Cairene children sold during the Mamluk period.[39] Another of his works, *Kitāb al-Sulūk li-Maʿrifat Duwal al-Mulūk*, is a chronicle of the Ayyubid and Mamluk dynasties up until 844/1440.[40] It gives us actual accounts of social and economic activities related to sugar production and consumption in Egypt. Moreover, al-Maqrīzī wrote a small book entitled *Kitāb Ighāthat al-Umma bi-Kashf al-Ghumma*, which criticizes the Mamluk regime by revealing flaws in both *iqṭāʿ* holdings and monetary systems closely tied to the sugar economy in medieval Egyptian society.[41]

From around the tenth century, the Islamic world came to know various travel accounts (*riḥla*) of pilgrimages to Mecca. For example, two well-known travelers, Muḥammad Ibn Jubayr al-Andalusī[42] (540–614/1145–1217) and Abū ʿAbd Allāh Muḥammad Ibn Baṭṭūṭa al-Lawātī [43] (703–770 or 779/1304–1368–9 or 1377), initially intended to make the pilgrimage to Mecca, but expanded their travels to include other Islamic lands. Their travel accounts are also quite useful in helping us understand sugarcane cultivation and sugar production as practiced in thirteenth-fourteenth century Egypt and Syria. Abū Muʿīn Nāṣir Khusraw (394 – between 465 and 471/1004 – between 1072 and 78) from Balkh, who visited Cairo under the Fatimids in 439/1047, wrote a travel account upon

---

38 Al-Maqrīzī, *Kitāb al-Mawāʿiẓ wal-Iʿtibār bi-Dhikr al-Khiṭaṭ wal-Āthār*, 2 vols., Bulaq, 1270H.; repr. Baghdad, 1970. *Fihrist Khiṭaṭ Miṣr* by A.A. Harīdī, 3 vols., Cairo, 1983–84.

39 For works by al-Maqrīzī, see the following references. ʿInān, *Miṣr al-Islāmīya wa-Taʾrīkh al-Khiṭaṭ al-Miṣrīya*, pp. 49–63; D.P. Little, *An Introduction to Mamluk Historiography*, Wiesbaden, 1970, pp. 76–80; M.M. Ziyāda etc., *Dirāsāt ʿan al-Maqrīzī*, Cairo, 1971; N.O. Rabbat, "al-Maqrizi's Khitat, an Egyptian *Lieu de Mémoire*," D. Behrens-Abouseif ed., *The Cairo Heritage*, Cairo, 2000, pp. 17–30.

40 Al-Maqrīzī, *Kitāb al-Sulūk li-Maʿrifat Duwal al-Mulūk*, ed. M.M. Ziyāda, vols. 1–2, Cairo, 1939–58; ed. S.A. ʿĀshūr, vols. 3–4, Cairo, 1970–73.

41 Al-Maqrīzī, *Kitāb Ighāthat al-Umma bi-Kashf al-Ghumma*, ed. M.M. Ziyāda and J. al-Shayyāl, Cairo, 1940; English tr. by A. Allouche, *Mamluk Economics*, Salt Lake City, 1994. For al-Maqrīzī's argument, see Sato, *State and Rural Society*, pp.237–239.

42 Ibn Jubayr, *Riḥlat Ibn Jubayr*, Beirut, 1964; English tr. by R. Broadhurst, *The Travels of Ibn Jubayr*, London, 1952.

43 Ibn Baṭṭūṭa, *Tuḥfat al-Nuẓẓār fī Gharāʾib al-Amṣār*, Arabic text and French tr. by C. Défremery and B.R. Sanguinetti, *Voyages d'Ibn Battûta*, 4 vols., Paris, 1854; repr. Paris, 1969; English tr. by H.A.R. Gibb, *The Travels of Ibn Baṭṭūṭa*, 3 vols., Cambridge, 1956–71.

returning home under the Persian title *Safar Nāma*.[44] The book vividly relates how the Fatimid Caliph, al-Mustanṣir (reigned 427–487/1036–94), used large quantities of sugar for festivals during Ramaḍān.

In regards to the fiscal régime of Egypt, we can first cite *Minhāj fī ʿIlm Kharāj Miṣr* by Abū al-Ḥasan ʿAlī al-Makhzūmī (d. 585/1189).[45] According to Claude Cahen,[46] al-Makhzūmī presents more useful information from his firsthand experience in the fiscal administration of Egypt than does his contemporary, Asʿad Ibn Mammātī (d. 606/1209), who provides a rather methodical account in his *Kitāb Qawānīn al-Dawāwīn*.[47] After completing a detailed survey of al-Fayyūm province in Upper Egypt in the years 641–642/1243–44, Ayyubid government official Abū ʿAmr ʿUthmān al-Nābulusī (d. 660/1261)[48] submitted a report entitled *Taʾrīkh al-Fayyūm wa-Bilādih* to Sultan al-Ṣāliḥ (reigned 637–647/1240–49). This book provides us with uniquely specific insights into one hundred villages in the province, including the amount of sugarcane grown, the revenues generated, the other kinds of crops grown, the irrigation rights granted, and depictions of rural districts.

Among the Arabic chronicles, al-Maqrīzī's above-mentioned *Kitāb al-Sulūk* provides the most information on sugarcane, sugar production, and the sugar trade. Islamic historical chronicles generally focus on the achievements of caliphs and sultans; but Maqrīzī's chronicle is abundant in its accounts of social life in fourteenth-fifteenth century Egypt. Having worked repeatedly as a market inspector (*muḥtasib*) in Cairo, al-Maqrīzī can provide us with detailed descriptions of sales and purchases of sugar and sugar candies. The chronicles of Abū al-Maḥāsin Ibn Taghrībirdī (ca. 812–874/ca. 1409–1470),[49] a member of the *awlād al-nās* (the male progeny of *mamlūk* military elite), and Badr al-Dīn al-ʿAynī (762–855/1361–1451)[50] from the town of ʿAynṭāb also give useful information on the production of sugar in Mamluk Egypt and Syria. We further note

44 Nāṣir Khusraw, *Safar Nāma*, Berlin, 1340 H. For the career and works of Nāṣir Khusraw, see A.C. Hunsberger, *Nasir Khusraw, The Ruby of Badakhshan: A Portrait of the Persian Poet, Traveller and Philosopher*, London, 2000.

45 Al-Makhzūmī, *Minhāj fī ʿIlm Kharāj Miṣr*, London, British Library, MS. Add. 23483. Partly ed. by Cl. Cahen, *al-Muntaqā min Kitāb al-Minhāj fī ʿIlm Kharāj Miṣr*, Cairo, 1986.

46 *EI*², s.v. al-Makhzūmī. See also Cl. Cahen, *Makhzūmiyyāt*, Leiden, 1977.

47 Ibn Mammātī, *Kitāb Qawānīn al-Dawāwīn*, ed. A.S. Atiya, Cairo, 1943.

48 Al-Nābulusī, *Taʾrīkh al-Fayyūm wa-Bilādih*, ed. B. Moritz, Cairo, 1898; repr. Beirut, 1974.

49 Ibn Taghrībirdī, *al-Nujūm al-Zāhira fī Mulūk Miṣr wal-Qāhira*, vols. 1–12, Cairo, 1963; vols. 13–16, ed. F.M. Shaltūt etc., Cairo, 1970–72; English tr. by W. Popper, *History of Egypt 1382–1469 AD*, 10 vols., Berkeley, 1954–63.

50 Al-ʿAynī, *ʿIqd al-Jumān fī Taʾrīkh Ahl al-Zamān: ʿAṣr Salāṭīn al-Mamālīk*, ed. M.M. Amīn, 4 vols., Cairo, 1987–1992.

that the chronicle of Shams al-Dīn Ibn al-Jazarī (d. 738/1338)[51] provides us with various accounts of sugar production and consumption in Syria during the early Mamluk period. The biographical chronicle of Sultan al-Nāṣir's reign was penned by Mūsā al-Yūsufī (d. 759/1358),[52] a commander in the al-Ḥalqa al-Manṣūra army under the Mamluks. This is also quite notable for providing us with reliable information on the production and commerce of sugar at the apex of the Mamluk state.

Among the encyclopedists living in the Mamluk period, I will first cite Aḥmad al-Nuwayrī (677–733/1279–1333). His major work *Nihāyat al-Arab fī Funūn al-Adab* took seventeen years to complete and was divided into five parts: (1) Heaven and Earth, (2) Human Beings, (3) Animals, (4) Plants, and (5) History.[53] One chapter in the second part (vol. 8 in the edited book) thoroughly recounts observations of sugarcane grown and sugar produced in the district of Qūṣ in Upper Egypt, making this a unique and important account of the sugar industry in thirteenth-fourteenth century Egypt. A couple other encyclopedias, *Masālik al-Abṣār fī Mamālik al-Amṣār* by Ibn Faḍl Allāh al-ʿUmarī (700–749/1301–49)[54] and *Ṣubh al-Aʿshā fī Ṣināʿat al-Inshāʾ* by Shihāb al-Dīn al-Qalqashandī (756–821/1355–1418),[55] both of which were used to educate Mamluk bureaucrats, give us still more accounts of sugar production and sugar trade in Egypt and Syria. Moreover, we should consult biographical dictionaries to examine the careers of sugar traders and *Kārimī* merchants. For example, *Kitāb al-Wāfī bil-Wafayāt* by Ibn Aybak al-Ṣafadī (696–764/1297–1363),[56] *al-Durar al-Kāmina fī Aʿyān al-Miʾat al-Thāmina* by Ibn Ḥajar al-ʿAsqalānī (773–852/1372–1449),[57] and *al-Manhal al-Ṣāfī wal-Mustawfī baʿda al-Wāfī* by Ibn

51 Ibn al-Jazarī, *Taʾrīkh Ḥawādith al-Zamān*.

52 Al-Yūsufī, *Nuzhat al-Nāẓir fī Sīrat al-Malik al-Nāṣir*, ed. A. Ḥuṭayṭ, Beirut, 1986.

53 Al-Nuwayrī, *Nihāyat al-Arab fī Funūn al-Adab*, vols. 1–18, Cairo, 1954; ed. M.M. Amīn etc., vols. 19–33, Cairo, 1975–97.

54 Al-ʿUmarī, *Masālik al-Abṣār fī Mamālik al-Amṣār*, Istanbul, Topı Kapı Saray Müzesi, Yeni Kütüphanesi, MS. Ahmed III 2797-a3; *Masālik al-Abṣār fī Mamālik al-Amṣār: Mamālik Miṣr wal-Shām wal-Ḥijāz wal-Yaman*, ed. A.F. Sayyid, Cairo, 1985; *Masālik al-Abṣār fī Mamālik al-Amṣār: Qabāʾil al-ʿArab fī al-Qarnayn al-Sābiʿ wal-Thāmin al-Hijrīyayn*, ed. D. Krawulsky, Beirut, 1985; *Masālik al-Abṣār fī Mamālik al-Amṣār: Dawlat al-Mamālīk al-Ūlā*, ed. D. Krawulsky, Beirut, 1986.

55 Al-Qalqashandī, *Ṣubḥ al-Aʿshā fī Ṣināʿat al-Inshāʾ*, 14 vols., Cairo, 1963; *Fahāris Kitāb Ṣubḥ al-Aʿshāʾ*, Cairo, 1972.

56 Al-Ṣafadī, *Kitāb al-Wāfī bil-Wafayāt*, ed. S. Dedering etc., vols. 31vols., Wiesbaden, 1949–2010.

57 Ibn Ḥajar, *al-Durar al-Kāmina fī Aʿyān al-Miʾat al-Thāmina*, ed. M.S. Jād al-Ḥaqq, 5 vols., Cairo, 1966–67.

Taghrībirdī.[58] These provide us with ample information on mosques, schools, hospitals, and sufi convents built by wealthy merchants to promote social welfare (*maṣlaḥa*).

And finally, I will cite several works on agriculture, medicine, pharmacology, nutrition, and health maintenance. *Kitāb al-Filāḥat al-Nabaṭīya* was originally translated from Syriac into Arabic, and Ibn Waḥshīya (4/10 c.) subsequently added accounts of conditions in Syria and Iraq. More recently, Tawfīq Fahd published a critical edition in three volumes, mainly based on manuscripts from Istanbul.[59] The book has plenty of information about sugar production, but its generalized descriptions make it difficult to identify the exact locations where sugarcane was grown and sugar was made. *Kitāb al-Filāḥat al-Musulimīn al-Andalusīyīn* by Abū Zakariyā Yaḥyā Ibn al-ʿAwwām (6–7/12–13 c.) from Sevilla is also quite a useful reference on the realities of sugarcane cultivation in Islamic Andalusia.[60] ʿAbd Allāh Ibn al-Bayṭār al-Andalusī (d. 646/1248) was born in Málaga at the end of the twelfth century, and in around 617/1220 travelled across North Africa to the eastern Islamic world. Upon his arrival in Cairo, he was appointed as the head of all Egyptian pharmocologists by Sultan al-Kāmil al-Ayyūbī (reigned 615–635/1218–38). His major pharmacopoeial work *al-Jāmiʿ li-Mufradāt al-Adwiya* includes an entry for "*sukkar*" wherein the various medical effects of sugar are explained citing the views of authoritative medical doctors through history.[61] Ibn al-Nafīs al-Dimashqī (d. 687/1288), personal physician to Sultan Baybars I (reigned 658–676 /1260–77) and known as "a second Ibn Sīnā," wrote a voluminous work entitled *Shāmil fī al-Ṣināʿat al-Ṭibbīya*, in which he gives systematic and specific descriptions of sugar as a medicine in the medieval Islamic world. He is also unique in explaining the production processes for various kinds of sugar more precisely than the previous Arab authorities.[62]

Regarding works on sugar for nourishment and to maintain health, Ibn Buṭlān (d. 458/1066), a Christian physician in Baghdad, is noted for compiling

---

58 Ibn Taghrībirdī, *al-Manhal al-Ṣāfī wal-Mustawfī baʿda al-Wāfī*, ed. M.M. Amīn etc. 12 vols., Cairo, 1956–2006.

59 Ibn Waḥshīya, *al-Filāḥat al-Nabaṭīya*, ed. T. Fahd, 3 vols., Damascus, 1993–98.

60 Ibn al-ʿAwwām, *Kitāb al-Filāḥat al-Musulimīn al-Andalusīyīn*, Paris, Bibliothèque Nationale, MS. Arabe 2804.

61 Ibn al-Bayṭār, *al-Jāmiʿ li Mufradāt al-Adwiya wal-Aghdhiya*, 4 vols., Bulaq, 1874; repr. Baghdad, n. d.

62 Ibn al-Nafīs, *al-Shāmil fī al-Ṣināʿat al-Ṭibbīya*, 30 vols., Abu Dhabi, n.d. For the life of Ibn al-Nafīs, see *EI*^{2}, s.v. Ibn al-Nafīs (M. Meyerhof-[J. Schacht]); M. Ulmann, *Islamic Medicine*, Edinburgh, 1978, pp. 68–69; L. Chipman, *The World of Pharmacy and Pharmacists in Mamlūk Cairo*, Leiden, 2010, pp. 123–124.

a basic manual on health maintenance (*Taqwīm al-Ṣiḥḥa*) that includes an index of 280 health-related items such as edibles, dishes, drinks, spices, lifestyles, and living enviroments. H. Elkhadem edited the Arabic text and translated it into French with careful annotations.[63] Ibn Riḍwān al-Miṣrī (388–460/998–1068), a suitable rival to Ibn Buṭlān, composed *The Prevention of Bodily Ills* (*Kitāb Dafʿ Maḍār al-Abdān*), which provides us with the valuable insight that the common people of Upper Egypt became consumers of sweets produced from cheap raw sugar (*qand*) and molasses (*ʿasal*) in the early eleventh century.[64] And, Ibn al-Quff al-Karakī (630–685/1233–86), who was born in the citadel city of al-Karak in south Syria, compiled a book on health maintenance and disease prevention entitled *Jāmiʿ al-Gharaḍ fī Ḥifẓ al-Ṣiḥḥa wa-Dafʿ al-Maraḍ*, wherein he presents more than 250 recipes, including those for many kinds of sweets and sweetened meat dishes.[65] We can compare the accounts provided by these authors with those in *The Book of Nourishments* (*Kitāb al-Aghdhiya*) by Ibn Khalṣūn al-Andalusī (7/13 c.) in almost the same period.[66]

63 Ibn Buṭlān, *Taqwīm al-Ṣiḥḥa*, Arabic text and French tr. by H. Elkhadem, *Le Taqwīm al-Ṣiḥḥa* (*Tacuini Sanitatis*) *d'Ibn Buṭlān*, Leuven, 1990.

64 Ibn Riḍwān, ʿAlī b. Riḍwān al-Ṭabīb al-Miṣrī, *Kitāb Dafʿ Maḍār al-Abdān*, Arabic text ed. by A.S. Gamal and English tr. by M.W. Dols, London, 1984.

65 Ibn al-Quff, *Jāmiʿ al-Gharaḍ fī Ḥifẓ al-Ṣiḥḥa wa-Dafʿ al-Maraḍ*, ed. S. Kh. al-Ḥamārna, Amman, 1989. For the career and works of Ibn al-Quff, see S. Kh. Hamarneh, *The Physician, Therapist and Surgeon Ibn al-Quff*, Cairo, 1974.

66 Ibn Khalṣūn, *Kitāb al-Aghdhiya*, Arabic text and French tr. by S. Gigandet, Damascus, 1996.

CHAPTER 1

The Origin and Expansion of Sugar Production in the Islamic World

The Origin of Sugar Production and its Expansion to West Asia

The Origin of Sugarcane Cultivation

Wild sugarcane plants, indigwenous to India and Southeast Asia, were hybridized in New Guinea to create a domesticated plant variety called *Saccharum Officinarum* in Latin (denoting "sugar of a druggist"). Sugarcane is a perennial large grass, two to four meters high, with its widest stalks up to four centimeters in diameter. Domesticated sugarcane plants hybridized in New Guinea were introduced into Indonesia, Malaysia, India, and South China during the last several centuries BC. This type of sugarcane, which was previously thought to have first appeared in India and then spread to neighboring regions, is now thought to have originated in southern New Guinea.

Allow me to quote some viewpoints on this issue. E.O. von Lippmann, who pioneered the historical study of global sugar production, has said that sugarcane clearly originated from Northeast India, specifically from the Bengal province.[1] Yet, Sucheta Mazumdar, an historian of sugar production in modern China, is careful not to identify a point of origin, stating that sugarcane growing was introduced into South China sometime after the third century BC by way of Southeast Asia or East India.[2]

However, Noel Deerr, the author of *The History of Sugar*, believed that sugarcane originated in New Guinea and spread to Southeast Asia, India, and China.[3] Andrew M. Watson also held that early domestication and hybridization may have occurred in the New Guinea region,[4] while Christian Daniels says that shifting agriculturalists of Southeast Asia, Indonesia, Melanesia, and Polynesia planted sugarcane in mixed gardens in prehistoric times.[5] Although its true origin is still uncertain, sugarcane cultivation is generally considered to have originated somewhere between New Guinea and Indonesia, a few centuries BC. From these early times, through long after the systemization of sugar

1 Lippmann, *Geschichte des Zuckers*, p. 39.
2 Mazumdar, *Sugar and Society in China*, p. 15.
3 Deerr, *The History of Sugar*, vol. 1, p. 16.
4 Watson, *Agricultural Innovation*, p. 24.
5 Daniels, *Agro-Industries: Sugarcane Technology*, p. 191.

 | DOI 10.1163/9789004281561_003

manufacturing, raw sugarcane was chewed and sucked for its sweet taste, or cooked and eaten.[6]

The Origin of Sugar Production

So then, when and where did sugarcane cultivation for sugar production originate? First, Deerr refers to *The Geography of Strabo*: He (Nearchus – an admiral in Alexander the Great's army) also states, concerning the reeds, that they produce honey, although there are no bees, and in fact that there is a fruit-bearing tree from the fruit of which honey is compounded, but that those who eat the fruit raw become intoxicated.[7] Minoru Kawakita, based on this description, further explained that Alexander's soldiers were delighted when they discovered this solid honey, not made by bees, in North India.[8] But it should be noted that Nearchus only states "reeds that produce honey", not referring to "solid honey" or "sugar candy". Furthermore, Sidney W. Mintz, in his book *Sweetness and Power*, raises serious questions about Deerr's interpretation of this (Nearchus's statement) as a reference to sugar cane, but his citations of Greek and Roman authorities are not entirely convincing.[9]

According to Mintz, *Materia Medica* by Dioscorides (a Roman herbalist in the first century) reads: "There is a kind of concreted honey, called saccharon, found in reeds in India and Arabia Felix (now Yemen), like in consistence to salt, and brittle to be broken between the teeth, as salt is. It is good for the belly and the stomach being dissolved in water and so drank, helping the pained bladder and the reins."[10] However, Mintz also notes: "Some students of sugar history suppose that saccharon referred to an entirely different substance, the so-called sugar of bamboo, a gum that accumulates in the stems of certain bamboos and has a sweet taste."[11] When we re-read this sentence in *Materia Medica*, it describes "a kind of concreted honey, called saccharon, found in reeds", not saccharon made of reeds. So, this description is not enough to lead to the conclusion that a method for producing granulated sugar crystals from boiled sugar juice originated around the first century AD.

---

6 Watson, *Agricultural Innovation*, p. 24.

7 Deerr, *The History of Sugar*, vol. 1, p. 63. For an English translation of the geographic book by Strabo (64 or 63 BC–ca. 23 AD), see *The Geography of Strabo*, ed. & tr. H.L. Jones, London and New York, 1917–32, vol. 7, p. 33.

8 M. Kawakita, *A World History of Sugar*, p. 14.

9 Mintz, *Sweetness and Power*, p. 20.

10 Mintz, *Sweetness and Power*, p. 20. See also English translation by R.T. Gunther, *The Greek Herbal of Dioscorides*, London, 1968, p. 125.

11 Mintz, *Sweetness and Power*, p. 20.

On the other hand, von Lippmann, based on an account that the Funan Kingdom at the south end of the Ganges River forwarded sugarcane [not sugar] to the Chinese Emperor in the year 286 AD, speculates that sugar production originated in India after the third century.[12] However, Funan was not actually located at the south end of the Ganges River in India, but rather at the lower reaches of Mekong in Viet Nam. Daniels does not draw a clear conclusion on this point, stating that sugarcane cultivation for sugar production seems to have initiated in northern India.[13]

Thus, although the precise time when sugar production originated also remains uncertain, we may conclude that a method for manufacturing crystal-form sugar began in north India sometime after the first century, and after Dioscorides.

The Eastward Route: Expansion from India to China and Okinawa

Sugarcane cultivation for sugar production expanded from North India to both the East and the West. Eastward, sugarcane was centered in southern China, in such regions as Kuang-tung, Kuang Xi, and Annan, in the early fourth century BC. It was during the Tang dynasty that the process for making granulated sugar crystals *sha tang* 沙糖 was introduced from India into China. Previously, solidified molasses *shi mi* 石蜜 had been made by simply setting the boiled juice in direct sunlight.[14] Legend says, "In Samarqand, when a child is born, his parents put solidified molasses in his mouth and glue on his hand. The parents do this so that when the child becomes an adult, he will use sweet words, and will always have coins in his hand."

Daniels relates that this is also extremely important for the light it sheds upon the transmission of sugar production technology from India to China via the medium of Buddhist monks during the Tang dynasty (ninth–tenth centuries).[15] Mazumdar has the same view, stating that commercial sugar production for wide circulation started during the Song dynasty, while in the preceding Tang dynasty, sugar was used exclusively for medicine and festival goods.[16]

It is said that sugar was first introduced to Japan by the Chinese Buddhist priest, Jianzhen 鑑真 (688–763); however, we lack the exact source materials to confirm this fact. Regardless, it is certain that ambassadors to the Tang dynasty

---

12 Lippmann, *Geschichte des Zuckers*, p. 49.

13 Daniels, *Agro-Industries: Sugarcane Technology*, p. 191.

14 Tai, *The Evolution of Sugar Production in China*, pp. 9–23.

15 Daniels, *Agro-Industries: Sugarcane Technology*, p. 288.

16 Mazumdar, *Sugar and Society in China*, pp. 15–33.

and Buddhist priests brought some amount of Chinese-produced sugar with them to Japan. During the Muromachi period (fourteenth–fifteenth centuries), sugar imports from Ming China flourished, and as the Japanese tea ceremony gained popularity among the upper classes, the use of sugar in confections also increased. However, growing sugarcane for sugar in Okinawa and the Amami Islands only began after the formation of the Tokugawa Shogunate. It is likely that Gima Shinjo 儀間真常 , a farmer of royal descent, who had learned how to make sugar in the Fujian province of China, began producing brown sugar (sugar with molasses content) in Ryukyu (now Okinawa) in 1623, using techniques that were brought to the Amami Islands at the end of the seventeenth century. In any case, white sugar separated from molasses was not produced in Okinawa or the Amami Islands, even after the Meiji Restoration in the latter half of the nineteenth century.[17]

The Westward Route: Expansion from India to Iran

Westward, sugarcane was grown for sugar beginning in pre-Islamic Iran under the rule of the Sasanid dynasty (226–651). However, the available source materials are not necessarily sufficient to verify this fact, as von Lippmann supposes that Christians in Gundishapur (an old city in south-west Iran during the Sasanids) expanded sugarcane cultivation and developed sugar production there.[18] But, Berthold Laufer contradicts this sharply, "This is no more than an ingenious speculation, which, however, is not substantiated by any documents."[19] Yet, al-Muqaddasī, an Arab geographer in the tenth century, states, "Jundīsābūr (Gundishapur) was the prosperous, old capital city of the province, but now it has perished. The Kurds overcame it, bringing discrimination and disturbances; as before, there is still abundant sugar (*kathīrat al-sukkar*) in this province."[20] This clearly shows that Gundishapur had a long-standing tradition of making sugar since, at least, the early Islamic period.

Laufer, who criticized von Lippmann, takes the Sui Annals compiled in seventh century China as reliable source material, which attributes *shi-mi* (hard sugar, literally "stone honey") and *ban-mi* ("half honey") to Sasanian Persia and

17 For the history of sugar in Japan, see the following works. Matsuura, *Wind and Earthenware*; S. Naga, *A History of Black Sugar as Seen from the Source Materials in Okinawa and Amami* (*Okinawa-Amami no Bunken kara mita Kurozato no Rekishi*, in Japanese), Naha, 2003; H. Hashimoto and A. Takada ed., *Science of Sugar* (*Sato no Kagaku*, in Japanese), Tokyo, 2006.

18 Lippmann,*Geschichte des Zuckers*, p. 93.

19 B. Laufer, *Sino-Iranica: Chinese Contributions to the History of Civilization in Ancient Iran*, Chicago, 1919; repr. Taipei, 1973, p. 376.

20 Al-Muqaddasī, *Aḥsan al-Taqāsīm*, 408.

to Ts'ao.[21] *Ban-mi* probably refers to a half-dried, soft sugar. Watson also considers the accounts in the Sui Annals reliable, and concludes that sugarcane was probably grown in Iran for some decades before the Arab conquest in 642.[22] On the other hand, Mintz refers to a report by the Byzantine emperor Heraclius in 627, where sugar is described as an "Indian" luxury. But, Mintz vaguely suggests, "Between the fourth and eighth centuries, the major sugar production centers seem to have been the coast to the west of the Indus delta, and the head of the Persian Gulf, on the Tigris-Euphrates delta."[23] I note the following account by Abū al-ʿAbbās Aḥmad al-Balādhurī (d. ca. 279/892).

> When Caliph ʿUmar b. al-Khaṭṭāb conquered al-Sawād (Iraq) in 16/637, ʿUthmān b. Ḥunayḥ surveyed the cultivated fields, and levied 10 dirhams on each jarīb (about 1600 m^2) of date palms (*nakhl*), 10 dirhams on each jarīb of grapes (*karm*), 6 dirhams on each jarīb of sugarcane (*qaṣab*), 4 dirhams on each jarīb of wheat (*burr*), and 2 dirhams on each jarīb of barley (*qamḥ*). ʿUthmān wrote this to ʿUmar, who approved it.[24]

This account demonstrates that sugarcane for making sugar had been grown in the province of al-Sawād before the Arab conquest in the first half of the seventh century. As the tax revenue on sugarcane was higher than that on the important crop of wheat, we can infer that sugarcane in Iraq was cultivated not to obtain juice for drinking, but for making sugar.

The Expansion of Sugarcane Cultivation from Iran to Egypt

The Expansion from Iran to Iraq

Little is known about sugarcane cultivation during the Sasanid Dynasty period. However, as the Islamic period began, accounts of sugarcane in Iran and Iraq increased considerably. Legend says that the Muslims of the Arabian Peninsula brought sugarcane to the lands they invaded in the seventh and eighth centuries, introducing the plant in Iraq, Syria, Maghrib, Andalusia, and the Mediterranean islands. However, as Watson notes, though this legend may be true, no

21 Laufer, *Sino-Iranica*, p. 376. Ts'ao was a union of states formed in Samarqand by the Sogdians.

22 Watson, *Agricultural Innovation*, p. 160.

23 Mintz, *Sweetness and Power*, p. 23.

24 Al-Balādhurī, *Futūḥ al-Buldān*, ed. A.A. al-Ṭabbāʿ and U.A. al-Ṭabbāʿ, Beirut, 1957, 376.

part of it seems to be based on established facts.[25] Here, based on geographical works compiled in Arabic and Persian from around the tenth century, we will describe the expansion of sugarcane grown for making sugar from Iran to Iraq.

Sugarcane was called *qaṣab al-sukkar*, and also *al-qaṣab al-fārisī*[26] in Arabic, which suggests that the Arabs considered sugarcane a plant inherited from Persia. In the early Islamic period, *Tabaṣṣur bil-Tijāra* written by Abū ʿUthmān ʿAmr al-Jāḥiẓ (ca. 160–255/ca.776–868–9) gives us the first account of sugar production in Iran. He notes special products in the province of Ahwāz such as sugar (*sukkar*), dates (*tamr*), fruit-based syrup (*dibs*), and raw sugar (*qand*).[27] Ahwāz in the district of Khūzistān was favored with ample irrigation water for sugarcane cultivation coming from the Dujayl River, and a suitable climate with high temperatures and high humidity.[28] Abū al-Ṭayyib Aḥmad al-Mutanabbī (303–354/915–965), a famous Arab poet born in al-Kūfa, praises the hard sugar crystal produced in Ahwāz.

> Even though our enemies could crush coal and iron,
> They can never crush sugar crystal made in Ahwāz.[29]

Abū ʿAbd Allāh Muḥammad al-Jahshiyārī (d. 331/942), a politician who had a role in the ʿAbbasid administraion, reports in his *Kitāb al-Wuzarāʾ wal-Kuttāb* the annual state income of each province during the reign of Hārūn al-Rashīd (reigned 170–193/786–809).[30] According to that source, two Persian provinces paid sugar in kind: 30,000 raṭl (68,250 kilograms) of sugar (*sukkar*) from Ahwāz, and 20,000 raṭl (45,500 kilograms) of white sugar (*fānīdh*) from Sijistān.[31] In addition, *Kitāb Ṣūrat al-Arḍ* by Ibn Ḥawqal (fourth/tenth century) and *Aḥsan al-Taqāsīm* by al-Muqaddasī both relate that sugarcane cultivation was particularly brisk in Jubba and Sūs in the province of Khūzistān, as well as in the province of Fārs.[32] *Ḥudūd al-ʿĀlam* (compiled in 372/982), an anonymous work in Persian, states that ʿAskar Mukram is a prosperous town, where enough red and white sugar (*shakar*) and raw sugar (*qand*) are produced to meet the de-

---

25 Watson, *Agricultural Innovation*, p. 160.

26 For example, see al-Muqaddasī, *Aḥsan al-Taqāsīm*, 188.

27 Al-Jāḥiẓ, *Tabaṣṣur bil-Tijāra*, 32–33.

28 For the sugar production in Ahwāz, see also P. Schwarz, "Die Zuckerpressen von Ahwāz," *Der Islam*, 6 (1916), pp. 269–279.

29 Al-Mutanabbī, *Dīwān Abī al-Ṭayyib al-Mutanabbī*, ed. A. ʿAzzām, Cairo, 1944, 189.

30 Al-Jahshiyārī, *Kitāb al-Wuzarāʾ wal-Kuttāb*, ed. M. al-Saqā, I. al-Abyārī, and A. Shalabī, Cairo, 1938, 281–288.

31 Al-Jahshiyārī, *Kitāb al-Wuzarāʾ*, 282–283.

32 Ibn Ḥawqal, *Kitāb Ṣūrat al-Arḍ*, 254, 257; al-Muqaddasī, *Aḥsan al-Taqāsīm*, 402, 405, 424.

mands of the entire world.[33] According to Yāqūt al-Rūmī al-Ḥamawī (d. 626/1229), an ex-slave geographer born in Byzantine territory, "'Māsakān white sugar' (*al-fānīdh al-māsakānī*) was named after the province of Māsakān adjacent to Mukrān beyond Sijistān. This is praised as the highest quality white sugar, and *fānīdh* is a type of sugar not produced outside Mukrān, from where this sugar is distributed throughout the country."[34]

Thus, sugar production in Iran from the ninth to the twelfth centuries was concentrated from south-western to southern and south-eastern Iran in Khūzistān, Sijistān, Fārs, Māsakān, and Mukrān.

But what about sugar production in Iraq? As mentioned above, sugar production had already begun in the province of al-Sawād at the end of the Sasanid dynasty. Ibn Ḥawqal in the tenth century stated that there was no village in Iraq without sugarcane crops,[35] and al-Muqaddasī in the same period also reported that Sinjār produces commercial goods such as almonds (*lawz*), pomegranates (*rummān*), sugarcane (*qaṣab*), and sumac (*summāq*).[36] As Sinjār is near Mosul, that area may be the northern limit for sugarcane growing in Iraq. *Al-Filāḥat al-Nabaṭīya* by Ibn Wahshīya (fourth/tenth century) gives no account of sugarcane crops in Iraq, but does list various ways that sugar is used in cooking and medical treatment. For example, Ibn Wahshīya explains that the green seeds of terebinth (*buṭm*) are crushed and drunk together with sugar and wine to greatly increase sexual desire.[37]

According to Zakariyā' al-Qazwīnī (d. 682/1283), an Arab geographer in the thirteenth century, Ṭīzanabād (west to al-Kūfa) was surrounded by grape and fruit tree orchards, caravansaries (*khān*), and sugar pressing factories (*maʿṣara*).[38] Further, Ibn Saʿīd al-Maghribī (d. 673/1274 or 685/1286), born in Granada, compiled accounts of his travels in the Eastern world, in which he describes dates from al-Baṣra, and rice (*aruzz*) and sugarcane from al-Baṭā'iḥ (the great swamp) as being particularly cheap in Baghdad (before the Mongol invasion).[39] To sum up, in Iraqi plains irrigated by the Tigris and the Euphrates, sugarcane cultivation expanded considerably from the seventh century, centering on the fertile regions of al-Sawād.

---

33 Anon., *Ḥudūd al-ʿĀlam*, Tehran, 1962, 138; English translation and commentary V. Minorsky, *Ḥudūd al-ʿĀlam: The Regions of the World*, London, 1970, 130. Here Minorsky mistranslates the Arabic and Persian term '*qand*' as 'refined sugar.'

34 Yāqūt, *Muʿjam al-Buldān*, 5vols., Beirut, 1957, V, 42.

35 Ibn Ḥawqal, *Kitāb Ṣūrat al-Arḍ*, 254.

36 Al-Muqaddasī, *Aḥsan al-Taqāsīm*, 145.

37 Ibn Waḥshīya, *al-Filāḥat al-Nabaṭīya*, I, 162.

38 Al-Qazwīnī, *Āthār al-Bilād wa-Akhbār al-ʿIbād*, Beirut, 1960, 417–418.

39 Ibn Saʿīd al-Maghribī, *Kitāb al-Jughrāfiyā*, ed. I. al-ʿArabī, Beirut, 1970, 158.

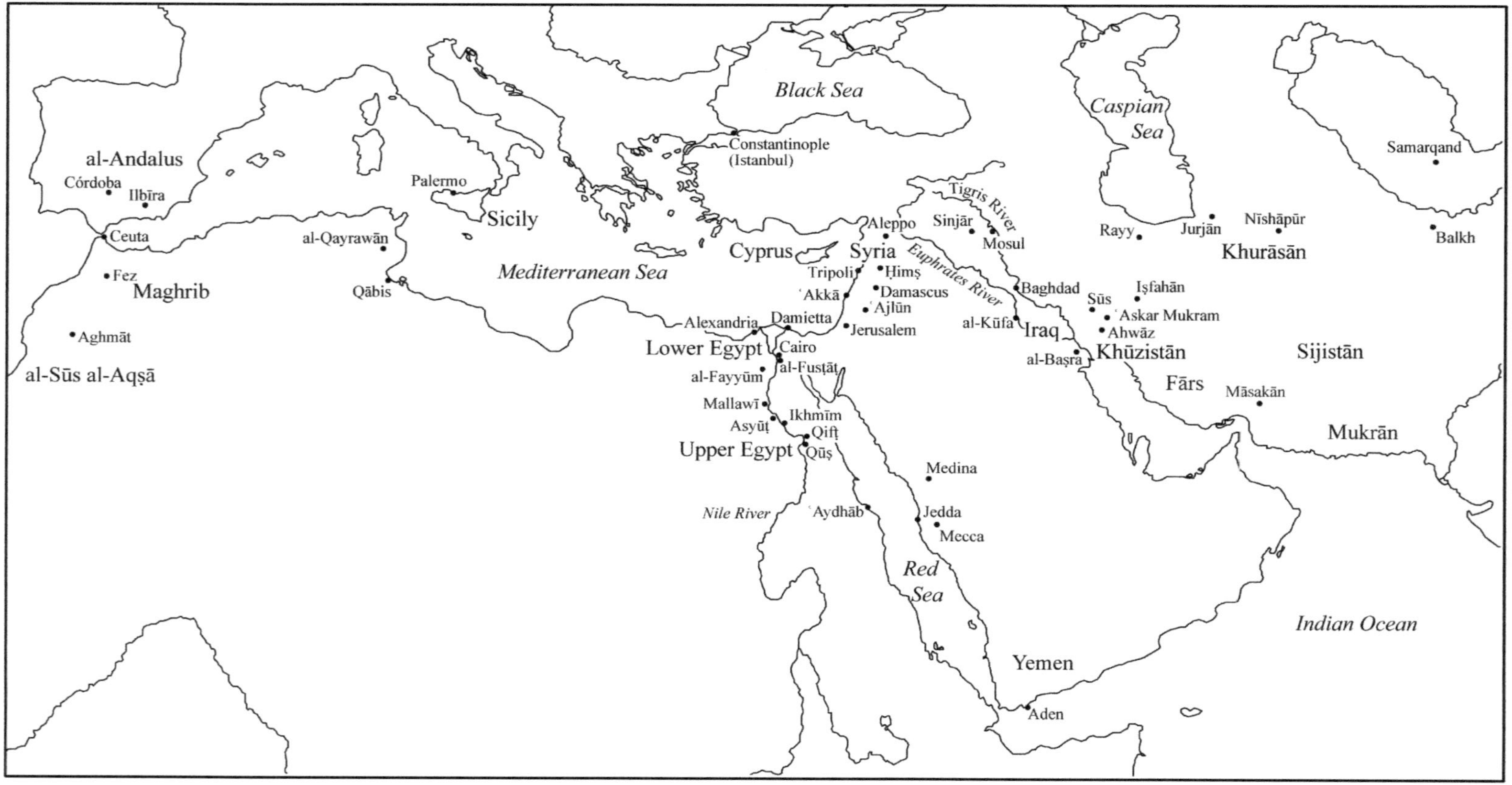

MAP 1 *The medieval Islamic world*

Expansion to Syria (Bilād al-Shām)

In historical Syria (Bilād al-Shām), sugarcane cultivation expanded not to the Orontes valley, which included the provinces of Ḥimṣ and Ḥamā, but to the coastal regions (al-Sāḥil) and to the Jordan valley (al-Ghawr). Helmut Blume erroneously states that this type of agricultural-industrial enterprise (sugar production) developed neither in Khūzistān, nor in the other medieval Arab sugarcane growing regions, but in the medieval Levant only after its conquest by the Crusaders.[40] Since both the coastal regions and the Jordan valley were irrigated by small rivers, springs, and wells, we can see, contrary to Blume's view, that sugarcane was also grown in Syria, although on a smaller scale than in Iran, Iraq, and Egypt.

It is within reason to speculate that sugarcane cultivation was brought from Iraq into southern Syria sometime before the tenth century, and subsequently expanded into other areas. Arabic sources list a number of cities as centers of sugarcane production, such as 'Akkā, Sūr, Bayrūt, Ṭarābulus, Markab, and Bāniyās in the coastal regions, Arīḥā and Baysān in the Jordan valley, and Ṭabarīya at the source of the river Jordan.[41] According to R. Ellenblum, in the Latin Kingdom of Jerusalem, the Franks learned how to grow crops unknown in their homelands, such as sugarcane.[42] Further, citing historical documents, he shows the economic importance of sugar production in the Frankish Kingdom during the twelfth century.[43]

Among the production centers in Syria, Tripoli (Ṭarābulus) and its surroundings were the most important to sugarcane harvesting and sugar production from the tenth to the fourteenth centuries. Al-Iṣṭakhrī, a tenth century geographer and the predecessor of Ibn Ḥawqal, states that Ṭarābulus was a prosperous town, with date trees and sugarcane in its environs.[44] This may be the oldest account of sugarcane in the district of Ṭarābulus, where the Qadīsha

40 Blume, *Geography of Sugar Cane*, p. 164.

41 Al-Muqaddasī, *Aḥsan al-Taqāsīm*, 161, 176, 180–181; Ibn Ḥawqal, *Kitāb Ṣūrat al-Arḍ*, 176; al-Iṣṭakhrī, *Kitāb Masālik al-Mamālik*, ed. M.J. de Goeje, Leiden, 1967, 46; Banyāmīn al-Tuṭīlī, *Riḥlat Banyāmīn (1165–1173)*, Arabic tr. by I. Ḥaddād, Baghdad, 1945, 92; Ibn Shaddād, *al-A'lāq al-Khaṭīra fī Dhikr Umarā' al-Shām wal-Jazīra: Lubnān*, Damascus, 1963, 92, 104; al-Idrīsī, *Kitāb Nuzhat al-Mushtāq*, IV, 372, 374; Ibn Sa'īd, *Kitāb al-Jughrāfiyā*, 152; al-Qazwīnī, *Āthār al-Bilād*, 142; Yāqūt, *Mu'jam al-Buldān*, IV, 217; Abū al-Fidā', *Taqwīm al-Buldān*, ed. M. Reinaud and M. de Slane, Paris, 1840, 255. See also Ouerfelli, *Le sucre*, pp. 31–46.

42 R. Ellenblum, *Frankish Rural Settlement in the Latin Kingdom of Jerusalem*, Cambridge, 1998, p. 213; Ouerfelli, *Le sucre*, pp. 45–52.

43 Ellenblum, *Frankish Rural Settlement*, p. 176.

44 Al-Iṣṭakhrī, *Kitāb Masālik al-Mamālik*, 46.

River quenched its fertile crop lands. It is said that in 1182, the general assembly of the Hospitallers instructed the head of their order in Tripoli to send sugar to their main headquarters in Jerusalem for the preparation of syrups and medications for sick patients.[45] Ibn Shaddād (d. 684/1285) also states that sugarcane was grown in abundance in the low lands of Ṭarābulus.[46] Al-Sakhāwī (d. 902/1497) also gives another account that sugarcane was cultivated in Aṭrābulus (Tripoli).[47]

Shihāb al-Dīn Aḥmad al-Nuwayrī, who was posted in Ṭarābulus as the superintendent of military affairs (*nāẓir al-jaysh*), meticulously reported the results of the cadastral survey (*rawk*) of Ṭarābulus in 717/1317. At the conclusion of the survey, the *kharāj* year changed from 716 to 717 and miscellaneous taxes on certain items (nine in total) were abolished according to the *rawk*'s standing tradition. The sultan's decree regarding this tax exemption for sugarcane growers in Ṭarāulus is cited by al-Nuwayrī as follows:

> Sultan al-Malik al-Nāṣir (reigned 693–694/1293–94, 698–708/1299–1309, 709–741/1310–41) ordered that the following miscellaneous taxes (*muʿāmala*) be abolished in the region of Ṭarābulus.
>
> *The peasants (*fallāḥ*) in the region of Ṭarābulus were exempted from forced labor in the sugarcane fields belonging to the government. Instead, a tax in kind equal to 2,000 dirhams was levied on them.
>
> *Tax on the sugarcane of amirs (*aqṣāb al-umarāʾ*). Some amirs overseeing districts where sugarcane was grown had demanded labor from their peasants in lieu of taxes, or had imposed a 3,000 dirhams labor rental tax (*ujrat al-ʿamal*).[48]

That is, the 2,000 dirhams levied on peasants who were forced to work in sugarcane fields belonging to the government, and the 3,000 dirhams levied on peasants who worked in the fields of *iqṭāʿ*s held by amirs, were both abolished by Sultan al-Nāṣir's decree in 717/1317.[49] The total exemption for the nine items listed came to 109,000 dirhams annually, or roughly the 110,000 dirhams that al-Nuwayrī mentioned elsewhere.[50] The 5,000 dirhams tax exemption for

---

45 E. Lev and Z. Amar, *Practical Materia Medica of the Medieval Eastern Mediterranean according to the Cairo Genizah*, Leiden and Boston, 2008, p. 296.

46 Ibn Shaddād, *al-Aʿlāq al-Khaṭīra: Lubnān*, 104.

47 Al-Sakhāwī, *al-Buldānīyāt*, ed. H.M. al-Qaṭṭān, Riyad, 2001, 82.

48 Al-Nuwayrī, *Nihāyat al-Arab*, XXXII, 260.

49 T. Sato, "Fiscal Administration in Syria during the Reign of Sultan al-Nāṣir Muḥammad," *Mamlūk Studies Review*, 11–1 (2007), pp. 31–33.

50 Al-Nuwayrī, *Nihāyat al-Arab*, XXXII, 255–56.

sugarcane cultivation in Ṭarābulus was around 4.5% of the 110,000 dirhams total. According to E. Ashtor, in the latter half of the fourteenth century, sugar production in Syria, including Ṭarābulus, gradually declined for a variety of reasons: the exploitation of peasants by the Mamluks in power, repeated outbreaks of plague, technological stagnation, and other factors.[51]

Expansion to Lower Egypt

As mentioned above, the emergence of sugarcane in Syria cannot be traced back beyond the tenth century. But, papyrus documents show sugarcane in Egypt during the middle of the eighth century.[52] However, the scale of this sugarcane cultivation must have been limited, and it would have been mostly restricted to Lower Egypt. For example, al-Muqaddasī states that in the province of al-Fayyūm in Upper Egypt, rice (*aruzz*) and flax (*kattān*) were the main crops,[53] excluding the sugarcane that would later flourish there.

Furthermore, the sugarcane districts mentioned by such geographers as al-Masʿūdī (d. 346/956) and Ibn Ḥawqal were Alexandria, Sanhūr, al-Sāfiya, and Dumā Jumūl, which were all located in Lower Egypt.[54] Nāṣir Khusraw also refers to the outskirts of al-Fusṭāṭ as Egypt's only sugar producing district,[55] and al-Idrīsī relates that sugarcane in Egypt was grown in Ḥimā al-Kabīr at the outskirts of al-Fusṭāṭ, Minyat Badr adjacent to Tinnīs, and Minyat al-ʿUlūq near Damietta.[56] Also, Ibn Mammātī, who regarded sugarcane as the most profitable crop, tells us that it was planted in the province of al-Buḥayra in Lower Egypt.[57] However, ʿAbd Allāh al-Bakrī (d. 487/1094) was probably the first to describe in detail the sugarcane cultivation in such districts as Asyūṭ and Qūṣ in Upper Egypt.[58]

---

51 Ashtor, "Levantine Sugar Industry in the Late Middle Ages," pp. 112–120.

52 D. Müller-Wodarg, "Die Landwirtschaft Ägyptens in der frühen ʿAbbāsidenzeit," *Der Islam*, 32 (1956), pp. 47–48; Watson, *Agricultural Innovation*, p. 28; Abū Sadīra, *al-Ḥiraf wal-Ṣināʿāt fī Miṣr al-Islāmīya*, pp. 354–355.

53 Al-Muqaddasī, *Aḥsan al-Taqāsīm*, 201, 208.

54 Al-Masʿūdī, *al-Tanbīh wal-Ashrāf*, ed. A.I. al-Ṣāwī, Cairo, 1938; repr. Baghdad, n.d., 20; Ibn Ḥawqal, *Kitāb Ṣūrat al-Arḍ*, 131, 134.

55 Nāṣir Khusraw, *Safar Nāma*, 79.

56 Al-Idrīsī, *Kitāb Nuzhat al-Mushtāq*, III, 329, 335, 339.

57 Ibn Mammātī, *Kitāb Qawānīn al-Dawāwīn*, Damascus, Maktabat al-Asad, MS. Microfilm No. 672, fols. 30, 221.

58 Al-Bakrī, *Kitāb al-Masālik wal-Mamālik*, Wien, Österreichische Nationalbibliothek, MS. Cod Mixt 779, fols. 19–20; al-Bakrī, *Jughrāfiyat Miṣr min Kitāb al-Mamālik wal-Masālik*, ed. A.Y. al-Ghānim, Kuwait, 1980, 81, 83.

In other words, the main sugarcane producing districts documented in Arabic source materials up to the end of the eleventh century are mostly restricted to the outskirts of al-Fusṭāṭ and the villages of Lower Egypt. This may show that conditions were better in Lower Egypt than in Upper Egypt, both for digging new canals and for setting up the waterwheels required for sugarcane.[59] We may therefore conclude that sugarcane spread to Upper Egypt on a large scale around the eleventh or twelfth century. Both al-Makhzūmī and Ibn Mammātī give detailed accounts of how sugarcane was grown in Egypt,[60] which indicates that sugarcane had gained public attention as a commercial product at the time.

The Expansion of Sugar Production to Upper Egypt, Maghrib, and Andalusia

Expansion from Lower Egypt to Upper Egypt

Both Muḥammad al-Musabbiḥī (366–420/977–1029) and Ibn al-Maʾmūn al-Baṭāʾiḥī (d. 588/1192) repeatedly refer to sugar consumption in the Fatimid court of Cairo,[61] but do not refer to the districts in Egypt where sugarcane was grown. As mentioned above, al-Bakrī in the eleventh century is probably the first geographer to give a reliable account of sugarcane cultivation in Upper Egypt. His main work, *Kitāb al-Masālik wal-Mamālik*, relates that Asyūṭ was a district of Upper Egypt with the most plentiful and finest sugarcane, and that the upriver district of Qūṣ had markets (*sūq*), public baths (*ḥammām*), and sugarcane pressing factories (*maʿṣara lil-sukkar*), each with about one hundred workers (*rajul*).[62] This account shows that sugar production throve in the districts of Upper Egypt in the around the eleventh century. We should also note that the workers in the sugar pressing factories were referred to only as "men" (*rajul*), not "slaves" (*ʿabd*). European scholars have generally believed that the

59 Ibn Iyās says, "Most of the large canals (*khalīj*), small canals (*turʿa*), irrigation dikes (*jisr*), and inlets (*khawr*) are found in Lower Egypt, while they are scarce in Upper Egypt" (*Kitāb Nuzhat al-Umam fī ʿAjāʾib wal-Ḥikam*, Istanbul, Süleymaniye Kütüphanesi, MS. Ayasofya 3500, fol. 95r-v).

60 Al-Makhzūmī, *Minhāj fī ʿIlm Kharāj Miṣr*, fols. 32r-33v; Ibn Mammātī, *Kitāb Qawānīn al-Dawāwīn*, 366–367.

61 Al-Musabbihī, *Akhbār Miṣr*, ed. A.F. Sayyid, T. Bianquis, and H. Naṣṣār, 2vols., Cairo, 1978–84, I, 65, 79–80; Ibn al-Maʾmūn, *Nuṣūṣ min Akhbār Miṣr*, ed. A.F. Sayyid, Cairo, 1983, 26, 31, 35–36, 42, 63.

62 Al-Bakrī, *Jughrāfiyat Miṣr*, 81, 83.

main workforces in sugar production in the Islamic world were slaves, just as on sugar plantations in the New World.[63]

Thereafter, sugarcane as commercial crop expanded from Lower Egypt into Upper Egypt. Here, we take up the case of al-Fayyūm, a fertile province in Upper Egypt irrigated by the Yusuf Canal (Baḥr Yūsuf). In 641/1243, ʿUthmān al-Nābulusī, under an order from the Ayyubid Sultan al-Malik al-Ṣāliḥ Ayyūb, visited the province of al-Fayyūm to survey the entire area over two years. Upon finishing his survey, al-Nābulusī compiled a book entitled *Taʾrīkh al-Fayyūm wa-Bilādih*, and dedicated it to Sultan al-Sāliḥ. *Taʾrīkh al-Fayyūm* vividly details the expansion of sugarcane crops into the province of al-Fayyūm during the twelfth -thirteenth centuries:

1. The village of Dahmā (*iqṭāʿ*)
   In this village, cotton (*quṭn*) was grown until irrigation water was diverted to sugarcane. As sugarcane spread, all the water was devoted to its irrigation, which led to [the village] ceasing cotton cultivation.[64]
2. The village of Dhāt al-Ṣafāʾ (*iqṭāʿ*)
   In this village, sesame (*simsim*) was grown, and then, as soil fertility declined, rice (*aruzz*) was introduced. But rice was also eventually abandoned, and water diverted, in favor of the village's new sugarcane crops.[65]
3. The village of Shāna (*iqṭāʿ*)
   As the population of this village increased, many residents relocated to the village of Lawāsī to grow crops there. But, because Lawāsī was quite far, others relocated to closer places. However, it is also said that this migration (*intiqāl*) was caused by a lack of irrigation water, due to the increase of sugarcane plantations in the province of al-Fayyūm.[66]
4. The village of Shadamūh (*iqṭāʿ*)
   This village had fruit orchards with dates, grapes, and sycamore. Mainly winter crops were grown there. Summer crops were also grown, until sugarcane took over.[67]

---

63 For example, Mintz states, "Slavery played a part in the Moroccan sugar industry and probably elsewhere" (*Sweetness and Power*, p. 27). Based on this account, Minoru Kawakita furthered the misunderstanding that a connection between sugar and slavery was established when the Muslims had a monopoly on global sugar production (*A World History of Sugar*, in Japanese, p. 16).

64 Al-Nābulusī, *Taʾrīkh al-Fayyūm*, 100–101.

65 Al-Nābulusī, *Taʾrīkh al-Fayyūm*, 102.

66 Al-Nābulusī, *Taʾrīkh al-Fayyūm*, 122–123.

67 Al-Nābulusī, *Taʾrīkh al-Fayyūm*, 125–126.

These instances show that sugarcane plantations expanded to the extent of replacing such summer crops as rice, cotton, and sesame, because cultivation required a great deal of water even after the Nile had receded. All the cases mentioned above were villages granted as *iqṭāʿ* to amirs and soldiers. However, sugarcane was also grown in the sultan's domain, including such villages as al-ʿUdwa, Sinnūris, Fānū, and Maṭar Ṭāris. According to a survey in 1243, the total land area used for sugarcane crops in the province of al-Fayyūm amounted to 1,468 *faddāns* (about 881 hectares), while the land area for wheat, for example, was 29,000 *faddāns* (about 17,400 hectares) in total.[68]

The following accounts confirm that in the first half of the Mamluk period sugarcane plantations were already popular in other districts of Upper Egypt besides the province of al-Fayyūm. We find an account of the year 697/1298 in *Kitāb al-Sulūk* by Taqī al-Dīn Aḥmad al-Maqrīzī, an Egyptian historian in the Mamluk period:

> [After the Ḥusāmī cadastral survey (*al-Rawk al-Ḥusāmī*) in 697/1298] Mankūtamur, *nā'ib al-salṭna*, was granted vast *iqṭā*ʿs in Upper Egypt; that is to say, Marj Banū Humaym and its surroundings, Samhūd and its surroundings, Ḥarajat Qūṣ, Madīnat Udfū, and waterwheels (*dūlāb*)[69] in these districts. The revenues consisted of over 110,000 *ardabb*s of crops, raw sugar (*qand*), molasses (*ʿasal*), dates, sheep, and firewood. He owned 27 sugarcane pressing factories (*maʿṣara li-qaṣab al-sukkar*) in these areas.[70]

Al-Maqrīzī gives another account of Mallawī in Upper Egypt:

> During the reign of Sultan al-Nāṣir, the land area for sugarcane crops increased to 1,500 *faddāns* (about 955 hectares) annually in this district. Al-Nashw, superintendent of the sultan's treasury (*nāẓir al-khāṣṣ*), seized all the sugar produced there in 738/1337–8 to send 14,000 *qinṭār*s [*jarwī*] (1,260,000 kilograms) of raw sugar, not including molasses, to the Dār al-Qand (the storehouse for raw sugar) in al-Fusṭāṭ. Later, he forced the

68 Al-Nābulusī, *Ta'rīkh al-Fayyūm*, 23. See also Cl. Cahen, "Le régime des impôts dans le Fayyūm ayyūbide," *Arabica*, 3 (1956), p. 15; Sato, *State and Rural Society*, p. 213.

69 H. Rabie explains that the *dūlāb* was a Persian word for the waterwheels commonly used on the banks of the Nile as described by al-Muqaddasī ("Some Technical Aspects of Agriculture in Medieval Egypt," A.L. Udovitch ed., *The Islamic Middle East, 700–1900*, Princeton, 1981, pp. 70–71).

70 Al-Maqrīzī, *Kitāb al-Sulūk*, 1, 843–844.

> people in the district to deliver an additional 8,000 *qinṭārs* (720,000 kilograms) of raw sugar.[71]

Ibn Baṭṭūṭa, who visited Mallawī at the beginning of the fourteenth century, states:

> The town has 11 sugarcane pressing factories (*maʿṣara li-sukkar*) where even beggars or sufi mendicants (*faqīr*) can enter freely. They come to the factories with warm bread, put it into pots boiling pressed juice, and go out with bread steeped plentifully in sugar juice.[72]

According to Abū al-Fidāʾ(d. 732/1331), Qamūla, a village located south of Qūṣ in Upper Egypt, also had many sugarcane fields.[73] Abū al-Faḍl al-Udfuwī (d. 748/1347) further relates that he found forty sugar factories (*maṭbakh li-sukkar*) and six sugarcane pressing factories (*maʿṣara li-qaṣab al-sukkar*) in Qifṭ, and in Samhūd he found many such factories and a total of seventeen stone mills (*ḥajar*).[74] Al-Udfuwī's description shows that during the thirteenth and fourteenth centuries, Qifṭ was a particularly important center for sugar production in Egypt. *Al-sukkar al-qifṭī* was widely known in the Islamic world for its puri-

71 Al-Maqrīzī, *al-Khiṭaṭ*, I, 204. Ibn Iyās says that after al-Nashw's seizures (*ḥawṭa*), sugarcane planting in this district declined (*Nashq al-Azhār fī ʿAjāʾib al-Aqṭār*, Istanbul, Süleymaniye Kütüphanesi, MS. Haci Beşir Ağa 497–498, fol. 114r-v; id., *Nuzhat al-Umam*, fols. 177v-178r). See also Ashtor, "Levantine Sugar Industry in the Late Middle Ages," p. 99; A. Levanoni, *A Turning Point in Mamluk History: The Third Reign of al-Nāṣir Muḥammad Ibn Qalāwūn 1310–1341*, Leiden, 1995, p. 150; Sato, *State and Rural Society*, pp. 214–215. Al-Nashw's seizures of sugar in Mallawī will be discussed in detail later.

72 Ibn Baṭṭūṭa, *Tuḥfat al-Nuẓẓār*, I, 100–101. Ibn Baṭṭūṭa calls the town 'Manlawī'. It was also known as 'Mallawī' and 'Maltawī' (M. Ramzī, *al-Qāmūs al-Jughrāfī lil-Bilād al-Miṣrīya*, 6 vols., Cairo, 1953–68, II-4, pp. 68–69).

73 Abū al-Fidāʾ, *Taqwīm al-Buldān*, 103–104. Yāqūt says that Qamūla had many date trees and vegetable gardens (*Muʿjam al-Buldān*, IV, 398–399).

74 Al-Udfuwī, *al-Ṭāliʿ al-Saʿīd al-Jāmiʿ li-Asmāʾ al-Fuḍalāʾ wal-Ruwāt*, Cairo, 1914, 7–8, 9, 18; Yāqūt also states that sugarcane cultivation was common in Bahjūra in Upper Egypt (*Muʿjam al-Buldān*, I, 514). In 742/1341–42 Amir Qūṣūn was able to make numerous grants to his *mamlūks*, partly because he held 500 *faddāns* of privately owned land in Upper Egypt for sugarcane cultivation (al-Maqrīzī, *Kitāb al-Sulūk*, II, 561; al-Yūsufī, *Nuzhat al-Nāẓir*, 370–371). See also S.D. Goitein, *A Mediterranean Society*, 6vols., Berkeley and Los Angeles, 1967–93, vol. 1, pp. 125–126.

ty.[75] These accounts show that sugarcane had become a major crop in the districts of Upper Egypt by around the thirteenth or fourteenth century.

Expansion to the Mediterranean Islands, Maghrib, and Andalusia

In 647, Muʿāwiya, govenor of Syria, sent his Arab fleet to Cyprus and, after a severe plundering by the Arab Muslims, assumed joint rule over the island together with the Byzantine emperor. Further, in 655, with the aid of the Arab-Muslim army stationed in Egypt, Muʿāwiya secured nearly complete control of the Eastern Mediterranean Sea upon defeating the Byzantine fleet in the Battle of the Masts (*Dhū al-Ṣawārī*). At the beginning of the ninth century, Arabs sent from Andalusia set out to overtake Crete, and in 878, the Aghlabids in Tunisia took control of Sicily, which remained under Muslim rule until the Norman Conquest in the latter half of the eleventh century.

The influence of Arab-Muslim culture gradually permeated these Mediterranean islands now under Arab rule, with sugar production being an important example. However, there are few accounts in Arabic on sugarcane in the Mediterranean islands. Ibn Ḥawqal in the tenth century briefly states that sugarcane (*qaṣab fārisī*) was grown in the marshlands near Palermo in Sicily.[76] Abū ʿAbd Allāh Muḥammad al-Idrīsī (d. 560/1165) relates that both Lafqasīya (Lefkosa, or Nicosia) and Karīnīya (Kyrenia) in Cyprus were beautiful towns with markets and sugarcane,[77] but gives no account of sugarcane crops in Sicily, where he lived for quite a while.

According to Deerr, by the end of the ninth century, Sicily was exporting sugar to Africa, but after the Norman Conquest, the industry suffered, and recovery was slowed by taxes and duties.[78] Watson as well says that around the tenth century, sugar produced in districts including Palermo was exported to North Africa. When the Normans overtook the island, the sugar industry still existed, but its fortunes fluctuated.[79]

However, according to M. Ouerfelli, it wasn't until the end of the thirteenth century that sugar production began to flourish on Mediterranean islands like Cyprus and Sicily. When the town of ʿAkkā was fell in 1291, the Crusaders, members of religious orders, merchants, and artisans immigrated to Cyprus, where

---

75 Ibn al-Ḥājj, *al-Madkhal ilā Tanmiyat al-Aʿmāl bi-Taḥsīn al-Nīyāt*, 4 vols., Beirut, 1981, IV, 154; Labib, *Handelsgeschichte Ägyptens*, p. 320; E. Ashtor, *A Social and Economic History of the Near East in the Middle Ages*, Berkeley and Los Angeles, 1976, p. 243.

76 Ibn Ḥawqal, *Kitāb Ṣūrat al-Arḍ*, 122.

77 Al-Idrīsī, *Kitāb Nuzhat al-Mushtāq*, VI, 644.

78 Deerr, *The History of Sugar*, vol. 1, pp. 76–79.

79 Watson, *Agricultural Innovation*, p. 29.

they, particularly the Lusignan royal family, the Hospitallers, and the Venetian merchants, began cultivating sugarcane based on their experience producing sugar in the Holy Land of Palestine.[80]

Regarding districts in Maghrib, Ibn Ḥawqal states that in al-Sūs al-Aqṣā there were citron (*utrujj*), walnut (*jawz*), almond (*lawz*), and date trees (*nakhl*), sugarcane (*qaṣab al-sukkar*), sesame (*simsim*), hemp (*qunnab*), and many other kinds of herbs.[81] This description shows that already in the tenth century, sugarcane was grown in districts as remote as al-Sūs al-Aqṣā near Agadir. Ibn Ḥawqal gives no account of sugarcane in the other districts of Maghrib, where wheat, barley, cotton, and flax were abundant. Thus, we need further research on whether al-Sūs al-Aqṣā was the first example of reclaimed land used for sugarcane crops in the Maghrib area.

The same applies to the districts of Andalusia. *Le calendrier de Cordoue*, compiled in 961, relates, "On 31 January, an early-ripening variety of purslane (*rijla bakīra*) is seeded, and sugarcane (*qaṣab al-sukkar*) is harvested. People produce jam (*mirabba*) from citrons (*utrujj*) and carrots (*jizar*), and acidic drinks from citrons."[82] *Le calendrier de Cordoue* was originally titled *Kitāb al-Anwāʾ* in Arabic, which was a combination of both the traditional calendar of the Arabs and the social customs of Andalusia.[83] This account seems to suggest that sugarcane was already being grown in the outskirts of Córdoba in the mid tenth century. Based on this account, M. Ouerfelli also states that sugarcane cultivation was established in Andalusia in the tenth century, though still limited in scale.[84] However, as *Le calendrier de Cordoue* was compiled from the books of *Anwāʾ* in the eastern Islamic world, its accounts of sugarcane cultivation might have been taken from these Arabic books.

The mid eleventh century finally brought us reliable information on sugarcane growing and sugar production in Maghrib and Andalusia. According to al-Bakrī, an Arab geographer in the eleventh century, fruit trees (*thamar*) and sugarcane (*qaṣab al-sukkar*) were widely grown on the expansive riverside land in Sūs, and sugar produced there was exported to all the countries of the Maghrib.[85] During the twelfth and thirteenth centuries, sugarcane expanded from al-Sūs al-Aqṣā to Aghmāt, Sabta (Ceuta), Qābis in Maghrib, and Ilbīra in

80 Ouerfelli, *Le sucre*, pp. 102–121.

81 Ibn Ḥawqal, *Kitāb Ṣūrat al-Arḍ*, 91.

82 Anon., *Le calendrier de Cordoue*, new ed. by Ch. Pella, Leiden, 1961, pp. 36–37.

83 Ch. Pellat, *Le calendrier de Cordoue*, Avant-propos, pp. VII-XI; *EI*², s.v. Anwāʾ (Ch. Pellat).

84 Ouerfelli, *Le sucre*, p. 181.

85 Al-Bakrī, *Kitāb al-Masālik wal-Mamālik*, ed. A. P. van Leeuwen and A. Ferre, 2 vols., Tunis, 1992, II, 853.

Andalusia.[86] Al-Idrīsī commented that the refined sugar produced in al-Sūs al-Aqṣā was the same as Sulaymānī white sugar (*al-sukkar al-sulaymānī*) and solid white sugar (*tabarzad*).[87] Ibn al-ʿAwwām (6–7/12–13c.) explained the growing cycle of sugarcane in detail, from planting in the spring, to periodic irrigation, to harvesting in winter,[88] which shows that sugarcane crops had already become commonplace in Andalusia during that period.

In the mid fifteenth century, the Portuguese, who had learned to grow sugarcane and produce sugar from the Muslims in Andalusia, began growing sugarcane in the Madeira Islands and the Açores Islands. And then, the Spanish followed suit in the Canary Islands. In 1493, emulating these examples, Christopher Columbus (ca. 1451–1506) is said to have brought sugarcane to the New World on his second voyage with the financial support of Ferdinand and Isabella, which led to large-scale sugarcane plantations in the Caribbean Islands and Brazil, beginning in the early sixteenth century.[89]

---

86 Al-Idrīsī, *Kitāb Nuzhat al-Mushtāq*, III, 230; V, 528; Ibn Saʿīd, *Kitāb al-Jughrāfiyā*, 123; Yāqūt, *Muʿjam al-Buldān*, IV, 289; al-Qazwīnī, *Āthār al-Bilād*, 502.

87 Al-Idrīsī, *Kitāb Nuzhat al-Mushtāq*, III, 227.

88 Ibn al-ʿAwwām, *Kitāb al-Filāḥat al-Muslimīn al-Andalusīyīn*, fols. 164b-165b.

89 Deerr, *A History of Sugar*, vol. 1, pp. 100–104, 116–117; Mintz, *Sweetness and Power*, p. 32.

CHAPTER 2

From Red Sugar to White Sugar: Sugar Production Technology

Sugarcane Cultivation as Described by al-Nuwayrī

Al-Nuwayrī, an Encyclopedist from Upper Egypt

Shihāb al-Dīn Aḥmad b. ʿAbd al-Wahhāb al-Nuwayrī, a leading encyclopedist of the Mamluk period, was born in the village of al-Nuwayra in Ikhmīm in Upper Egypt. He grew up in Qūṣ, one of the cultural centers in Mamluk Egypt, under the protection of his father, who served as a government official in that district. In 698/1298, at the age of twenty, al-Nuwayrī traveled with his father to Cairo, where he mastered Islamic learning – hadith, history, and geography – under instructors Badr al-Dīn Muḥammad Ibn Jamāʿa (639–733/1241–1333), Shaykha Zaynab bint Munajjā (d.715/1316),[1] a female hadith scholar, and others. His earliest official post was as a scribe of *dīwān al-khāṣṣ* that managed the sultan's domain (*khāṣṣ al-sulṭān*). In 701/1301, Sultan al-Nāṣir appointed al-Nuwayrī to a new post managing the sultan's domain in Syria. In 710/1310, he was transferred to the Syrian coastal town of Tripoli, where he remained for about two years, overseeing a military office (*dīwān al-jaysh*), and giving *iqṭāʿ* assignments to the Mamluk cavalrymen. He held several other official posts after returning to Cairo, but retired in 716/1316 at the age of thirty-seven to devote his time to completing what became his various important literary works.[2]

As I mentioned, his main work, *Nihāyat al-Arab fī Funūn al-Adab*, consists of five sections in thirty-one volumes[3]: (1) Heaven and Earth, (2) Human Beings, (3) Animals, (4) Plants, and (5) History. This organization shows that the work is a systematic compilation of the common knowledge of the Mamluk scholars. The first four sections are covered in ten volumes, but the remaining

1 M. Chapoutot-Remadi states one of his teachers as Shaykha Wazīra bint Munajjā (*EI*², s.v. al-Nuwayrī), but based on the contemporary biographical dictionaries, not Wazīra but Zaynab is correct. See al-Udfuwī, *al-Ṭāliʿ al-Saʿīd*, 46–47; al-Maqrīzī, *Kitāb al-Muqaffā al-Kabīr*, ed. M. al-Yaʿlānī, 8 vols., Beirut, 1991, I, 521–522; Ibn Ḥajar, *al-Durar al-Kāmina*, I, 209–210; Ibn Taghrībirdī, *al-Manhal al-Ṣāfī*, I, 361–362.

2 For more on al-Nuwayrī's life and works, see *EI*², s.v. al-Nuwayrī (M. Chapoutot-Remadi); A.M. Jamāl al-Dīn, *al-Nuwayrī wa-Kitābuh Nihāyat al-Arab fī Funūn al-Adab*, Cairo, 1984; A. al-Nadawī, *Minhaj al-Nuwayrī fī Kitābih Nihāyat al-Arab fī Funūn al-Adab*, Damascus, 1987.

3 The edited book consists of thirty-three volumes in total.

 | DOI 10.1163/9789004281561_004

twenty-one volumes are all devoted to history. This ratio shows the emphasis that al-Nuwayrī placed on history, from the creation of human beings, right up to the events of 731/1331, leaving off only two years before his death.[4] A reliable reporter on Egypt and Syria, al-Nuwayrī provides us with the most detailed and specific accounts of sugarcane growing and sugar production in the medieval Islamic world.

The cultivation of sugarcane and production of sugar are explained in the second section, Human Beings (VIII, pp. 264–272 in the edited book). Al-Nuwayrī notes that the below descriptions of sugarcane cultivation, crops, and the related technologies use terminology from the Qūṣ district in Upper Egypt, but that these terms are not much different from those used in other districts.[5] In the following section, I will attempt a faithful translation of this invaluable account provided by al-Nuwayrī. The titles in angle brackets are added for ease of reference.

Sugarcane Cultivation as Seen in Nihāyat al-Arab

Al-Nuwayrī describes the growing and harvesting of sugarcane as follows:

> <Plowing and Planting>
> Sugarcane (*qaṣab al-sukkar*) and its pressing factories (*maʿṣara*) differ according to location, district, and between the countries of Egypt and Syria. Even within Egypt, they vary by province, district, and area. However, a common principle (*qāʿidat kullīya*) throughout Egypt is that premium quality soft fields, well-irrigated by the Nile, are chosen. After the esparto grass (*ḥalfāʾ*) is weeded out, the cleanly cut field is plowed six times with a *muqalqila*, a large plow (*miḥrāth kabīr*),[6] and smoothed flat. Then, the field is cultivated six more times and smoothed with harrows. This process is known as "*al-barsh al-ḥarth*."[7] After the field is tilled with

4 Al-Nuwayrī notes that we describe not only history, but all the literary (*adab*) fields (*Nihāyat al-Arab*, XIII, 5).

5 Al-Nuwayrī, *Nihāyat al-Arab*, VIII, 271. Based on the account of al-Nuwayrī, Ibn Iyās also relates the sugarcane cultivation process in medieval Egypt (*Nuzhat al-Umam fī al-ʿAjāʾib wal-Ḥikam*, ed. M.Z.M. ʿAzab, Cairo, 1995, 139–140).

6 Al-Makhzūmī (d. 585/1189) and Ibn Mammātī (d. 606/1209), who describe sugarcane cultivation in great detail, give no account of *muqalqila*. We can therefore conclude that the *muqalqila* was probably invented for sugarcane cultivation or for irrigation work in the twelfth or thirteenth centuries. H. Rabie and Mohamed Ouerfelli transcribe the term as "*muqalqala*" (Rabie, "Some Technical Aspects," p. 64; Ouerfelli, *Le sucre*, p. 231).

7 *Al-barsh al-ḥarth* probably means the work of plowing the *barsh* (fields uncultivated due to surplus water in the previous year). See Sato, *State and Rural Society*, p. 216.

the *muqalqila*, sugarcane stalks with one or two joints are planted. The planting is done after water flows into the basin (*ḥawḍ*) through irrigation channels. The length of each sugarcane stalk (*qiṭʿa*) is three complete joints (*unbūb*). Full-length stalks with many buds are selected for planting.[8]

<Irrigation and Soil Loosening>
When planting is finished, the stalks are covered with soil, which is distributed horizontally, not vertically. After planting in the early spring, the field is irrigated weekly. As sugarcane buds and leaves break through the field's surface, they are accompanied by esparto grass and purslane. The field is then loosened to weed out the accompanying plants and grasses. This soil loosening is called "*ʿazq*." The *ʿazq* is repeated until the sugarcane eventually becomes so strong and dense that the field workers (*ʿuzzāq*) can no longer enter the field. It is said that the projections of the sugarcane stalks expel the field workers. Irrigation with water-wheel buckets (*qādūs*) is done a total of twenty-eight times.[9]

<Irrigation Customs>
The traditions of sugarcane cultivation with waterwheels (*maḥāla*)[10] on the Nile are as follows: If the field is near the Nile, eight *faddāns*[11] are irrigated [per day] with eight oxen. But if the field is far from the Nile, no more than four to six *faddāns* are irrigated. When the Nile rises, the field is irrigated with the so-called "water of repose" (*māʾ al-rāḥa*). That is, one side of the irrigation dike (*jisr*) that prevents flooding is cut open to allow water into the fields through channels (*jadwal*). The depth of the water is maintained at around one *shibr* (twenty-three centimeters). The water is left to warm up for two or three hours, and then drained from the other side of dike. This irrigation process is repeated in the same way on certain days to introduce new water at determined intervals. Next, the sugarcane is weaned. The preceding passages describe plowing, planting, irrigation, soil loosening, and other issues. If these are not carried out in full, the

8 Al-Nuwayrī, *Nihāyat al-Arab*, VIII, 264–265.

9 Al-Nuwayrī, *Nihāyat al-Arab*, VIII, 265.

10 A water wheel operated with oxen, donkeys, or camels has been called *sāqiya* or *maḥāla* in Egypt. See Rabie, "Some Technical Aspects," p. 71; Sato, *State and Rural Society*, p. 255.

11 W. Hinz, relying on the account of al-Qalqashandī, estimates a *faddān* at 6,368m² (*Islamische Masse und Gewichte*, Leiden, 1955, p. 65).

> crop failure can be attributed to the officials in charge (*mubāshir*).[12] The water supply, on the other hand, is a matter of God's will, and beyond the purview of the officials.[13]
>
> <Pest Control>
> Tar (*qaṭrān*) must be applied to the sugarcane before it becomes sweet in order to prevent damage from insects (*sūs*). The explanation given is that farmers pour tar into a waterwheel bucket (*qādūs*) with a hole in the bottom, which is plugged with esparto grass. The bucket is hung over the water channel, and a tar and water mixture is dripped onto the sugarcane. Also, if the officials fear damage from mice (*fa'r*), they must set up a thin, backward-arching mud wall around the fields. This wall, made of mud and straw, is called "*ḥīṭān al-fa'r*" and prevents mice from climbing onto the sugarcane fields. If a mouse tries to climb the mud wall, the arch of its design sends the mouse falling back to the ground. These are what the officials in charge must do to attentively and reliably manage sugarcane crops.[14]
>
> <Harvesting>
> At the beginning of Kīhak (the fourth Coptic month, 27 November-26 December), the leaves are cut, and the sugarcane is harvested and carried to the pressing factories. When the planting season begins the following year, the cut sugarcane leaves remaining on the fields are burned, and the soil is loosened and irrigated, as explained above. The next generation of sugarcane appears, which in Egypt is called the "*khilfa*" (sugarcane of the second year). Raw sugar (*qand*) made from the *khilfa* is more valuable than that made from the "*ra's*" (sugarcane of the first year).[15]

In the passages above, al-Nuwayrī systematically explains the workings of sugarcane cultivation in order: plowing, planting, soil loosening, irrigation, pest control, and harvesting. His account shows that, as growing sugarcane requires periodic irrigation and soil loosening, and brisk harvesting within about ten

---

12 *Mubāshirs* denote bureaucrats working in the central and regional offices (*dīwān*). According to al-Qalqashandī, the *mubāshirs* were actually superintendents (*nāẓir*), financiers (*mustawfī*), representatives (*shādd*), and so on (*Ṣubḥ al-A'shā*, III, 452). See Sato, *State and Rural Society*, pp. 192–193.

13 Al-Nuwayrī, *Nihāyat al-Arab*, VIII, 266.

14 Al-Nuwayrī, *Nihāyat al-Arab*, VIII, 267.

15 Al-Nuwayrī, *Nihāyat al-Arab*, VIII, 267.

months, it must have been more complicated work and required a great deal more labor than cultivating wheat and barley. So, we can see that sugarcane was a new commercial crop in the medieval ages, requiring significant capital and advanced farming techniques. The introduction of the *muqalqila* large plow for deep plowing is particularly noteworthy. Although the term *muqalqila* had already been used to describe an agricultural device used in creating irrigation dikes, al-Nuwayrī is the first to cite the use of *muqalqila* in sugarcane cultivation in Upper Egypt.[16]

As growing sugarcane consumes a considerable amount of soil, after the harvest of the *khilfa* (the second-year sugarcane), growers had to either plant other rotation crops or leave the field fallow. Al-Makhzūmī (d. 585/1189) says the following about this:

> Sugarcane prefers [the optimal soil of] *al-bāq* – land left fallow for over four years. It should be also planted after broad beans and sesame, or land called "*al-barsh*," which was uncultivated [due to a surplus of water in the previous year].[17]

Sugarcane, therefore, needs to be planted on uncultivated and well-irrigated, soft soil of good quality.

Sugarcane Growers and Sugar Factory Workers

Setting aside al-Nuwayrī's account for a while, let's look at the people who grew the sugarcane and worked at the sugarcane pressing factories. In regards to the sugarcane growers, *Ta'rīkh al-Fayyūm* by 'Uthmān al-Nābulusī provides us with valuable accounts:

1. Sugarcane in the Village of al-'Udwa (80 *faddāns*)[18]
   80 *faddāns* cultivated by *murābi'ūn*
2. Sugarcane in the Village of Sinnūris (318 *faddāns*)[19]
   222 *faddāns* cultivated by *muzāri'ūn*
   96 *faddāns* cultivated by *murābi'ūn*
3. Sugarcane in the Village of Fānū (268 *faddāns*)[20]

16 Sato, *State and Rural Society*, p. 207.
17 Al-Makhzūmī, *Minhāj fī 'Ilm Kharāj Miṣr*, fol. 32r-v.
18 Al-Nābulusī, *Ta'rīkh al-Fayyūm*, 32–34.
19 Al-Nābulusī, *Ta'rīkh al-Fayyūm*, 107–110.
20 Al-Nābulusī, *Ta'rīkh al-Fayyūm*, 156–159.

95 *faddāns* cultivated by *murābiʿūn*
173 *faddāns* cultivated by (not identified, *muzāriʿūn*?)

"*Muzāriʿūn*" were peasants who cultivated land allotted under *qabāla* contracts[21] concluded with the government or with *iqṭāʿ* holders (*muqṭaʿ*) after the Nile flood. In contrast, "*murābiʿūn*," according to Cl. Cahen, meant peasants who had the rather insubstantial right to one-fourth (*rubʿ*) of what they produced, being levied the standard tax in cash on their cultivation of sugarcane.[22] While *muzāriʿūn* grew wheat and barley rather than sugarcane, *murābiʿūn* grew only sugarcane, and did so in the royal farms (*awāsī*) controlled directly by the government or the sultan.[23] Nevertheless, we note that both *muzāriʿūn* and *murābiʿūn* were free tenant farmers, and by no means slaves according to Islamic law.

There are no other sources in Arabic to indicate that slaves grew sugarcane in Egypt or Syria. The slaves of Islamic societies are mainly house slaves (*ʿabd*, *jāriya*) and military slaves (*mamlūk*), rarely used for farming. The black slaves of Zanj, who rebelled against the ʿAbbasid caliphate during 255–270/869–883, had been employed solely to improve the salt-damaged lands (*sibākh*) of South Iraq.[24] Moreover, we find no account in al-Ṭabarī's contemporary chronicle, *Taʾrīkh al-Rusul wal-Mulūk*, that the Zanj were forced to cultivate sugarcane in ʿAbbasid Iraq.

Regarding the workers in the Egyptian pressing factories, a papyrus document in Arabic from the early ninth century provides important information. It reads…

1. …[ ]…..
2. sugarcane cutters (*qaṭṭāʿīn*)
3. peelers (*muqashshirīn*)
4. stackers and tanners of sugarcane (*raṣṣāṣ wal-dabbāgh*)[25]
5. carriers of sugarcane (*naqqālīn*)

---

21 *Qabālas* are annual contracts made between proprietors (the government or *muqṭaʿ*) and peasants after the flood of the Nile in autumn. See Sato, *State and Rural Society*, pp. 192–197.

22 Cl. Cahen, "Le régime des impôts dans le Fayyūm ayyūbide," p.23.

23 Regarding *awāsī*, see Sato, *State and Rural Society*, pp. 217–218.

24 Al-Ṭabarī, *Taʾrīkh al-Rusul wal-Mulūk*, ed. M.J. de Goeje, 15 vols., Leiden, 1879–1901; repr. Leiden, 1964, III, 1742.

25 The *dabbāgh* literally means "tanner," but his actual role is unclear. Ouerfelli explains this as a person who carries the harvested sugarcane, but without indicating any reliable source (*Le sucre*, p. 70).

6. throwers [of small pieces of sugarcane into the stone mill] (*ṭarrāḥ*)
7. drivers of oxen [that rotate the stone mill] (*nakhkhās*)
8. stone mill foremen (*ḥajjārīn*)
9. cooks of pressed juice (*ṭabbākh*)
10. laborers of raw sugar (*ghilmān al-qand*)
11. caldron supervisor (*ṣāḥib al-dast*)
12. diggers of cone-shaped earthenware moulds (*daffān*)
13. laborers of cone-shaped earthenware moulds (*ghilmān al-abālīj*)[26]

The above text lists the thirteen types of workers in a sugar factory. J. Sauvaget, who re-examined the text, interpreted *ghilmān* (no. 10, 13) as slaves,[27] and P. Berthier, based on Sauvaget's interpretation, supposes that slaves were likewise employed in the sugar production factories of medieval Morocco.[28]

But, it is difficult to believe that slaves would only be employed for two out of thirteen different types of work. So, the word *ghilmān* in this text would be better translated as "youths," "mates," or "laborers."[29] Also, Ibn Iyās, an Egyptian historian in the later Mamluk period, relates, "In the Coptic month of Kīhak (27 November–26 December) sugarcane is harvested, pressed, and cooks (*ṭabbākh*) are employed for sugar production."[30] It is noteworthy that the term "cooks" (*ṭabbākh*) rather than "slaves" (*ghulām* or *ʿabd*) is used to describe the sugar workers. As I mentioned in the prologue, S.W. Mintz, based on Berthier's unlikely supposition, came to the conclusion that slavery played a role in the sugar industry in Morocco, and probably elsewhere.[31] This view, however, has no proper sources, and is a mistake based on the assumption that slaves were employed in the sugar industry throughout the world.

---

26 A. Grohmann ed., *Arabic Papyri in the Egyptian Library*, 6vols., Cairo, 1934–62, vol. 3, pp. 227–229. We find many mistakes in his reading of the original Arabic text and its translation into English, reflecting a lack of knowledge of sugar production technology. See also Ouerfelli, *Le sucre*, p. 70.

27 J. Sauvaget, "Sur un papyrus arabe de la Bibliothèque Égyptienne," *Annales de l'Institut d'Études Orientales* (Alger), 7 (1948), pp. 31, 37–38. *Ublūj* (pl. *abālīj*) will be discussed later in greater detail.

28 Berthier, *Les anciennes sucreries du Maroc*, vol. 1, p. 236. Deerr also supposes that the intimate connection between sugar and slavery may be looked on as having its roots in the wave of Arab expansion which spread over North Africa from the seventh century onwards (*The History of Sugar*, vol. 2, p. 259).

29 I agree with Ouerfelli's view that the *ghilmān* in the text does not necessarily refer to slaves, but rather youths or boys (*Le sucre*, p. 70, note 187).

30 Ibn Iyās, *Nuzhat al-Umam*, 247.

31 Mintz, *Sweetness and Power*, p. 27.

Sugar Production as Described by al-Nuwayrī

The following passages taken from al-Nuwayrī are considered the most detailed accounts of sugar production in the Islamic, Chinese, and other worlds.[32]

<Cleaning the Sugarcane>
The custom of sugar production in Egypt is as follows: the cane is carried on the backs of camels or donkeys from the harvest fields to the pressing factory (*maʿṣara*), and unloaded at the cane house (*dār al-qaṣab*). [In the cane house] are tables (*watara*), firewood (*ḥaṭab*),[33] and men (*rajul*) with great knives – knives 2/3 *dhirāʿ* (about 50 centimeters) long, and 1/6 *dhirāʿ* (11 centimeters) wide. With these knives they clean the cane stalks and cut off the non-sweet top part. They call this part "*luklūk* (good-for-nothing)." They remove the roots and mud from the lower part of the stalks. This is called "cleaning" (*taṭhīr*).[34]

<Cutting the Sugarcane into Small Pieces>
Stalks are taken from the table and put with other stalks lined up against a long wall. One side abuts the cane house, and the other, the "band" house (*bayt al-nuwab*).[35] Men seated in front of the table hold in their

32 C. Daniels, "The Adoption and Transfer of New Sugarmaking Technology within South China during the Late Ming – Early Qing Period (Minmatsu Shinsho ni okeru shin seito gijutsu taikei no saiyo oyobi kokunai iten, in Japanese)," *Shujitsu Joshi Daigaku Shigaku Ronshu*, 3 (1988), p. 104.

33 This indicates that, in addition to leaves cut from sugarcane, firewood was also used in the boiling of pressed juice at sugar factories in medieval Egypt. The *sanṭ* trees in Upper Egypt, particularly in the province of Qifṭ, were commonly used as firewood in Egypt. Al-Dīnawarī relates, "The *sanṭ* are trees that grow in Upper Egypt, customarily used as people's firewood (*ḥaṭab*). The trees have been regarded as the best kind of firewood among them" (*Kitāb al-Nabāt*, II, 50). Al-Bakrī also says, "Qifṭ has thick *sanṭ* trees which are used as firewood in Egypt" (*Jughrāfiyat Miṣr*, 83). Furthermore Ibn Mammātī relates, "In this month [Barmūda (27 March–25 April)] it is important to cut down *sanṭ* trees [in Upper Egypt] and carry them to the shore of al-Fusṭāṭ via the Nile" (*Kitāb Qawānīn al-Dawāwīn*, 250). See also Ouerfelli, *Le sucre*, pp. 268–270.

34 Al-Nuwayrī, *Nihāyat al-Arab*, VIII, 267–268. Deerr's translation of al-Nuwayrī's text into English also has many mistakes reflecting his lack of knowledge of sugar production technology (*The History of Sugar*, vol. 1, pp. 90–92).

35 The term *nuwab* (sing. *nawba*) is obscure in meaning. The editor of *Nihāyat al-Arab* supposes it may denote the house where the canes are washed (Al-Nuwayrī, *Nihāyat al-Arab*, VIII, 268, note 3). However, I suppose that *nuwab* means "band", owing to the rhythmical sound of the cane cutting works.

hands the knives that are used to cut the cane. Each man takes a number of stalks, places them on the table, and cuts them into small pieces, which he then throws into the band house. Then the small pieces, all the same size, are placed in baskets called "*ʿiyāras*," to be carried to the stone mill (*ḥajar*).[36]

<Pressing the Sugarcane with a Stone Mill>
The cut cane stalks are laid under a stone mill that is turned by powerful oxen (*baqar jayyid*). The juice is pressed out and flows through openings in the base to a narrow collector. After the stalks have been pressed at the stone mill, they are taken to another location, where they are placed in baskets weaved from esparto grass. These baskets are laid under a wheel on a beam (*takht*) that rolls over them until it has crushed out the remainder of the juice.[37]

As these passages show, after the harvest and the cleaning, the cane is cut into small pieces to be pressed with a stone mill. The passages explain that the stone mill was not a roller-type pressing machine that crushed long canes inserted between two horizontal or vertical rollers, but an edge-type machine that crushed small pieces of sugarcane under a stone (Figure 1). According to Daniels, the wooden or stone roller mill for sugar production was introduced in China sometime after the sixteenth century.[38] So, the horizontal roller mill, which was illustrated by Napoléon's science team, must have first appeared in Egypt sometime during the Ottoman era. Let us resume al-Nuwayrī's account of sugar production.

<Filtration of the Pressed Juice>
The pressed juice is carried to another place, and passed through a sieve (*munkhul*), which is placed in a prepared cage. From here, the juice flows to a hall (*bahw*) where a collection vessel is placed. When the vessel is filled with strained juice, it is brought to the sugar refinery (*maṭbakh*). It is then strained a second time in a large boiler (*khābiya*), into which all the juice in the hall (*bahw*) is poured and strained. The *khābiya* holds 60 *maṭar*s of juice. Each *maṭar* is half an *al-qinṭār al-laythī*. An *al-qinṭār*

36 Al-Nuwayrī, *Nihāyat al-Arab*, VIII, 268.

37 Al-Nuwayrī, *Nihāyat al-Arab*, VIII, 268–269.

38 Daniels, "The Adoption and Transfer of New Sugarmaking Technology," pp. 108–113.

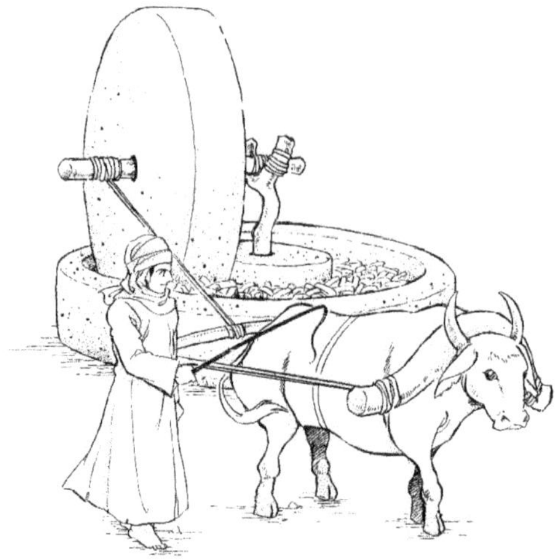

FIGURE 1 *A presumed edge-mill* (ḥajar) *for pressing sugarcane* (ILLUSTRATION BY SAEKO TAKISHITA)

> *al-laythī* is 200 dirhams. So, the *khābiya* holds 3,000 *raṭls*. This is the capacity of the *khābiya*.[39]

According to this, since a *maṭar* is 48 kilograms, the *khābiya* holds 2,880 kilograms of juice. If we assume a cylinder with a diameter of 1.5 meters, the height would be about 1.6 meters. By the way, Marco Polo relates in his travel diaries, which we will refer to later, that ash had already been used to neutralize the pressed juice in the Islamic world, something al-Nuwayrī does not refer to in this text.

> <Boiling of the Pressed Juice>
> The *khābiya* is fired up outside the refinery, and brought to a brisk boil until the volume of juice has decreased, and the fire is then removed. When the boiling has ceased, the liquid is carried to large vessels (*yaqṭīn*). In the handle of each *yaqṭīn* there is a large piece of wood the length of a man's forearm. The liquid is poured into another large vessel (*dann*) at the bottom through a wool filter. This is the third straining. After the liquid has settled there for a while, it is transported from the *danns* to another boiler (*qidr*) with caldrons (*dast*), where it is further boiled down.[40]

39 Al-Nuwayrī, *Nihāyat al-Arab*, VIII, 269.

40 Al-Nuwayrī, *Nihāyat al-Arab*, VIII, 269–270.

<*Ublūj*, pl. *Abālīj*>
For each stone mill, one *khābiya* and eight *qidr*s are used to boil the juice produced at the stone mill and the *takht*. After boiling, the juice is carried with copper vessels (*dast*), on the upper edge of which are two wooden handles. The workers hold the vessel by the handles to avoid being burned. The boiled juice, called "*maḥlab*" (milk), is poured into cone-shaped earthenware moulds (*ublūj*, pl. *abālīj*), which are wide at the top and narrow at the bottom. In the bottom of each *ublūj* are three holes, which are plugged with cane stalks. These *ublūj*s are placed in the drip house (*bayt al-ṣabb*), in which there are long benches like mangers. Under each *ublūj* is a vessel (*qādūs*) into which drips the molasses (*ʿasal al-qaṭr*) as it separates from the *maḥlab*. The workers use large spoons to fill the *ublūj*s one after another. The *ublūj*s are of two different sizes; one holds more than a *qinṭār* [*jarwī*][41] and the other less. When all the *ublūj*s are full and prepared, they are brought from the drip house to the burial house (*bayt al-dafn*). They are placed over the vessels, into which drips any remaining molasses. The by-products of the canes that were cleaned are pressed and boiled separately. These are called "*khābiya*," and produce low-grade molasses (*ʿasal*).[42]

The above passage explains the most important processes in separating the raw sugar (*qand*) from the black molasses (*ʿasal*) with cone-shaped earthenware moulds (*ublūj*s). Nowadays, actual *ublūj*s are hard to find. But as I mentioned in the preface, in 2006, I found an *ublūj* on display at the ʿAjlūn Castle Museum in North Jordan (Figure 2). The accompanying description explains that the *ublūj* has three small holes in the bottom, which exactly matches al-Nuwayrī's account above.[43] Mutsuo Kawatoko, who excavated at the al-Fusṭāṭ site for more than ten years, discovered a slender cone-shaped earthenware object (Figure 3) from the middle of the Mamluk period. The lower part is missing, but, as the figure shows, this must have been the kind of *ublūj* used in the sugar refineries in al-Fusṭāṭ.

M. Ouerfelli, based on the same account by al-Nuwayrī, explains the process of refining sugar. However, his explanation doesn't mention the Arabic term *ublūj*, or the separation of the raw sugar (*qand*) from the molasses (*ʿasal*). He translates the text as, "Ces pots sont placés sur des récipients également en

41 The *qinṭār jarwī* (96.7 kilograms) was used for sugar weight in medieval Egypt.

42 Al-Nuwayrī, *Nihāyat al-Arab*, VIII, 270–271.

43 Several clear photographs of the *ublūj*s excavated at several sites in Morocco are illustrated in Berthier's *Les anciennes sucreries du Maroc*, vol. 2.

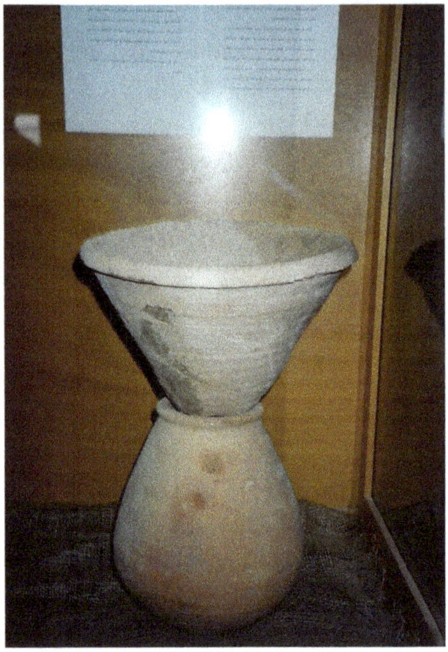

FIGURE 2 *The* ublūj *at the ʿAjlūn Castle Museum*

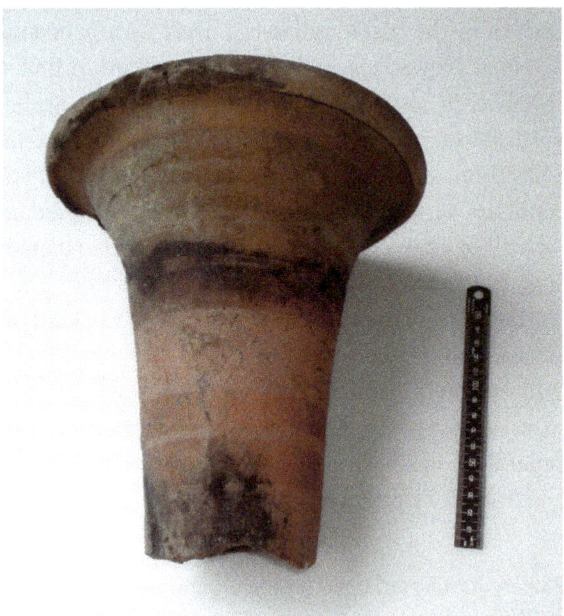

FIGURE 3 *The* ublūj *excavated in al-Fusṭāṭ (The Institute of Egyptology at Waseda University, Tokyo;* PHOTO TAKEN BY MUTSUO KAWATOKO)

terre cuite pour permettre au sirop de s'égoutter."[44] But this literal translation fails to clearly explain the *ublūj*'s function in separating the black molasses from the boiled sugar juice.

According to al-Nuwayrī, when the *ublūj*s are full of boiled juice, they are brought from the drip house to the burial house (*bayt al-dafn*). The word *dafn* indicates that the surface of the *ublūj* was covered with earth. When water was sprinkled on the surface, the molasses flowed down slowly, causing a cone-shaped solidification of the sugar (raw sugar at the first stage) in the *ublūj*. In China, this process was known as *fu tu fa* 覆土法, or the process of covering a surface with earth. *Tien-kung kai-wu* (天工開物), published in the early seventeenth century, also refers to the *ublūj* as "*wa liu*" (瓦溜, earthenware).[45] Daniels supposes that this technique of sugar production came to China from Egypt or other Arab countries during the Yüan Dynasty (1271–1368).[46]

I have doubts about al-Nuwayrī's explanation that the *ublūj*s are of different sizes, one holding more than a *qinṭ*ār [*jarwī*] (96.7 kilograms) and the other less.[47] Another historian, al-Maqrīzī, relates that one *ublūja* (*ublūj*) is equal to 1/9 of a *qinṭār* [*jarwī*], or about ten kilograms, far smaller than of the size given by al-Nuwayrī.[48] On the other hand, E. Ashtor, in discussing the technological decline of Levantine sugar production in the later Mamluk period, reads al-Maqrīzī's sentence as "one *ublūja* is equal to 9 *qinṭār*s."[49] This is clearly a misreading, which leads to the incredible conclusion that one *ublūj* is equal to over 870 kilograms.

Anyhow, if one *ublūj* is nearly 100 kilograms, as al-Nuwayrī relates, it would be nearly impossible for one person to carry. From my visual inspection, the *ublūj* at the ʿAjlūn Castle Museum was about 30 centimeters in both height and maximum diameter. Based on these measurements, when we calculate the cubic volume, it holds 7,065 cm^3. As the specific gravity of sugar is 1.59, this *ublūj* would hold about 11.2 kilograms of sugar, which corresponds to the numbers given by al-Maqrīzī, not by al-Nuwayrī. The size and weight of an *ublūj* vary by

44 Ouerfelli, *Le sucre*, p. 245.

45 Song Yingxing (宋應星), *Tenko Kaibutsu* (*Tien-kung kai-wu*), Japanese tr. by K. Yabuuchi, Tokyo, 1969, p. 125.

46 Daniels, "The Adoption and Transfer of New Sugarmaking Technology," p. 106.

47 If al-Nuwayrī uses the ordinary *qinṭār*, which was not the standard in medieval Egypt, it holds 45 kilograms and is the smaller of the two.

48 Al-Maqrīzī, *al-Khiṭaṭ*, I, 103.

49 Ashtor, "Levantine Sugar Industry in the Late Middle Ages," p. 123. Ouerfelli also makes the same mistake as Ashtor (*Le sucre*, p. 262, note 199).

district and period.[50] However, the *ublūj* I saw in ʿAjlūn would hold over 10 kilograms, which could be carried by one person.

> <The Yield of Sugar>
> The yields that come from the presses have different names, such as *ḍarība*, *waḍʿa*, and *yad*. One *ḍarība* is 8 *yad*s, one *yad* is a full *khābiya*, and as mentioned above, one *khābiya* is 3,000 *raṭl*s *laythī* of pressed juice. Therefore, one *ḍarība* is 24,000 *raṭls* of juice. One *ḍarība* of juice, if the cane is good quality, yields 15–25 *qinṭār*s of raw sugar (*qand*) and 8–12 *qinṭār*s of molasses (*ʿasal*). The maximum yield from a *faddān* of cane is 3 *ḍarība*s; namely 2+1/2 *ḍarība*s of raw sugar and molasses (*qaṭr*) and 1/2 *ḍarība* of low-grade molasses (*ʿasal*). The total of 3 *ḍarība*s is equal to 24 *qinṭār*s *miṣrī*. There are some sugarcanes of inferior quality, the juice of which does not solidify to raw sugar. These are boiled to produce a low-grade molasses, which is called "[liquid] discharge" (*mursal*).[51]

In medieval Egypt, the weight of sugar was measured in *qinṭārs jarwī*, units of 96.7 kilograms.[52] According to al-Nuwayrī, the raw sugar yielded from a *faddān* (0.637 hectare) of good cane is 15–25 *qinṭārs jarwī*, or 1,450–2,418 kilograms. This amount nearly matches al-Nuwayrī's accounting that the total yield of sugar is 3 *ḍarība*s, that is 24 *qinṭār*s *miṣrī* (*jarwī*), or 2,321 kilograms. If we add the raw sugar and molasses yields together, the total rises to 2,224–3,578 kilograms. According to H.A. Rivlin, the yield of sugar in Egypt during the reign of Muḥammad ʿAli was almost 2,500 kilograms per *faddān* (0.44 hectare).[53]

> <From Red Sugar to White Sugar and Rock Sugar>
> When the raw sugar (*qand*) is dried and starts to turn white, it is brought to the sugar refinery (*maṭbakh al-sukkar*), dissolved in water with clean milk added (*laban ḥalīb*), and boiled. It then becomes white sugar (*sukkar bayāḍ*) and fine molasses (*quṭāra*). Each *qinṭār* of raw sugar yields 5 parts white sugar and 7 parts fine molasses. When the process is repeated, one gets a pure white refined sugar, and the trickle of fine molasses begins

50 According to Ouerfelli, three kinds of earthenware objects (forme de terre) were used in the medieval Mediterranean world; the biggest one for the first refinery was 24.66 litres (*Le sucre*, pp. 276–277).

51 Al-Nuwayrī, *Nihāyat al-Arab*, VIII, 271.

52 Hinz, *Islamische Masse und Gewichte*, p. 25.

53 H.A. Rivlin, *The Agricultural Policy of Muḥammad ʿAlī in Egypt*, Cambridge, Mass., 1961, p. 146.

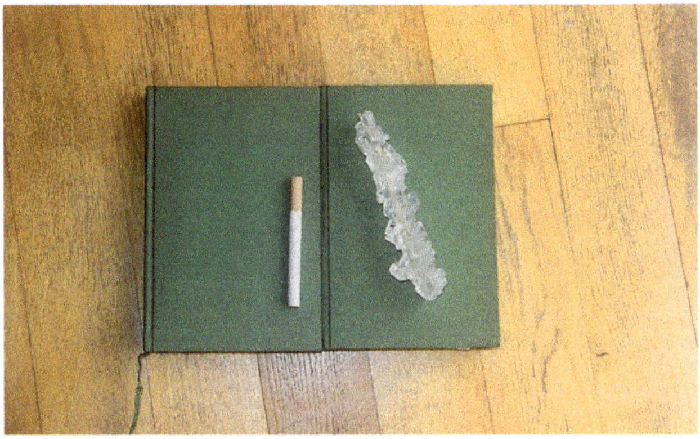

FIGURE 4 *The* nabāt *found at a market in Damascus*

> to form rock sugar (*qaṭr al-nabāt*), which, once boiled again, becomes pure rock sugar (*nabāt*).[54]

Raw sugar (*qand*) is often called "red sugar" (*sukkar aḥmar*) in Arabic sources.[55] As al-Nuwayrī relates, dried raw sugar is dissolved in water with fresh milk added, and one uses an *ublūj* to get white sugar and fine molasses. He goes on to explain that the fine molasses (*quṭāra*), once again boiled, becomes rock sugar (*sukkar al-nabāt*). The word "*nabāt*" means plant. How do we conclude that "plant" means rock sugar? When I walked around the markets in Damascus, I found ranged rock sugar crystallized around the stalks of a certain plant they called "*nabāt*" (Figure 4). Ibn al-Nafīs al-Dimashqī, the personal physician of Sultan Baybars I, gives an interesting account of the process of manufacturing rock sugar.

> There are various kinds of sugar. Among these, *ṭabarzad* sugar[56] is the most popular in Egypt and Syria. It is also called "*sukkar ublūj*," formed in

54 Al-Nuwayrī, *Nihāyat al-Arab*, VIII, 272.

55 For examples, see the following sources; Ibn al-Ḥājj, *al-Madkhal*, IV, 149, 152; al-Dimashqī, *Kitāb al-Ishāra ilā Maḥāsin al-Tijāra*, Cairo, 1900, 32; Ibn al-Nafīs, *al-Shāmil*, XV, 115–116, 126; Abū Sahl, *Kitāb al-Mi'a fī al-Ṭibb*, ed. F. Sanagustin, 2 vols., Damascus, 2000, I, 139. It was also called *sukkar khām* in Ottoman Egypt (N. Hanna, *Making Big Money in 1600: The Life and Times of Isma'il Abu Taqiyya, Egyptian Merchant*, New York, 1998, p. 88).

56 According to Lippmann, *ṭabarzad* was a kind of pure and crystallized solid sugar originally produced in Persia (*Geschichte des Zuckers*, pp. 101–102). See also M. Ahsan, *Social Life under the Abbasids*, London and New York, 1979, p. 102; Sato, "Sugar in the Economic Life of Mamluk Egypt," p. 96. However, based on Ibn al-Nafīs's account above, *ṭabarzad* was not rock sugar, but refined solid sugar, different from *sukkar al-nabāt*. See also Ibn

> a cone shape. The *mukarrar* (repeatedly refined sugar) is dissolved in water, refined with an *ublūj*, and then refined once again. As it is repeatedly refined, it becomes whiter and purer, but both the sweetness and taste suffer. The *sukkar al-nabāt* is another kind of sugar that is boiled repeatedly. After the boiled juice is solidified using an *ublūj*, it is dissolved in water, and left in a vessel (*qidr*). When the twigs from a date palm are thrown in the vessel, small rock sugar (*ḥajar ṣaghīr*) crystallizes on them.[57]

The above account shows that "*nabāt*" indicates twigs from a date palm used to accelerate the crystallization of refined sugar. This explains why rock sugar has been called "*sukkar al-nabāt*" since the medieval Islamic ages. The red sugar, white sugar, and rock sugar are named according to various districts and times, which are explained in the Glossary.

The Spread of Sugar Production Technology from Egypt to China

The Travels of Marco Polo

Marco Polo (1254–1324), who visited Fujian under Yüan rule in 1290, relates the following in his travelogues.

> At the end of the three days, and proceeding another fifteen miles, one comes to the city of Unken, where they have an enormous quantity of sugar. From this city the Great Kaan gets all the sugar that is used at his court – enough to represent a considerable sum in value. You must also know that in these parts, before the Great Kaan subjected them to his lordship, the people did not know how to prepare and refine sugar so well as is done at Babylon. They did not let it congeal and solidify in moulds, but merely boiled and skimmed it, so that it hardened into a kind of paste, and was black in color. But after the country had been conquered by the Great Kaan, there came into these regions some men of Babylon, who had been at the court of the Great Kaan and who taught them how to refine it with the ashes of certain trees.[58]

Sayyār, *Annals of the Caliphs' Kitchens: Ibn Sayyār al-Warrāq's Tenth-Century Baghdadi Cookbook*, English tr. by N. Nasrallah, Leiden, 2007, pp. 601–602.

57 Ibn al-Nafīs, *al-Shāmil*, xv, 115–116.

58 Marco Polo, *The Travels of Marco Polo*, English tr. from the text of L.F. Benedetto by A. Ricci, London, 1931, p. 258.

The Babylon cited here is identified by most scholars as the Babylon of al-Fusṭāṭ in Egypt, not that of Iraq.[59] Evidently, we can take this to mean that the Babylonian method of refining sugar by congealing and solidifying it in moulds did not differ from the separation of molasses from boiled juice with the *ublūj*s as explained by al-Nuwayrī. As mentioned above, the *ublūj* cone-shaped earthenware moulds were the equivalent of *wa liu* (瓦溜) in China. The above account relates that some men from Babylon taught the Chinese how to refine the boiled juice using the ashes of certain trees, which is a significantly different method of sugar production than separating the molasses from the boiled juice with an *ublūj*.

Matsuo Otagi, who translated *The Travels of Marco Polo* into Japanese, notes that the refining techniques for producing crystal sugar had already been brought to Tang Dynasty China from India during the first half of the seventh century. He therefore concludes that Marco Polo was mistaken in assuming a new technique from Egypt was introduced during the Yüan period.[60] However, according to Tai, in the Tang period, crystal sugar was acquired with the use of a bamboo spatula,[61] which was a significantly different technique than using *ublūj*s. Otagi, whose principle specialization was Chinese history, had little knowledge of just how much sugar production technologies had progressed from Fatimid to Mamluk Egypt. Tai states that *wa liu* equivalent to *ublūj*s were first brought to China under the Yüan rule in the second half of the thirteenth century.[62] Daniels also notes that at present, most scholars regard Marco Polo's account as accurate, rejecting S. Mazumdar's skepticism.[63]

Technology Transfer between East and West

Accordingly, based on Marco Polo's account above, we can conclude that an important transfer of sugar technology transpired between the Islamic world and China. It is widely known that beginning in the eighth century, Chinese paper manufacturing, gunpowder, and compasses were brought to the Islamic

59 Yule and Cordier note that the Babylonia of the passage is Cairo, –Babylon of Egypt, the sugar of which was very famous in the Middle Ages (*The Book of Ser Marco Polo*, 2 vols., 3rd ed., London, 1929, vol. 2, p. 230, note 8).

60 *Toho Kenbunroku*, Japanese tr. by M. Otagi, 2 vols., Tokyo, 1970–71, vol. 2, p. 104, note 12.

61 Tai, *The Evolution of Sugar Production in China*, p. 93. See also E.H. Schafer, *The Golden Peaches of Samarqand*, Berkeley, Los Angeles, and London, 1963, pp. 153–154.

62 Tai, *The Evolution of Sugar Production in China*, pp. 99–103.

63 Daniels, *Agro-Industries: Sugarcane Technology*, pp. 351–352. Mazumdar relates, "Marco Polo was of course an unabashed propagandist for the Mongols, so it is difficult to judge whether the Chinese cane sugar was indeed of such poor quality" (*Sugar and Society in China*, p. 36).

world, which initiated the development of Islamic civilization in the ʿAbbasid periods. The introduction and expansion of paper manufacturing were especially useful in the development of Islamic sciences like law, theology, hadith studies, history, medicine, mathematics, and geography. Some brands of paper, such as *Sulaymānī* from Persia, *Jaʿfarī* from Iraq, and *Firʿawnī* from Egypt, were valued throughout the Islamic world for their quality. When inexpensive paper spread in the tenth century, the use of light and flexible paper (*kāghad, waraqa*) replaced parchment and papyrus in academic activities, central and regional bureaucracies, and the court records of Muslim societies.[64]

Marco Polo said that several people from Babylon (i.e. al-Fusṭāṭ) taught the Chinese a new technology for sugar production that had been developed in Islamic Egypt. When the Crusaders under Amalric, King of Jerusalem, approached Cairo in *Ṣafar* 564/November 1168, the Fatimid wazir Shāwar issued an order to set the commercial center of al-Fusṭāṭ on fire to prevent supplying the raiding Crusaders with provisions.[65] However, after it was burned down, sultans, amirs, and major merchants began reconstructing the sugar refineries (*maṭbakh al-sukkar*) in al-Fusṭāṭ during the Ayyubid and Mamluk periods.[66] As mentioned above, after the harvest, the sugarcane was pressed and boiled at pressing factories (*maʿṣara li-qaṣab al-sukkar*) adjacent to the sugarcane fields in local provinces. The raw sugar produced there was mostly transported to the sugar refineries (*maṭbakh al-sukkar*) of al-Fusṭāṭ, where it was refined to white and rock sugar, and sold commercially in domestic and international markets. We can therefore conclude that the sugar production techniques that had substantially evolved in medieval Egypt were brought to China, in contrast to techniques for paper manufacturing, gunpowder, and compasses, which moved from the East to the West.

64 For the development of paper manufacturing in the Islamic world, see the following works. J. Pedersen, *The Arabic Book*, English tr. by G. French, Princeton, 1984, pp. 54–71; J.M. Bloom, *Paper before Print: The History and Impact of Paper in the Islamic World*, New Haven and London, 2001.

65 *EI*², s.v. al-Fusṭāṭ (J. Jomier); S. Lane-Poole, *Saladin and the Fall of the Kingdom of Jerusalem*, London, 1898; repr. Beirut, 1964, p. 93; A.S. Ehrenkreutz, *Saladin*, Albany, 1972, p. 49; M.C. Lyons and D.E.P. Jackson, *Saladin: The Politics of the Holy War*, Cambridge, 1982, p. 22.

66 Ibn Duqmāq, *Kitāb al-Intiṣār*, I, 41–46.

CHAPTER 3

On Camels and Ships: Sugar as Commodity

The Prosperity of al-Karkh in Baghdad

The Establishment of Baghdad

In 136/754, as is widely known, the second ʿAbbasid caliph, Abū Jaʿfar al-Manṣūr (reigned 136–158/754–775), decided to establish a capital city suitable for the new state (*dawla*). He himself searched for an adequate place, and eventually selected Baghdad, on the west bank of the Tigris river. The chronicle by al-Ṭabarī (d. 310/923) relates al-Manṣūr's opinion as follows.

> The place is suitable for the army post, and there is no obstacle that separates us from China. We get all the provisions from the sea through the Tigris, and any kinds of food from al-Jazīra and Armenia. The Euphrates brings us any kinds of provision from al-Shām and Raqqa.[1]

This account shows that in selecting Baghdad, al-Manṣūr carefully considered the supply of provisions from surrounding countries. When the new capital was completed in 146/766, it was officially named Madīnat al-Salām (City of Peace), but people nevertheless continued to refer to it as Baghdad. The city layout was round, with a diameter of 2.35 kilometers, and surrounded by three concentric circular walls, the second main wall being 34 meters high. In the center of the city was the Golden Gate Castle (*Qaṣr Bāb al-Dhahab*), which served as the caliph's residence with an adjacent mosque. Around them stood the mansions of the caliph's family, the stations for over four thousand guards, and government offices, like the *dīwān al-kharāj*, *dīwān al-rasāʾil*, *dīwān al-jaysh*, and so on. That is, the privileged class (*khāṣṣa*) resided within the round city, while the common people (*ʿāmma*) such as merchants, artisans, ʿulama, and others, lived outside the city walls.[2]

1 Al-Ṭabarī, *Taʾrīkh al-Rusul wal-Mulūk*, III, 272.

2 For the establishment and development of Baghdad, see the following works. *EI*², s.v. Baghdād (A.A. Duri); G. Le Strange, *Baghdad during the Abbasid Caliphate*, Oxford, 1900; repr. New York, 1972; J. Lassner, *The Topography of Baghdad in the Early Middle Ages*, Detroit, 1970; S.A. al-ʿAlī, *Baghdād Madīnat al-Salām: al-Jānib al-Gharbī*, 2 vols., Baghdad, 1985.

 | DOI 10.1163/9789004281561_005

The round city had four evenly spaced gates, named the Khorasan Gate, the Basra Gate, the Kufa Gate, and the Syria (or Damascus) Gate. The use of these names reflected the aspirational view of Baghdad as a grand international city. Departing from the Khorasan Gate, one crossed the Tigris River, followed the Khorasan road to the East, and finally arrived at Chang'an, the capital of the Tang dynasty. From the Basra Gate, one went down the Tigris to the port city of Basra, from where one sailed the Persian Gulf and the Indian Ocean to get to India and Southeast Asia. From the Kufa Gate, one went south and reached the city of al-Kūfa, where *ḥajj* pilgrims from the eastern countries gathered, and beyond which lied Mecca, the central city of the Islamic world. And finally, from the Syria Gate, one went up along the Euphrates to arrive at the old city of Damascus, or beyond to Constantinople, the terminus of the Silk Road.

On both sides of the arcades at the four gates, markets (*sūq*) were set up for trading daily goods. In the center of these four gates, as mentioned above, resided the caliph, his family, and other high officials. As these markets were located near the castle, it was difficult to guard the caliph and other important persons. In 157/774, all the markets from the arcades were therefore relocated to the district of al-Karkh, two kilometers south of the round city.[3]

Al-Karkh as Commerce and Industry Center

Al-Karkh was conveniently located between the Salat and Isa canals. At that time, it was well known that as the riverbed of the Euphrates was higher than that of the Tigris, when a canal was dug between two rivers, water naturally flowed from the Euphrates to the Tigris.[4] Taking advantage of this situation, many canals were constructed between the two rivers in the eighth and ninth centuries, providing water used for drinking, irrigation, and transportation. We may presume that the prosperity of Baghdad during the ʿAbbasid period was primarily based on the development of an irrigation agriculture utilizing these canal systems, and on the commercial activities of the East-West caravan route and North-South river route.

From the end of the eighth century, as economic activities developed, Baghdad began to import expensive commercial goods, including silk textiles and pottery produced in China, spices and timbers from Southeast Asia and India, woolen goods and Turkic and Slavic slaves from Central Asia, and black slaves and gold from Africa. It exported to the surrounding Islamic countries and the Byzantine Empire the special products of Iraq, such as silk and cotton textiles,

---

3 *EI*^{2}, s.v. al-Karkh (M. Streck-[J. Lassner]); Le Strange, *Baghdad*, pp. 57–68; Lassner, *The Topography of Baghdad*, pp. 60–63.

4 H.Q. el-Sāmarrāie, *Agriculture in Iraq during the 3rd Century AH*, Beirut, 1972, p. 12.

precious metals, glassware, and papers. Al-Yaʿqūbī (d. 284/897), in his geography book, gives the oldest surviving account of the prosperity of Baghdad.

> Through the two big rivers near Baghdad, the Tigris and the Euphrates, various kinds of commercial goods and provisions are easily brought in. Even non-Islamic countries, such as India, Sind, China, Tibet, Turk, Daylam, Khazar, and Ethiopia, provide us with every kind of commercial good. In Baghdad, there are six thousand roads (*darb*) and lanes (*sikka*), thirty thousand mosques (*masjid*), and ten thousand public baths (*ḥammām*), and those numbers are increasing even now. The Chicken Canal, which took its name from the residence of chicken owners, was dug for Karkh and adjacent districts. Moreover, large ships (*safīna kabīra*) sail in the Great Isa Canal, and bring barley and other goods from Syria and Egypt through Raqqa to the shore, where markets and stores (*khānāt*) stand in a row. As the provision of water improved, the cultivated fields and orchards expanded around the city. Numerous artisans from various countries gathered and produced every kind of provision.[5]

This account confirms that Baghdad prospered in the ninth and tenth centuries because of commercial trade with other countries, fertile agricultural production, and the immigration of artisans. The district of al-Karkh, which came to be known as "home to great merchants and Shiʿites,"[6] was the center of these commercial and industrial activities. Next, we will look at the connection between the rising commercial center of al-Karkh and sugar as a new commercial product.

From Dibs *to Sugar: A Change in the Production of Sweeteners*

But before that, we will look at changes in sweeteners production in ʿAbbasid Iraq. In ancient Mesopotamia, before sugar production, sweeteners were made from ripe fruits, like apricots, grapes, and dates. Even in Islamic times, these ripe fruits were used to make a traditional, thick, condensed juice known in Arabic as *dibs*.[7] Even after sugar became the preferred source of sweetener among the ʿAbbasid court and the wealthier families, *dibs* remained popular among the common people. For example, the district of Arrajān in Fārs was

---

5 Al-Yaʿqūbī, *Kitāb al-Buldān*, BGA, VII, ed. M.J. de Goeje, Leiden, 1967, 234, 250–251.

6 Ibn al-Athīr states that before the civil strife of 361/971, al-Karkh was home to great merchants (*tājir*) and Shiʿites (*al-Kāmil*, VIII, 619).

7 Ahsan, *Social Life under the Abbasids*, pp. 100–101.

particularly noted for producing *dibs* made from dried grapes.[8] It is said that *sikbāj*, a well-known dish, was cooked with fatty meat, carrots or eggplants, almonds, currants, dried figs, a mixture of date juice and vinegar, and the usual spices.[9]

As mentioned above, when the pressed juice is boiled and refined with an *ublūj*, one gets raw sugar and molasses (*ʿasal*), which originally meant honey. Egyptian historian al-Maqrīzī wrote an unusual book entitled *Niḥal ʿIbar al-Naḥl* (*A Gift Essay on Honeybees*), in which he compiles the Arabic traditions relating to bees and honey, and describes the various kinds of honey and their respective colors and medicinal effects. According to his account, the following was custom in Mamluk Egypt.

> In the Coptic month of Amshīr (26 January-24 February), female bees (worker bees) gather, and in Barmūda (27 March-25 April), they begin to collect honey. The best flowers are the trefoil (*qurṭ*) and the grass pea (*julubbān*). Also, mothers often drink honey dissolved in water when the weather gets cold or the wind is blowing hard.[10]

Al-Maqrīzī gives yet another account.

> The best honey smells sweet, tastes bitter, and is stimulating and sticky. Honey prevents meat from rotting, and if one puts honey on his body, it both guards against lice and kills them. Moreover, one can preserve the remains of food by putting them in honey. Honey preserves meat for three months and fruits for six months.[11]

The above accounts clearly show that after sugar production began, honey still continued to play an important role in the everyday life of Muslim societies. However, sugar was superior to honey for its exquisite taste, ease of transport, and medicinal effects. This increased the demand for sugar considerably, leading to a flourishing sugar industry. As Ibn Ḥawqal (fourth/tenth century) states, there was no village in Iraq without sugarcane crops.[12]

---

8 Al-Thaʿālibī, *Laṭāʾif al-Maʿārif*, ed. I. al-Abyārī and H.K. al-Ṣayrafī, Cairo, 1960, 237. See also G. Le Strange, *The Lands of the Eastern Caliphate*, London, 1905; repr. London, 1966, p. 294.

9 Ahsan, *Social Life under the Abbasids*, p. 83.

10 Al-Maqrīzī, *Niḥal ʿIbar al-Naḥl*, ed. J. al-Shayyāl, Cairo, 1946, 30.

11 Al-Maqrīzī, *Niḥal ʿIbar al-Naḥl*, 40–42.

12 Ibn Ḥawqal, *Kitāb Ṣūrat al-Arḍ*, 254.

Sugar Distribution in the Eastern Islamic World

During the tenth century, as I mentioned in Chapter One, Ahwāz in the district of Khūzistān was well known as a center for sugar production in the eastern Islamic world. Al-Thaʿālibī (350–429/961–1038) from Nīshāpūr describes the following in a chapter detailing to the features of each district of Persia.

> <Description of Ahwāz>
> ʿAskar Mukram produces sugar that is unequaled in both quality and quantity. Although more sugarcane is cultivated in Iraq, Jurjān, and India, the sugar from ʿAskar Mukram is the best for commercial goods (*matjar*). Every year 50,000 *raṭl*s (113,700 kilograms) of sugar from ʿAskar Mukram are transported to the sultan (caliph) in Baghdad in addition to the *kharāj* tax.[13]

ʿAskar Mukram, a province north of Ahwāz with ample water, extended along the Dujayl river. Al-Jahshiyārī states that 30,000 *raṭl*s (68,250 kilograms) of sugar were levied in kind as an annual tax on Ahwāz.[14] According to al-Thaʿālibī, over 100,000 kilograms of sugar, in addition to the *kharāj* tax payments, were annually transported to the capital city of Baghdad. Al-Thaʿālibī goes on to list the fruits, other crops, and processed goods specific to each district in the Islamic world.

> Apples (*tuffāḥ*) in Syria, ripe dates (*ruṭab*) in Iraq, bananas (*mawz*) in Yemen, walnuts (*jawz*) in India, fava beans (*bāqillā*) in al-Kūfa, sugar (*sukkar*) in Ahwāz, honey (*ʿasal*) in Iṣfahān, white sugar (*fānīdh*) in Māsakān, dates (*tamr*) in Kirmān, fruit-based syrup (*dibs*) in Arrajān, figs (*tīn*) in Hulwān, grapes (*ʿinab*) in Baghdad, jujube fruits (*ʿunnāb*) in Jurjān, plums (*ijjāṣ*) in Bust, pomegranates (*rummān*) in Rayy, pears (*kummasrā*) in Nihāwand, quince (*safarjal*) in Nīshāpūr, apricots (*mishmish*) in Ṭūs, fruit cakes (*murabban*) in Marw, and melons (*baṭṭīkh*) in Khwārizm.[15]

We note that al-Thaʿālibī only notes Ahwāz and Māsakān in Persia as sugar producers, not mentioning the districts in Iraq. He says that sugar from ʿAskar Mukram was the best for commerce, so sugar from Ahwāz and Māsakān were probably superior in quality to sugar from Iraq.

---

13 Al-Thaʿālibī, *Laṭāʾif al-Maʿārif*, 174.

14 Al-Jahshiyārī, *Kitāb al-Wuzarāʾ*, 282–283.

15 Al-Thaʿālibī, *Laṭāʾif al-Maʿārif*, 237–238.

According to ʿAbd al-ʿAzīz al-Dūrī, in the ʿAbbasid period, these quality sugars were routinely transported to al-Karkh in Baghdad.[16] Al-Muqaddasī states that sugar was brought to Baghdad from Sūs (north of Ahwāz) for commerce.[17] Al-Idrīsī also states that sugarcane cultivation prospered in the twelfth century in the cities of Māsakān and Kaṣrān, which exported their sugar (*sukkar*) and white sugar (*fānīdh*) to countries east and west.[18] Moreover, Yāqūt al-Rūmī states that Māsakān was well known for producing white sugar (*fānīdh*) that was transported to various other countries.[19]

In the ninth and tenth centuries, Baghdad developed into a major city with a population of nearly one million. However, as economic activities advanced, the disparity in wealth increased, which brought about the appearance of rogue bandits (*ʿayyār*) from the lower class in Baghdad in the early ninth century. In groups of thirty or forty men, they attacked the caliph's court and the mansions of the leading merchants, repeatedly pillaging and starting fires that over time devastated al-Karkh and even Baghdad. Nevertheless, the common people thought well of the *ʿayyār*s, as they were chivalrous, generous, and sided with the weak.[20] Nonetheless, the people able to enjoy the sweetness of sugar were the caliphs and their families, the high-ranking officials and soldiers, and the major merchants. These were the privileged classes of *khāṣṣa* in Baghdad that the *ʿayyār*s repeatedly attacked.

The Growth of Sugar Production in Egypt

From Baghdad to Cairo: A Historical Change

As the economy in Baghdad prospered, the results of scholarly research came to be published in Arabic, one after another, in the fields of law, theology, hadith, history, medical science, mathematics, and geography. However, in contrast to the cultural prosperity of the day, the political authority of the ʿAbbasid caliphate began to decline in the ninth century.

16 A. al-Dūrī, *Taʾrīkh al-ʿIrāq al-Iqtiṣādī fī al-Qarn al-Rābiʿ al-Hijrī*, Baghdad, 1948, p. 135.

17 Al-Muqaddasī, *Aḥsan al-Taqāsīm*, 416.

18 Al-Idrīsī, *Kitāb Nuzhat al-Mushtāq*, II, 174.

19 Yāqūt, *Muʿjam al-Buldān*, V, 42.

20 Cl. Cahen, "Mouvements populaires et autonomisme urbain dans l'Asie musulman du moyen âge I-III." *Arabica*, 5 (1958), pp. 225–250; 6 (1959), pp. 25–56, 233–265; S. Sabari, *Mouvements populaires à Baghdad à l'époque ʿAbbaside*, Paris, 1981; M.R. al-Najjār, *Ḥikāyāt al-Shuṭṭār wal-ʿAyyārīn fī al-Turāth al-ʿArabī*, Kuwait, 1981. For the *ʿayyārs* in the Iranian cities, see D. Durand-Guédy, *Iranian Elites and Turkish Rulers: A History of Iṣfahān in the Saljūq Period*, London and New York, 2010, pp. 66, 162.

For example, in 205/821, Ṭāhir b. al-Ḥusayn, the governor of the Khurāsān region, founded the Ṭāhirid dynasty (205–278/821–873), who asserted their independance from Caliph al-Maʾmūn. Thereafter, Yaʿqūb b. al-Layth, who had risen from working as a coppersmith (*ṣaffār*) to found the Ṣaffārid dynasty (247–393/861–1003) in east Iran, advanced to Baghdad. Moreover, in the country of Māwarānnahr, Aḥmad b. Asad b. Sāmān, a local noble (*dihqān*), converted to Islam and then established in Balkh the Sāmānids (204–395/819–1005), who ruled over whole districts of Khurāsān. Around the same time, Aḥmad b. Ṭūlūn, the son of a Turkish *mamlūk*, founded in Egypt the Ṭūlūnids (254–292/868–905), refusing to pay taxes to Baghdad.

The appearance of these independent dynasties reduced the territory ruled by the ʿAbbasid caliphs, resulting in a significant decrease in state income. As the income decreased, the government was late paying its soldiers' salaries and could no longer retain control of them. The Turkish *mamlūk*s, originally employed to support the caliphate, consolidated their power in the latter half of the ninth century. According to Ibn al-Ṭiqṭaqā (seventh/thirteenth century), after the *mamlūk*s succeeded in killing Caliph al-Mutawakkil in 247/861, they retained, dethroned, or even killed subsequent caliphs as they pleased, as if the caliphs were their prisoners.[21]

In 324/936 Caliph al-Rāḍī (reigned 322–329/934–940) appointed Ibn Rāʾiq, co-governor of al-Baṣra and Wāsiṭ, to the position of great amir (*amīr al-umarāʾ*), and entrusted him with tax revenues and military affairs.[22] This was the first time in Islamic history that a caliph had entrusted another person with the ruling of a state. Ten years later, in Jumādā II 334/January 946, Muʿizz al-Dawla entered Baghdad with the Buwayhid army and established his own Shiʿite authority, putting the Sunnite caliphate under his protection. However, as he could not gather enough revenue to support his armies, Muʿizz al-Dawla assigned *iqṭāʿ*s in Lower Iraq (al-Sawād) to his commanders, his associates, and his Turkish slave soldiers. This was the creation of the so-called "military *iqṭāʿ* system", which was passed on to the Islamic dynasties that followed.[23] The ʿAbbasid caliphs, deprived of military power, retained only the nominal

21 Ibn al-Ṭiqṭaqā, *al-Fakhrī fī al-Ādāb al-Sulṭānīya*, Beirut, 1966.

22 For the appointment of Ibn Rāʾiq to *amīr al-umarāʾ*, see Miskawayh, *Kitāb Tajārib al-Umam*, Arabic text and English tr. by H.F. Amedroz and D.S. Margoliouth, *The Eclipse of the ʿAbbasid Caliphate*, 7 vols., London, 1920–21, I, 351.

23 For more about the *iqṭāʿ* system, see the following works. Cl. Cahen, "L'évolution de l'iqṭāʿ du IXe au XIIIe siècle," *Annales:ESC*, 8 (1953), pp. 25–52; A.K.S. Lambton, *Landlord and Peasant in Persia*, London, 1953; id., "Reflections on the IQṬĀʿ," G. Makdisi ed., *Arabic and Islamic Studies in Honor of Hamilton A.R. Gibb*, Leiden, 1965, pp. 358–376; I.A. Ṭurkhān, *al-Nuẓum al-Iqṭāʿīya fī al-Sharq al-Awsaṭ fī al-ʿUṣūr al-Wusṭā*, Cairo, 1963; A. al-Dūrī, "The

authority to acknowledge the rising military regimes of the Buwayhids and the Seljuqids.

In the western Islamic world, the Isma'ilites founded the Fatimid state in North Africa, advanced to Egypt in 358/969, and founded the new capital of Cairo (al-Qāhira) north of al-Fusṭāṭ. The Fatimid economy developed rapidly, benefiting from the use of Red Sea, rather than Persian Gulf trade routes. As mentioned above, the social order in Baghdad collapsed under the attacks of the *'ayyār* rogue bandits in the ninth and tenth centuries, which caused the merchants and 'ulama to flee to Damascus and Cairo. Thus, the economic and cultural forces that had grown in Baghdad shifted to Cairo in the eleventh and twelfth centuries.[24]

The Beginning of Prosperous Sugar Production in Fatimid Egypt

As explained in Chapter One, sugarcane cultivation was introduced in Lower Egypt in the eighth and ninth centuries. The cultivation then spread to Upper Egypt, where sugar production began to prosper in the late tenth century as the Fatimid rule of Egypt stabilized. Al-Musabbiḥī, raised in the old city of al-Fusṭāṭ, comments on a parade of sugar candy held by Caliph al-Ẓāhir (reigned 411–427/1021–36).

> On Friday at the end of Ramaḍān in 415/1024, a diorama, made of sugar candy and depicting a banquet (*simāṭ*) with figurines (*timthāl*), decorations (*tazwīn*), and castles (*qaṣr*), was paraded through the city streets. Wazir Najīb al-Dawla Abū al-Qāsim 'Alī al-Jarjalā'ī supervised the display, which boasted 152 figurines and 7 big castles. Officials on horseback and a Sudanese drum corps led the parade, and the people gathered to see it.[25]

This shows that at the festival of *'īd al-fiṭr*, the government held a parade of sugar candy to demonstrate the caliph's authority. The later Ayyubids and Mamluks continued this tradition of a sugar festival during Ramaḍān, which the Cairene people greatly enjoyed. According to P. Sanders, it was already common for castles made of sugar candy to be used for various courtesies and

Origins of Iqṭā' in Islam," *al-Abḥāth*, 22 (1969), pp. 3–22; H. Rabie, *The Financial System of Egypt AH 564–741/AD 1169–1341*, London, 1972; Sato, *State and Rural Society*.

24 E. Ashtor, "Un mouvement migratoire au haut moyen âge: Migrations de l'Irak vers les pays méditerranéens," *Annales: ESC*, 27 (1972), pp. 185–214.

25 Al-Musabbiḥī, *Akhbār Miṣr*, 65.

banquets in the Fatimid court.[26] Also, Ibn al-Ma'mūn al-Baṭā'iḥī, the son of a Fatimid wazir, gives the following account.

> On Thursday 12 of Muḥarram in 516/1122, which was the birthday of Caliph al-ʿĀmir bi-Aḥkām Allāh (reigned 495–524/1101–30), an order was given to prepare forty trays (*ṣīnīya*) of round cakes (*khushkanānij*), sweets (*ḥalwā*), and other kinds of cakes (*kaʿk*). In addition to these, sugar, honey, almonds, wheat flour, and sesame oil were by order of the caliph delivered to the tombs of prominent persons. Specifically, 500 *raṭl*s (484 kilograms) of sweets were distributed to mosque leaders (*mutaṣaddir*), Qur'an readers (*qāri'*), and sufi mendicants (*faqīr*).[27]

The word *ṣīnīya* literally meant "Chinese goods," but actually indicated round brass trays made in Egypt. And *khushkanānij* was a kind of round cake with almond and pistachio in the hollow center.[28] This account also reveals that on the caliph's birthday, various kinds of sugar-based sweets were given to the faithful. According to an account by Ibn al-Ma'mūn, in the year 517/1123 from the month of Rajab to Ramaḍān the caliph distributed sweets to the faithful at Azhar Mosque, ʿAmr Mosque, and other mosques in turn.[29]

Ibn al-Ma'mūn also provides the following account of a banquet held by his father, al-Ma'mūn, on the last day of *ʿīd al-naḥr* (*ʿīd al-aḍḥā*) in the month of Dhū al-Ḥijja 516/1122.

> The banquet expenses at the mansion of al-Ma'mūn were 1,326+5/12 dinars. And in addition to the sugar used in the kitchen, another 48 *qinṭār*s [*jarwī*] (4,600 kilograms) of sugar were used for both the castle of sweets (*qaṣr al-ḥalāwa*) and the leavened cakes (*qiṭaʿ manfūkh*).[30]

This account shows that on the last day of *ʿīd al-aḍḥā* in 516/1122, the Fatimid wazir, al-Ma'mūn, made sweets using a large amount of sugar for guests at his mansion. However, the several accounts cited above say nothing that clearly confirms the consumption of sugar by the common people of Fatimid Egypt.

---

26 P. Sanders, *Ritual, Politics, and the City in Fatimid Cairo*, Albany, 1994, pp. 78–79, 171.

27 Ibn al-Ma'mūn, *Nuṣūṣ min Akhbār Miṣr*, 35–36.

28 Ibn al-Ma'mūn, *Nuṣūṣ min Akhbār Miṣr*, 35. See also note 5 by the editor, A.F. Sayyid.

29 Ibn al-Ma'mūn, *Nuṣūṣ min Akhbār Miṣr*, 63. See also Ibn ʿAbd al-Ẓāhir, *al-Rawḍat al-Bahīyat al-Zāhira fī Khiṭaṭ al-Muʿizzīyat al-Qāhira*, ed. A.F. Sayyid, Cairo, 1996, 44.

30 Ibn al-Ma'mūn, *Akhbār Miṣr*, 42.

Sugar in the Age of Ṣalāḥ al-Dīn

What about the Ayyubid period? Ibn Duqmāq, a historian in Mamluk Egypt, states the following in his *Kitāb al-Intiṣār*.

> Sultan Ṣalāḥ al-Dīn Yūsuf b. Ayyūb endowed the twenty-four servants (*khādim*) of the Prophet's tomb with the village of Naqqāda (in the province of Qūṣ) along with 1/3 of the village of Sandabīs (in the province of Qalyūb) as *waqf.* They set up a waterwheel (*dūlāb*) in the village of Naqqāda and constructed a sugarcane pressing factory (*maʿṣara lil-qaṣab*) there. They entrusted a person to manage the waterwheel, staying on in the village.[31]

As mentioned above, it was well known that sugar production prospered in the province of Qūṣ from around the eleventh century. The twenty-four servants minding the Prophet's tomb in Medina, beneficiaries of a *waqf* grant of the village of Naqqāda in the province of Qūṣ, employed a person to manage the production and sale of sugar.

In regards to sugar during the reign of Ṣalāḥ al-Dīn, we find another account in a Syriac chronicle written by Bar Hebraeus (Abū al-Faraj Ibn al-ʿIbrī, d. 685/1286), a Jacobite bishop in Anatolia and Syria. In 588/1192, a Jewish merchant in Damascus went to ʿAkkā to make a complaint before Ṣalāḥ al-Dīn.

> I am a Jew and a merchant of Damascus. I was coming by sea from Alexandria, and I had with me twenty loads of sugar. And when I came to the port of ʿAkko thy servants plundered me, and they said unto me, "Thou art an infidel, and thy goods belong rightly to the Sūlṭān."[32]

When Ṣalāḥ al-Dīn heard this story and confirmed its veracity, he ordered his officials to recompense the merchant the price of the sugar. As one camel-load (*ḥiml*) is about 250 kilograms, twenty loads of sugar are equal to 5,000 kilograms. As the price of sugar in Syria at that time was 0.227 dinar per kilogram, the cost of 5,000 kilograms of sugar amounted to about 1,135 dinars. Assuming that 100 kilograms of wheat cost 1.56 dinars, almost 72,756 kilograms of wheat could be bought with 1,135 dinars.[33]

---

31 Ibn Duqmāq, *Kitāb al-Intiṣār*, II, 33.

32 Bar Hebraeus, *The Chronography of Gregory Abū'l Faraj commonly known as Bar Hebraeus*, Syrian text ed. and English tr. by E.A. Wallis Budge, 2 vols., London, 1932, II, 342.

33 For the price of wheat and sugar during the Ayyubid period, see E. Ashtor, *Histoire des prix et des salaires dans l'Orient médiéval*, Paris, 1969, pp. 245, 249.

In 619/1222, at the end of the Ayyubid period, Sultan al-Kāmil gave the entire province of al-Fayyūm to amir Fakhr al-Dīn ʿUthmān (d. 629/1232) as *iqṭāʿ darbastā* (complete *iqṭāʿ*), including its revenues, sugarcane, oxen, and farm implements.[34] Fakhr al-Dīn, who personally managed his own *iqṭāʿ*, did not always reside at al-Fayyūm, however. Al-Maqrīzī relates this in his *Khiṭaṭ*.

> In al-Barqīya outside Cairo, there is a tower known as the "Tower of al-Fayyūm" (*Burj al-Fayyūm*). This was constructed by amir Fakhr al-Dīn ʿUthmān b. Qizil, chief steward (*ustādār*) of al-Malik al-Kāmil. The name "Tower of al-Fayyūm" came from the fact that the whole province of al-Fayyūm was held by Ibn Qizil as *iqṭāʿ* [*darbastā*]. When he received a letter from al-Fayyūm, he would send a reply from the tower.[35]

Fakhr al-Dīn constructed a tower outside Cairo, and managed his *iqṭāʿ darbastā* using carrier pigeons, connecting about one hundred kilometers between Cairo and al-Fayyūm. He was praised as "a noble and great amir" for his distinguished service, constructing *masjids*, *madrasas*, and *maktabs* (schools) for infants, and supporting the sultan's state policies in his role as *ustādār*.[36] His son, Nūr al-Dīn ʿAlī b. ʿUthmān, was also an influential amir and managed a small sugar refinery (*maṭbakh al-sukkar*) in al-Fusṭāṭ in the middle of the thirteenth century.[37]

Ibn Mammātī, who was well acquainted with local administrative procedures in Egypt under the Ayyubids, explains the regulations for sugarcane cultivation by *iqṭāʿ* holders (*muqṭaʿ*) as follows.

> (1) When a district encompassing sugarcane fields that had been previously given to a soldier as *iqṭāʿ* in 588/1192 was granted to another soldier in the month before 589/December 1192, the first *muqṭaʿ* has the right to press the sugarcane.
> (2) If the land encompasses second-year sugarcane (*khilfa*), the land is to be vacated by the first *muqṭaʿ* on the tenth of Ṭūba (5 January 1193). And if the land encompasses first-year sugarcane (*raʾs*), the land is to be vacated on the tenth of Bashnas (6 May 1193).

34 Ibn al-ʿAmīd, *Akhbār al-Ayyūbīyīn*, ed. Cl. Cahen, *BEO*, 15 (1958), 134.

35 Al-Maqrīzī, *al-Khiṭaṭ*, II, 231.

36 Ibn al-ʿAmīd, *Akhbār al-Ayyūbīyīn*, 135. See also Sato, *State and Rural Society*, pp. 74–76.

37 Al-Maqrīzī, *Kitāb al-Sulūk*, I, 261, 281. For the career of amir Fakhr al-Dīn, see al-Ṣafadī, *Kitāb al-Wāfī bil-Wafayāt*, XIX, 503–504.

> (3) When the second *muqṭaʿ* has irrigated the sugarcane in the second year, whereas the first *muqṭaʿ* did not, the second *muqṭaʿ* has the right to harvest it, because the first *muqṭaʿ* has already been derelict in his military duty (*khidma*).
> (4) When the first *muqṭaʿ* still has an interest in the land after the determined term [according to (2) above] has already expired, he must pay the second *muqṭaʿ* 2+15/24 dinars per *faddān* as a levy. However, after paying this levy, he is free to press the sugarcane at the governmental pressing factory, and use its oxen, provisions, and tools.
> (5) When the first *muqṭaʿ* relinquishes the *iqṭāʿ*, he is obliged to restore it to the same state as when he assumed control of it, for example, returning equipment borrowed from the government.

These regulations show that the rights of the first *muqṭaʿ* who cultivated sugarcane in his *iqṭāʿ* were guaranteed for a certain period of time, even if he was replaced by a second *muqṭaʿ*. Further, it is interesting to note the fifth regulation, which obligated the *muqṭaʿ*, when leaving his *iqṭāʿ*, to restore it to its original state. This was a measure (*ʿimāra*) to maintain stable agricultural production, and also to facilitate the periodic reassignment of *iqṭāʿ*s to amirs and soldiers.[38]

The Managers of Sugar Production in al-Fusṭāṭ

As mentioned above, as sugarcane cultivation spread from Lower Egypt to Upper Egypt in the Fatimid and Ayyubid periods, sugar production peaked in the twelfth to thirteenth centuries. Al-Maqrīzī relates an incident that shows the prosperity of sugar production in Egypt.

> In this year (650/1252), news arrived at Cairo that the Mongol army had encountered a caravan (*qāfila*) headed for Baghdad from Harrān [near Aleppo] and plundered it of great assets, including 600 loads (*ḥiml*) of sugar made in Egypt, valued at 600,000 dinars.[39]

600 loads of sugar was equal to about 150,000 kilograms. According to Ibn Faḍl Allāh al-ʿUmarī (d. 749/1349), one kilogram of premium grade sugar was sold at 0.4 dinar in the early Mamluk period.[40] Based on this information, the cost of the stolen sugar would have amounted to just 60,000 dinars, not 600,000 dinars

38 See also Sato, *State and Rural Society*, p. 72.

39 Al-Maqrīzī, *Kitāb al-Sulūk*, I, 383–384.

40 Al-ʿUmarī, *Masālik al-Abṣār fī Mamālik al-Amṣār: Dawlat al-Mamālīk al-Ulā*, 84.

as al-Maqrīzī relates. However, 600 loads of sugar worth 60,000 dinars was still a considerable quantity, showing that great amounts of sugar were exported from Egypt to other regions of the Islamic world in the thirteenth century.

Here, let us cite a description of *maṭbakh al-sukkar*s given by Ibn Duqmāq in his *Kitāb al-Intiṣār.* The *maṭbakh al-sukkar* in Arabic sources refers to either a factory – adjacent to the sugarcane fields – that produces raw sugar (*qand*), or to a sugar refinery – separate from the sugarcane fields – that refines raw sugar through repeated boilings. Ibn Duqmāq provides an account of the 65 sugar refineries located in al-Fusṭāṭ.

(1) *Maṭbakh al-sukkar*s owned by the sultan …… 7
One of these is a government refinery (*maṭbakh al-dawla*) and the other six are the sultan's refineries (*maṭbakh al-khāṣṣ al-sulṭānī*). Each refinery has a manager (*shādd*) and other officials (*mubāshir*).

(2) *Maṭbakh al-sukkar*s owned by amirs …… 21
We can confirm that 12 of these refineries were built by the amirs themselves. The amirs brought the raw sugar from the *iqṭā*ʿs they held in local provinces to al-Fusṭāṭ for refining.

(3) *Maṭbakh al-sukkar*s owned by the leading merchants (*tājir*) …… 13
Three of these were originally constructed by amirs and then transferred to merchants. We can confirm that among these 13 refineries, three were managed by Jewish merchants and another four by the *Kārimī* merchants.[41]

(4) *Maṭbakh al-sukkar*s owned by persons not identified …… 27[42]

In this account, Ibn Duqmāq often says that the amirs (or merchants) managed their own refineries (*dawlaba maṭbakhahu*). The term "*dawlaba*" denotes the installation of equipment to refine sugar.[43] We can therefore presume that sultans, amirs, and merchants invested the capital needed to construct refineries, install equipment such as stone mills, large boilers, and *ublūj*s, and employ

41 The names of the refineries owned by the *Kārimī* merchants were as follows: Maṭbakh ʿUqbat al-Milḥ, Maṭbakh al-Kamāl ibn Marzūq, Maṭbakh Sirāj al-Dīn ibn al-Kharrūbī, and Maṭbakh Nūr al-Dīn ibn al-Kharrūbī.

42 Ibn Duqmāq, *Kitāb al-Intiṣār*, I, 41–46. Al-Maqrīzī states, quoting *Kitāb Ayqāẓ al-Mutaghaffil* by Ibn al-Mutawwaj al-Zubayrī (d. 730/1329), that in 725/1325, 66 sugar refineries (*maṭbakh al-sukkar*) were in operation in al-Fusṭāṭ (*al-Khiṭaṭ*, I, 343). See also Sato, "Sugar in the Economic Life of Mamluk Egypt," p. 99. Although the total number of *maṭbakh*s above is 68, three of them were counted twice as their ownership changed from amirs to merchants.

43 R. Dozy, *Supplément aux dictionnaires arabes*, 3rd ed., 2 vols., Paris, 1967, I, p. 477.

workers, and that they pursued profits through the trade of the white sugar and rock sugar produced in these refineries. Ibn Iyās (852–ca. 930/1448–ca.1524) gives an interesting account of a *mamlūk* amir producing sugar at his *iqṭāʿ* in Lower Egypt.

> In this year (726/1326) a village (*qarya*) called al-Naḥrīrīya was established in the province of al-Gharbīya. The reason was that amir Sunqur al-Saʿdī, head of the victorious army (*naqīb al-Jaysh al-Manṣūra*), had a *madrasa* adjacent to al-Nārqānī Bath, and the land of this village was in his *iqṭāʿ*. So, amir Sunqur therefore constructed there a mosque (*jāmiʿ*), a mill (*ṭāḥūn*), a caravansaray (*khān*), and a sugarcane pressing factory (*maʿṣara*).
>
> Then, as prosperity increased and many peasants (*fallāḥ*) migrated there, the annual *kharāj* tax grew to 15,000 dirhams. When the sultan [al-Nāṣir Muḥammad] heard this, he sent his representative to confiscate the *iqṭāʿ* from Sunqur. The village thereby became part of the sultan's domain, which annoyed Sunqur considerably. He nevertheless remained in the village and died there some years later.[44]

According to Ibn Ḥajar al-ʿAsqalānī, amir Sunqur had a strong interest in agriculture and established the village of al-Baḥribarāya (al-Naḥrīrīya).[45] As shown in these instances, both the sultans and the amirs willingly participated in the management of sugarcane pressing factories and sugar refineries during the Ayyubid and Mamluk periods. This clearly shows that sugar production and trade were "unfailingly profitable enterprises" at that time. In Syria also, as Ibn al-Furāt relates, during the reign of Qalāwūn (678–689/1279–90), amir Badr al-Dīn b. Dirbās showed special concern for the low-lying areas (al-Aghwār) in which sugarcane grew, as those resources were vital to the kingdoms and the ruling classes.[46]

---

44 Ibn Iyās, *Badāʾiʿ al-Zuhūr fī Waqāʾiʿ al-Duhūr*, ed. M. Muṣṭafā, 5 vols., Wiesbaden, 1960–75, I-1, 458.

45 Ibn Ḥajar, *al-Durar al-Kāmina*, II, 273. Ibn Ḥajar relates that amir Sunqur stayed at Tripoli and died there.

46 Ibn al-Furāt, *Taʾrīkh Ibn al-Furāt*, ed. Q. Zarīq, Beirut, 1936–42, VII, 191–192. See also L.S. Northrup, *From Slave to Sultan: The Career of al-Manṣūr Qalāwūn and the Consolidation of Mamluk Rule in Egypt and Syria (678–689 AH/1279–1290 AD)*, Stuttgart, 1998, p. 269.

Trade with Italian Merchants in Alexandria

Al-Maqrīzī describes in his *Khiṭaṭ* the situation seen in the districts of Egypt every June during the Mamluk period.

> In Ba'ūna (26 May-24 June), many ships (*markab*) set sail [to al-Fusṭāṭ] from Qūṣ [in Upper Egypt] and various towns in Lower Egypt, loaded with crops (*ghalla*), straw (*tibn*), raw sugar (*qand*), and molasses (*'asal*).[47]

According to this account, in the month of Ba'ūna, raw sugar and molasses were carried to al-Fusṭāṭ from both Upper and Lower Egypt. Al-Maqrīzī further relates as follows.

> When the water of the Nile flows into the Alexandria Canal during Misrā (25 July-23 August), ships (*markab*) loaded with various kinds of goods, like crops, spices (*bahār*), and sugar (*sukkar*), set sail.[48]

The above two accounts clearly show that refined sugar was transported to Alexandria, two months after raw sugar had been brought to al-Fusṭāṭ for refining. The Alexandria canal was a long canal connecting the area near Ṭanṭā with the coastal town of Alexandria, where Italian merchants, chiefly from Venice, Genoa, and Pisa, purchased various spices from Muslim merchants under the protection of their consulates.[49] However, as al-Maqrīzī relates, the Italians purchased sugar from Egypt, in addition to spices from the East.

Yutaka Horii, who has scrutinized the Arabic and Italian sources on commercial and diplomatic relations between the Egyptian sultan and the Venetians during the Mamluk and Ottoman periods, reaches the following conclusions: The fundamental rights that the Venetians had been granted by the sultan became standard in the fifteenth century – including: the consular jurisdiction inside the colony, the consul's right to negotiate with the sultan, the merchant's right to request the sultan's judgment in quarrels with Muslims, and the right not to be burdened with collective responsibility for debts.[50]

47 Al-Maqrīzī, *al-Khiṭaṭ*, I, 272. We find the same description in Ibn Iyās's *Nuzhat al-Umam*, 249.

48 Al-Maqrīzī, *al-Khiṭaṭ*, I, 273. See also Ibn Iyās, *Nuzhat al-Umam*, 250.

49 Ashtor, *A Social and Economic History*, states on page 299, "Even after the fall of Acre [in 1291] the trading nations sent ambassadors to the sultan of Cairo and concluded new commercial treaties, reducing customs duties and acquiring new rights." For the consulates in Alexandria, see Labib, *Handelsgeschichte Ägyptens*, pp. 198–203.

50 Y. Horii, "The Mamlūk Sultan Qānṣūh al-Ghawrī (1501–16) and the Venetians in Alexandria," *Orient*, 38 (2003), p. 181.

According to Horii's findings, the main goods the Venetians purchased from Egypt in the late fifteenth and early sixteenth centuries were spices from the East, such as pepper, ginger, clove, nutmeg, mace, cinnamon, and cassia, along with Egyptian products including fava beans and grains, such as wheat.[51] We note that sugar, one of the main commercial products of the previous centuries, is not found in the list of goods exported from Egypt. From the latter half of the fourteenth century, the Bedouins (*ʿUrbān*) repeatedly attacked sugar pressing factories and sugar refineries in Upper Egypt to steal raw sugar, white sugar, and oxen.[52] In addition to this political unrest, the intermittent spread of plague (*ṭāʿūn*) reduced the number of skilled artisans in Egyptian society, as al-Maqrīzī states in the following:

> Misfortunes (*miḥna*) occurred [intermittently]. The price of sugar increased due to the ruin of both waterwheels (*dūlāb*) in Upper Egypt and sugar refineries (*maṭbakh al-sukkar*) in the town of al-Fusṭāṭ. As many sugar candy artisans (*ṣāniʿ al-ḥalwā*) died off, production declined.[53]

As al-Maqrīzī clearly explains, several factors, including political corruption, social disorder, and natural disasters, caused the decline of the Egyptian sugar industry in the later Mamluk period. In the next chapter, we will revisit the decline of sugar production in Mamluk Egypt.

The Tricks of the Sugar Merchants in Mamluk Cairo

A Guidebook (al-Madkhal) *by Ibn al-Ḥājj*

Abū ʿAbd Allāh Muḥammad Ibn al-Ḥājj al-Mālikī (d. 737/1336) from Fās (Fez) was a well-known Mālikī jurist with a harsh view of the realities of Egyptian society under the Mamluks. After studying Islam in Fās, Ibn al-Ḥājj moved to Cairo to master *Muwaṭṭaʾ* – a collection of hadith complied by Mālik b. Anas (d. 179/796) – under the instruction of Abū Qāsim ʿUbayd al-Asʿardī (d. 692/1293). When Ibn al-Ḥājj died in 737/1336 at over eighty years of age, he was buried in al-Qarāfa, and the people of Cairo steadily began to visiting his tomb there to ask his blessing.[54]

51 Horii, "The Mamlūk Sultan Qānṣūh al-Ghawrī," p. 182.

52 For example, al-Maqrīzī, *Kitāb al-Sulūk*, II, 850, 896, 908.

53 Al-Maqrīzī, *al-Khiṭaṭ*, II, 99.

54 Al-Maqrīzī, *Kitāb al-Muqaffā al-Kabīr*, V, 90–91; Ibn Ḥajar, *al-Durar al-Kāmina*, IV, 355–356.

His main work was *al-Madkhal ilā Tanmiyat al-Aʿmāl bi-Taḥsīn al-Nīyāt* (*A Guidebook on the Promotion of Deeds with Proper Intentions*), completed in Cairo in 732/1332. As a brief overview, volume one includes the following sections: "The Search for Knowledge," "Ablutions," "The Feast of Breaking the Ramaḍān Fast," "The Feast of Immolation," etc. Volume two: "Mawlid al-Nabī," "Learning at Home and at School," and "Refraining from Ṣalāt at Tombs." Volume three: "Booty and Captives," "Interest," "The Asceticism of Ṣūfīs," "Muslim Rosaries," and "Funerals." And volume four: "Land Tax," "The Behavior Required of Druggists," "The Realities of Sugar Refineries," "Bakers," and "Water Carriers."

Ibn al-Ḥājj set out to explain the legal principles underlying all aspects of everyday life, and unintentionally provided us with a description of the realities of Egyptian societies in the fourteenth century. Here, let me examine the chapter on "The Realities of Sugar Refineries (*maṭbakh*)" from volume four. After pointing out the sanitary shortcomings of the refineries, Ibn al-Ḥājj makes specific suggestions to the Muslim brothers to resolve these issues. His *Madkhal* can therefore be seen as unique for its emphasis on detailed guidelines for the day-to-day lives of Muslim merchants and artisans.

Unsanitary Conditions in Sugar Refineries

First, regarding the sugar refining process of boiling *qand* and adding water, he points out the following problems[55]:

(1) Since the boiled juice is kept in uncovered jars (*jafna*), it is contaminated with insects and the urine of rats. In fact, insects swarm and crawl around in the jars for days on end.

(2) When the jars are placed in the burial house (*bayt al-dafn*), they are covered with soil. However, this soil is kept in a poor and open house, where artisans (*ṣāniʿ*) walk around with dirty feet over the jars covered with soil. Also, rats often live and breed in the soil.

The jars (*jafna*) in paragraph (1) above may indicate the cone-shaped *ublūj*s that were used for separating sugar from molasses. The second paragraph (2) clearly shows that the *ublūj*s were covered with soil in the burial house, although al-Nuwayrī did not mention this as a step of sugar refining in his explanation of *ublūj*s. Ibn al-Ḥājj, after pointing out these problems, makes some recommendations to the owners of sugar refineries, including putting covers

55 Ibn al-Ḥājj, *al-Madkhal*, IV, 150–151.

on the jars to protect them against rats and insects.[56] He then says the following regarding the refinery's large boilers (*khābiya*)[57]:

> (3) The artisans stand inside with bare feet, and even wash their feet as they clean the *khābiyas*. Quality molasses (*quṭāra*) is also kept in uncovered jars, where rats and insects have come to dwell. However, the artisans spray hot water on the *khābiyas* to clean off the clinging dirt, and they wipe the jars out completely.
> (4) After cleaning the *khābiyas*, when artisans boil the raw sugar with added water, they pour in a little milk (*laban*) to pick out the congealed dirt floating on the surface in the jars. As it continues to boil and the liquid begins to congeal, it is transferred to uncovered jars (*maṭara*) that often contain rat dung and insects.

As mentioned above, the *khābiya* was a large boiler holding nearly 3,000 kilograms of liquid. According to the third paragraph (3), the artisans cleaned the *khābiya* while standing inside it. It is also interesting to note that Ibn al-Ḥājj, just as al-Nuwayrī does, clearly mentions the technique of adding milk when refining sugar. Both *jafna* in (1) and *maṭara* in (4) may refer to a kind of jars similar to *ublūj*; however, we can find no other examples in the Arabic sources to support this assumption. Finally, Ibn al-Ḥājj gives a word of advice to employers (*mustaʾjir*),[58] suggesting if they increase the wages of the artisans (*ujrat al-ṣunnāʿ*), they can order the artisans to wash their feet and urge them to perform the requisite daily prayers and annual fasting during the month of Ramaḍān.[59]

The Tricks of the Sugar Merchants

Then Ibn al-Ḥājj criticizes the sugar merchants of Mamluk Cairo, accusing them of various deceptions.[60]

> (1) When the merchants sell fine molasses (*quṭāra*), they pour whey (*maṣl al-ʿuyūn*) into the jar, and stir it with a stick to mix them together. Then, yellow bubbles come up to the surface of the black molasses. When

56 Ibn al-Ḥājj, *al-Madkhal*, IV, 153.
57 Ibn al-Ḥājj, *al-Madkhal*, IV, 151.
58 Ibn al-Ḥājj also refers to "employers" as "refinery owners" (*ṣāḥib al-maṭbakh*) (*al-Madkhal*, IV, 153).
59 Ibn al-Ḥājj, *al-Madkhal*, IV, 153.
60 Ibn al-Ḥājj, *al-Madkhal*, IV, 151–153.

the buyers see the distinctive color, they assume the color indicates raw sugar (*ṣafā' al-qand*).

(2) Some sugar merchants employ a surprising technique. When a buyer purchases a loaf of white sugar and takes it home, upon breaking the loaf open, he finds red sugar inside. The buyers assume the whole loaf of sugar is white, without realizing that red sugar had been substituted for white sugar inside.

(3) When a buyer purchases premium grade molasses (*qaṭr al-nabāt*), some merchants replace it with older molasses. The merchants can repeat this deception (*tadlīs*) until their stock of older molasses is all sold. When selling old molasses, the merchants ought to tell their customers upfront that the molasses isn't fresh.

(4) When the lower part of a sugar loaf is red, some merchants coat it with white sugar to give the false impression that all sugar is white. The buyers assume both the inside and outside are of the same quality.

The Arabic sources from medieval times describe raw sugar as red (*sukkar aḥmar*) rather than brown.[61] A cone-shaped loaf of sugar, also called an *ublūj*, typically had a white upper section and a red or dark lower point.[62] Tricks (2) and (4) above were clearly employed by the sugar merchants to hide the red part, and present the illusion of an entire white cone.

Regarding these unfair practices by sugar merchants, Ibn al-Ḥājj says the following:

> The merchants might insist that they had to use such trickery because of lost capital or interest. But, they are responsible for their own debts (*dayn*), and if they follow the advice of the Muslim brothers to reduce their expenses, the grace of God will come to them one after another. "If they do what they are advised, it would, certainly, be better for them, and stronger in establishing their faith" (*al-Qur'ān*, IV/66).[63]

61 For example, see al-Dimashqī, *Kitāb al-Ishāra*, 32; Ibn al-Ḥājj, *al-Madkhal*, IV, 149, 152; Ibn al-Nafīs, *al-Shāmil*, XV, 116.

62 Daniels explains that the sugar at the top of the cone turned the whitest and that at the bottom, or narrow end, the darkest (*Agro-Industries: Sugarcane Technology*, pp. 377–379).

63 Ibn al-Ḥājj, *al-Madkhal*, IV, 154.

Reading the Books on *Ḥisba*

What is "Ḥisba"?

Next, we will discuss how the government dealt with the tricks of the sugar merchants during the Ayyubid and Mamluk periods. We find some important information on the official dealings with these deceptions in the books on *ḥisba*. In Arabic, *ḥisba* means "to promote good and forbid evil," or more specifically, "to maintain social order and improve people's standard of living in Muslim societies."[64] The person responsible for *ḥisba* was called the *muḥtasib*, who was appointed by the caliphs, the sultans, the local governors (*wālī*), or, starting in the ʿAbbasid period, judges (*qāḍī*). The books on *ḥisba* that we will look at here are manuals that provide the *muḥtasib*s with standards for their judgments, and rules for their conduct.

The origins of a governmental office of *ḥisba* in early Islamic history are unclear, but, in spirit, it apparently dates back to the time of the Prophet Muḥammad. During the ʿAbbasid period, *muḥtasib*s, or followers of the Umayyad *ʿāmil al-sūq*, were appointed for all the major cities, being particularly responsible for the inspection of markets (*sūq*). Their main duties were to detect fraud in the sale of commercial goods, incorrect weights and measures, loans with illegal interest (*ribā*), and overly strict lessons at schools. If they found such wrongdoings, they had the authority to confiscate weights and measures, and for particularly egregious violations, to beat violators and parade them through the streets in disgrace.[65] Moreover, when prices rose abnormally, the *muḥtasib*s were charged with telling the crop brokers and small-scale bazaar merchants to lower their prices.[66]

It is worth noting that al-Maqrīzī, an Egyptian historian in the Mamluk period, was appointed to the office of *ḥisba* in Cairo three times, in 801/1399, 802/1400, and 807/1404.[67] Although each time he only held the office for several months, at those times he was in a position to closely observe the social life of medieval Cairo, an opportunity he seems to have made great use of in the vivid descriptions in his written works, including *al-Khiṭaṭ* and *Kitāb al-Sulūk*.

---

64 EI², s.v. Ḥisba (Cl. Cahen and M. Talbi); J. Schacht, *An Introduction to Islamic Law*, Oxford, 1964, pp. 51–53.

65 EI², s.v. Ḥisba; R.P. Buckley, *The Book of the Islamic Market Inspector*, Oxford, 1999, pp. 1–24; A. Ghabin, *Ḥisba, Arts and Craft in Islam*, Wiesbaden, 2009, pp. 40–44.

66 Al-Maqrīzī, *Kitāb al-Sulūk*, II, 669.

67 Al-Maqrīzī himself affirms in his chronicle each time he was appointed to the office of *ḥisba*: *Kitāb al-Sulūk*, III, 969, 999, 1155. See also Ibn Taghrībirdī, *al-Manhal al-Ṣāfī*, I, 394–396; al-Sakhāwī, *al-Ḍawʾ al-Lāmiʿ li-Ahl al-Qarn al-Tāsiʿ*, 12 vols., Beirut, 1934–36, II, 21–25.

Here, let us choose two *ḥisba* books to cite from among the many *ḥisba* works written in the Islamic world since the eleventh century. The first is *Nihāyat al-Rutba fī Ṭalab al-Ḥisba* (*The Highest Stage in Pursuing Ḥisba*) by Jalāl al-Dīn ʿAbd al-Raḥmān al-Shayzarī (d. 589/1193), which is believed to be the earliest book on *ḥisba* written in the Eastern Islamic world. The author was probably from the small town of Shayzar in Northern Syria, but his life is completely unknown except that he lived in the age of Ṣalāḥ al-Dīn al-Ayyūbī. It is also unclear if he actually served as a *muḥtasib*, whether in Shayzar or in any other town in Syria.[68]

The book consists of forty chapters. To give some examples of the topics addressed, in Chapter 1: "The Conditions and Recommendations of *Ḥisba* imposed on *Muḥtasib*," Chapter 2: "Supervision of Markets (*sūq*) and Roads (*ṭarīqa*)," Chapter 3: "*Qinṭārs*, *Raṭls*, *Mithqāls* and *Dirhams*," Chapter 6: "Bakers (*khabbāz*)," Chapter 16: "Confectioners (*ḥalwānī*)," Chapter 18: "Druggists (*ʿaṭṭār*)," and Chapter 35: "Baths (*ḥammām*) and their Attendants."

The second book we will cite is *Maʿālim al-Qurba fī Aḥkām al-Ḥisba* (*Guideposts for Pious Deeds according to the Principles of Ḥisba*) by Ibn al-Ukhuwwa al-Qurashī (648–729/1250–1329). We have no exact information about the author except that he lived in Egypt during the early Mamluk period. This book consists of seventy chapters, and gives more detailed points for inspection than the aforementioned *Nihāyat al-Rutba* by al-Shayzarī. Examples of the subjects covered include, in Chapter 1: "The Conditions of *Ḥisba* and the Duties of *Muḥtasib*," Chapter 4: "The Inspection of *Ahl al-Dhimma*," Chapter 8: "Conduct Prohibited at Markets," Chapter 9: "*Qinṭārs*, *Raṭls* and *Mithqāls*," Chapter 16: "Butchers (*jazzār*)," Chapter 23: "Confectioners (*ḥalwānī*)," Chapter 24: "Syrup Dealers (*sharābī*)," Chapter 25: "Druggists," Chapter 37: "Jewelers (*ṣāʾigh*)," Chapter 48: "Preachers (*wāʿiẓ*)," Chapter 51: "Judges (*qāḍī*) and Notaries (*shāhid*)," and Chapter 69: "Carpenters (*najjār*) and Sawyers (*nashshār*)."

As mentioned above, this second book, *Maʿālim al-Qurba*, has more detailed points for inspection than the first one, *Nihāyat al-Rutba*; however, both books prescribe the inspection of merchant and artisan activities according to the points listed in *ḥisba* manuals. Here, we will compare these two books' handling of the inspection of sugar trade in the markets.

68 Buckley, *The Book of the Islamic Market Inspector*, pp. 12–13.

The Inspection of Sugar Trade

Since neither book has a separate chapter covering sugar merchants, we will discuss the chapters dealing with confectioners (*ḥalwānī*), which is closely related to sugar. Contrary to the simple accounting of confections given by al-Shayzarī, Ibn al-Ukhuwwa identifies 58 different types of confection, including "anemone (flower) candy" (*muqarraḍa sakab*), "soap candy" (*ṣābūnīya*), "minister sweets" (*wazīrīya*), "Cairo sweets" (*al-Qāhirīya*), "sparrow heads" (*ra's al-ʿuṣfūr*), "Turkish cakes" (*kaʿk Turkī*), and "sugar combs" (*amshāṭ sukkarī*).[69] After listing these, Ibn al-Ukhuwwa makes the following statement:

> Rather than honey (*ʿasal al-naḥl*), some confectioners add raw sugar to sweet pancakes (*mushabbak*) and Cairo sweets. This is plain deception (*ghishsh*). Others add starch (*nashā*) exceeding the allowed limit to soft sweets made from dates, and to soap candies. This trickery is easily detected by the impurities in the appearance of the sweets.[70]

Al-Shayzarī criticizes the use of flour (*daqīq*) or starch in producing sweets.[71] Ibn al-Ukhuwwa also regards the use of starch beyond a regulated level as deception. Also, according to Ibn al-Ukhuwwa, a penalty (*ḍarība*) or an obligation to improve product quality is to be imposed on a person who uses excessive flour in producing sweets. He recounts the following example.

> In regards to coloring, the obligation to improve product quality is as follows. Let's assume that a confectioner adds 5 *raṭl*s (1.5 kilograms) of starch to 10 *raṭl*s of flour, and fries it with sesame oil after baking, being careful to prevent stickage during the frying. The confectioner might call this "sugar bread (*sukkarī*)" despite having used raw sugar (*qand*) rather than [white] sugar (*sukkar*). The *muḥtasib* instructs the confectioner to decrease the amount of egg yokes used, and enhance the flavor, so as not to disappoint the customer. Every trick will be shown in the surface appearance of the sweets, which should be taken as a lesson.[72]

69 Ibn al-Ukhuwwa, *Kitāb Maʿālim al-Qurba fī Aḥkām al-Ḥisba*, ed. M.M. Shaʿbān and S.A. al-Muṭīʿī, Cairo, 1976, 181–183. Al-Shayzarī does not refer to any kind of sweets in Chapter 16: "Confectioners."

70 Ibn al-Ukhuwwa, *Kitāb Maʿālim al-Qurba*, 183.

71 Al-Shayzarī, *Nihāyat al-Rutba fī Ṭalab al-Ḥisba*, ed. S.B. al-ʿArīnī, Beirut, 1969, 40. He lists the types of *daqīq* as rice (*aruzz*), lentils (*ʿadas*), and sesame (*simsim*).

72 Ibn al-Ukhuwwa, *Kitāb Maʿālim al-Qurba*, 184.

Al-Shayzarī also states that the tricks concerning sweets (*ghushūsh al-ḥalāwa*) can be detected both in their surface appearance and in their taste, all of which the *muḥtasib* should teach the confectioners.[73] The examples mentioned above show that honey was sometimes seen as a better additive than raw sugar for making sweets, and the use of raw sugar instead of white sugar was a clear deception in the production of sweets known as *sukkarī*.

We also find some accounts of sugar in the chapter on syrup dealers (*sharābī*). I will take an example from the *ḥisba* book by al-Shayzarī.

> Many syrup dealers make a type of drink by mixing fresh milk (*laban ḥalīb*), vinegar (*khall*), and white lead (*isfīdāj*) with sugarcane juice (*ʿasal qaṣab al-sukkar*), which produces a pure color and a palatable taste. Also, some dealers add fruit juice or cream, instead of sugar and honey. The *muḥtasib* must urge the dealers to swear they will stop making the drinks this way, as it taints, contaminates, and degrades the mixture.[74]

This passage describes a kind of mixed syrup made of sugarcane juice, with additives, including white lead, that were known to worsen product quality. In Arabic medicine, white lead, which is only mentioned here in the *Nihāyat al-Rutba*, was used as an ointment to treat tumors.

As we will see later, druggists (*ʿaṭṭār*) sold sugar in markets as a medicine. However, we find no reference to this in *Nihāyat al-Rutba* or *Maʿālim al-Qurba*. Ibn al-Ḥājj sharply criticizes the tricks of sugar merchants, which would surely also apply to the conduct of druggists. Nevertheless, the real reason for this omission remains unclear.

---

73 Al-Shayzarī, *Nihāyat al-Rutba*, 41.

74 Al-Shayzarī, *Nihāyat al-Rutba*, 56–57; Buckley, *The Book of the Islamic Market Inspector*, 76.

CHAPTER 4

The Ups and Downs of the Sugar Merchants

The Jewish Sugar Merchants as Described in the Geniza Documents

The Discovery of the Cairo Geniza

First, we will summarize the history of the Cairo Geniza documents, based on several previous studies. In 1889, a large number of documents were found in an old synagogue in al-Fusṭāṭ that had long been used by Palestinian Jews. This collection of over 200,000 documents was named the "Cairo Geniza" after the storehouse (*geniza*) at the synagogue where they were kept. A considerable number of these documents were soon dispersed to various libraries in Europe and the United States. And within about ten years, the bulk of what remained was brought to the Cambridge University Library, and is presently known as the Taylor-Schechter Collection.[1]

In the medieval ages, there was Jewish custom of preserving any documents mentioning the name of God. These books and papers were stored in a *geniza* until they received a proper burial. A major part of the Cairo Geniza documents, considered the most important of the *geniza* materials, are written in the Arabic language using Hebrew script. The documents cover about three hundred years, from 354/965 to 663/1265, including business letters, court records, and other subjects related to religion and the life of the Jewish community. According to S.D. Goitein, if we count only the complete and significant Cairo Geniza fragments, they number about ten thousand.[2]

The documents of the Cairo Geniza reveal a range of transactions by the Jewish merchants, not just in Egypt, but from the Indian Ocean to the Red Sea, the Syrian Coast, Sicily, North Africa (Maghrib), and Andalusia. Goitein and other dedicated scholars studied the Cairo Geniza for over thirty years, meticulously investigating, classifying, and cataloging them. Accepting posts at Pennsylvania University in 1957 and Princeton University in 1971, Goitein devoted himself to the study and publication of the Geniza documents.

His main work, *A Mediterranean Society*, is seen as a monumental achievement, consisting of six volumes: (1) Economic Foundations, (2) The Community, (3) The Family, (4) Daily Life, (5) The Individual, and (6) Cumulative

1 S.D. Goitein, "The Documents of the Cairo Geniza as a Source for Mediterranean Social History," *JAOS*, 80 (1960), 91–100; *EI*², s.v. Geniza (S.D. Goitein).

2 *EI*², s.v. Geniza (S.D. Goitein).

 | DOI 10.1163/9789004281561_006

Indices.[3] He states that on one of his fifteen visits to the Cambridge University Library it became evident to him that the India trade, as far as reflected in the Geniza, was carried out largely by merchants based in the Mediterranean area.[4] Furthermore, Goitein explains, "the Fatimid conquest of Egypt in July, 969, marks the beginning of the classical Geniza period. The eclipse of their successors, the Ayyubids, in 1250, roughly coincides with its end."[5]

As mentioned previously, the Egyptian sugar industry reached its peak from the Fatimid to Ayyubid periods, as the cultivation of sugarcane expanded from Lower to Upper Egypt. We can see the prosperity of the Egyptian sugar industry in the Cairo Geniza documents brought forth by Goitein. Let us look at several documents on the Egyptian sugar industry and sugar trade, based on Goitein's works *A Mediterranean Society* and *Letters of Medieval Jewish Traders.*

The Jewish Sugar Merchants

The Management of Sugar Factories

As we saw in Chapter Three, of the 13 sugar refineries (*maṭbakh al-sukkar*) in al-Fusṭāṭ owned by merchants (*tājir*), three were managed by Jewish merchants. This indicates that Jewish merchants were also deeply involved with sugar production and trade, as were the sultans, amirs, and Muslim merchants. One document made known by Goitein reads:

> Joseph and his son Abū al-ʿAlā, both physicians, accept the scholar Mufaḍḍal as third partner in a sugar factory, each of them sharing one-third of profit and loss. Mufaḍḍal pays 50 dinars to his grandfather (probably a banker), which will be used for orders of payment for *kand*,[6] another 50 dinars he pays to the two partners directly (document number 23).[7]

This document is believed to have been written in 1229. According to Goitein, sugar factories – constructed in large numbers around al-Fusṭāṭ beginning in the eleventh and twelfth centuries – were managed mostly by the investors

---

3 Goitein, *A Mediterranean Society*. The author selected the documents describing the activities of the Jewish merchants from among the *Geniza* documents and compiled a volume entitled *Letters of Medieval Jewish Traders*, Princeton, 1973.

4 Goitein, *A Mediterranean Society*, vol. 1, Preface, pp. vii-viii.

5 Goitein, *A Mediterranean Society*, vol. 1, p. 29.

6 *Kand* probably indicates *qand* in the Arabic form, which means raw sugar.

7 Goitein, *A Mediterranean Society*, vol. 1, p. 366. See also *ibid.*, p. 89.

who shared in their profits and losses. This form of industrial cooperation was called "*shirka*" (partnership).[8]

The Sugar Merchants (*sukkarī*)

Goitein also states that *sukkarī*, or sugar-maker (and seller), is indeed one of the most common occupations and family names occurring in the Geniza documents from the beginning of the eleventh to the end of the thirteenth centuries.[9] He summarizes one document, dated 1142 that recounts the dealings between several *sukkarī*s, as follows:

> There is a deathbed declaration made by a *sukkarī* who had taken ill suddenly (and who died the day after making his declaration). In it, he records having received sugar worth 6 dinars from a *sukkarī* whom he refers to with the honorary epithet "the elder" (not applied to the dying man), and to whom he had paid one-third in cash; and he refers to still another *sukkarī* from whom he received sugar valued at 3 dinars. He himself sold much smaller amounts.[10]

These *sukkarī*s are small storekeepers who specialized in the sale of sugar worth only 3 to 6 dinars. As the price of one *qinṭār* of white sugar was about 9 dinars in Egypt during the twelfth century,[11] 3 dinars would have been worth 15 kilograms of white sugar. That was almost equal to the sugar of one *ublūj*.[12]

The Transactions between Yacob in al-Fusṭāṭ and Majjānī in al-Qayrawān

Next, allow me to cite a document from *Letters of Medieval Jewish Traders*. Two people, Yacob and Majjānī, were merchants engaged in large-scale trade between Egypt and Maghrib.

> First, there is a balance of an account which, according to his [Majjānī's] statement, amounted to 142 dinars. Then, in the year 429/1038, I [Yacob] sent him in the warship sugar, sal ammoniac, nutmeg paste, nutmeg,

8 Goitein, *A Mediterranean Society*, vol. 1, pp. 87, 170. For *shirka* or *sharika*, see also *A Mediterranean Society*, vol. 1, pp. 169f.; A. Udovitch, *Partnership and Profit in Medieval Islam*, Princeton, 1970, pp. 17–39.

9 Goitein, *A Mediterranean Society*, vol. 1, p. 126.

10 Goitein, *A Mediterranean Society*, vol. 1, p. 152.

11 Ashtor, *Histoire des prix et des salaires*, pp. 134–135.

12 See Chapter Two – Section 2.

> violet blossoms, rose marmalade, etc… In the same year, in the Sheikhi ship, which was bound for Tripoli but changed its course to al-Mahdiyya, I sent twenty-three bags of flax.[13]

The sugar forwarded to Majjānī in al-Qayrawān can surely be considered a commodity produced in Egypt. Goitein notes that these goods were sent from Egypt in a warship because of the Byzantine naval attack on Sicily that year.[14] The document, interestingly enough, relates that Yacob, a Jewish trader in al-Fusṭāṭ, sent personally selected goods, including Egyptian sugar, to his complaining partner, Majjānī in al-Qayrawān.

The *Kārimī* Merchants Versed in Sugar

The Appearance of the Kārimī *Merchants*

As mentioned in Chapter Three, from the end of the tenth century, the trade route between East and West began to shift from the Persian Gulf to the Red Sea due to political disturbances in Baghdad under ʿAbbasid rule. Commercial products such as spices, silk goods, and pottery were now transported from Aden to ʿAydhāb on the west coast of the Red Sea, then to Qūṣ in Upper Egypt, further down the Nile to the capital city of Cairo, and finally to Alexandria and Damascus. It was the *Kārimī* merchants who fostered commercial relations with India, Southeast Asia, and China on this Red Sea route.

The origins of the word *Kārimī* or *Kārim* have been variously argued to date.[15] Some assert that the name derives from *Kānim*, a territory in Western Sudan, and others believe it may be due to the fact that amber was known as *kārim* in Cairene markets. It is also said that the word *kārim* was used in Arabic documents to designate a fleet, especially a merchant fleet. In any case, according to S. Labib, the first usage of the term *Kārim* appears in a text handed down by al-Qalqashandī.[16] Yet, in his work *The Financial System of Egypt*, Hassanein Ra-

---

13 Goitein, *Letters of Medieval Jewish Traders*, pp. 98–99.

14 Goitein, *Letters of Medieval Jewish Traders*, p. 98, note 8.

15 For the *Kārimī* merchants, see the following works. W.J. Fischel, "Über die Gruppe der Kārimī-Kaufleute," *Analecta Orientalia*, 14 (1937), pp. 67–82; E. Ashtor, "The Kārimī Merchants," *Journal of the Royal Asiatic Society*, 1956, pp. 45–56; S.D. Goitein, *Studies in Islamic History and Institutions*, Leiden, 1966, pp. 351–360; Labib, *Handelsgeschichte Ägyptens*; Muḥammad A. al-Ashqar, *Tujjār al-Tawābil fī Miṣr fī al-ʿAṣr al-Mamlūkī*, Cairo, 1999; T. Sato, "Slave Traders and Kārimī Merchants during the Mamluk Period: A Comparative Study," *Mamlūk Studies Review*, 10–1 (2006), pp. 141–156.

16 *EI*², s.v. Kārimī (S.Y. Labib).

bie presents a new finding: the term *Kārim* first appears in the Arabic text of *Kanz al-Durar wa-Jāmiʿ al-Ghurar* by Ibn Aybak al-Dawādārī (d. 8/14 c.).[17]

Ibn Aybak al-Dawādārī gives an account that in 456/1064 the merchants (*tājir*) arrived late [in Cairo] because the *Kārim* was interrupted.[18] The *Kārim* in this case may indicate a merchant fleet. We find another account of the *Kārim* in *Nūr al-Maʿārif*, compiled during the reign of al-Muẓaffar Yūsuf (647–694/1250–95) in the Rasūlid dynasty.

> *Al-Raṭl al-Laytī* (*Laythī*) is equal to 200 *qaflas* (about 600 grams), a unit used by the people of Upper Egypt. This *raṭl* is also used in Qūṣ in weighing the *Kārimī*'s goods (*baḍāʾiʿ al-Kārim*) at the time of rental (*kirāʾ*) contracts.[19]

"The *Kārimī*'s goods" may not refer to amber, but rather to the commercial goods transported by a merchant fleet vessel named *al-Kārim*. On the other hand, al-Maqrīzī states that in 577/1181, there arrived in [Cairo] *Kārim* merchants on whom were levied a commercial tax (*zakāt*) for four years.[20] These instances show that, from the late twelfth century, a merchant group named *al-Kārim* or *al-Kārimī* participated in commerce, mainly between Yemen and Cairo (or Alexandria) via the Red Sea and the Nile.

In 569/1174, Ṣalāḥ al-Dīn sent the Ayyubid army and his brother Shams al-Dawla Tūrānshāh to Yemen,[21] mainly to reap commercial profits by providing protection for *Kārimī* merchants working in the port city of Aden. Based on the medieval sources, G.R. Smith proposed the following five possible explanations for Tūrānshāh's expedition to Yemen: (1) A religious motive/desire to get rid of the Kharijites positioned there, (2) Pressure from ʿUmārah, the Yemeni poet, on Tūrānshāh to unite Yemen with Ayyubid Egypt, (3) A desire to find a place of refuge for the Ayyubid house, (4) An economic intention to profit from Yemen's revenue, and (5) A desire to find a territory for Tūrānshāh himself.[22] After careful examination of these five ideas, he concludes that the two chief

17 Rabie, *The Financial System of Egypt*, p. 97, note 2.

18 Ibn Aybak al-Dawādārī, *Kanz al-Durar wa-Jāmiʿ al-Ghurar*, VI, ed. S. al-Munajjid, Cairo, 1961, 380.

19 Anon., *Nūr al-Maʿārif fī Nuẓum wa-Qawānīn wa-Aʿrāf al-Yaman fī al-ʿAhd al-Muẓaffarī al-Wārif*, 2 vols., Sanaa, 2003–05, II, 267–268.

20 Al-Maqrīzī, *Kitāb al-Sulūk*, I, 72–73.

21 Ibn al-Athīr, *al-Kāmil*, XI, 396f.

22 G.R. Smith, *The Ayyūbids and Early Rasūlids in the Yemen (567–694/1173–1295)*, London, 1978, pp. 32–35.

motives for embarking on the conquest appear to have been trade and finding a secure place of refuge should the dynasty meet with danger.[23]

Also, in 578/1183 Reginald of Chatillon, Lord of Karak and Shawbak, resolved to advance into Red Sea trade routes and eventually invade Mecca. If the operation succeeded, the Christians would rule over two sacred Muslim cities and break-up the trade monopoly on the Red Sea. The Muslims soon counterattacked, destroying Christian ships off the port town of ʿAydhāb. As A.S. Ehrenkreutz states, following the failure of the Christian naval raid, Salāḥ al-Dīn declared the Red Sea closed to non-Muslims to protect commercial profits, always an important source of Egyptian revenue.[24] So, we can conclude that the Red Sea, after Reginald's easy defeat, became literally "a sea of *Kārimī* merchants."

The Organization and Activities of the Kārimī *Merchants*

According to Muḥammad A. al-Ashqar, 201 of the *Kārimī* merchants are identifiable by their personal names and the sphere of their activities. Although a few Christian and Jewish merchants were found among the *Kārimī* groups, most of them were Muslims.[25] Here we will examine the strength of their organizational ties, and their relationship with the Mamluk sultans who protected and managed their commercial activities.

Generally speaking, the *Kārimī* merchants were a loose organization of interested partners sharing lodgings/stores (*funduq*) built along the commercial routes between Aden and Alexandria. Al-Qalqashandī, who compiled the *Ṣubḥ al-Aʿshā*, a voluminous encyclopedic secretarial manual, explains the governmental office overseeing the *Kārimī* merchants as follows:

> The office of spices and *Kārimī* merchants (*naẓar al-bahār wal-kārimī*) supervises the various kinds of spices and other goods transported from Yemen by the *Kārimī* merchants. This is an important office, sometimes attached to the ministry (*wizāra*), sometimes to the superintendence ([*naẓar*] *al-khāṣṣ*), and sometimes independent as the sultan pleases.[26]

---

23 Smith, *The Ayyūbids and Early Rasūlids*, p. 47.

24 Ehrenkreutz, *Saladin*, p. 180. He notes that in the long run this precautionary security measure produced adverse economic effects, because it eliminated Jewish and Coptic India merchants and their capital from direct participation in the Egyptian transit trade.

25 Al-Ashqar, *Tujjār al-Tawābil*, pp. 156, 467–539. For the Jews and Christians among the *Kārimī* merchants, see also Ashtor, "The Kārimī Merchants," p. 55; id., *A Social and Economic History*, p. 300.

26 Al-Qalqashandī, *Ṣubḥ al-Aʿshā*, IV, 32.

Moreover, al-Ashqar states that this office levied a 2.5% tax on commercial goods and issued transit permits (*jawāz*) to the *Kārimī* merchants.[27] During the Mamluk period, one influential merchant among them was officially appointed "chief of the merchants (*ra'īs al-tujjār* or *kabīr al-tujjār*)." Ira M. Lapidus believes that the merchants themselves were headed by *ra'īs*es who acted as liaisons between the merchants and the state in disciplinary, diplomatic, banking, and other interactions.[28] Ashtor, however, finds fault with the view of W. Fischel,[29] which is the same as that of Lapidus, arguing that the authority of the "chief of the *Kārimīs*", a title found in Arabic chronicles and biographical dictionaries, is perhaps not to be taken too literally.[30] For example, Ibn Ḥajar al-ʿAsqalānī relates that after Zakī al-Dīn al-Kharrūbī, a great *Kārimī* merchant, gained the title of *ra'īs al-tujjār* in 786/1384, his status in the government improved and he became preeminent among the *Kārimī* merchants.[31] This account shows that though Zakī al-Dīn gained the title of *ra'īs al-tujjār* and was to some extent influential with his *Kārimī* colleagues, he was never regarded as a state official with endorsed authority.[32]

Accordingly, the decisions as to how much the sphere of commercial activities would be expanded, and which kind of goods would be traded, fell upon the financial power and business acumen of each *Kārimī* merchant. Most of the *Kārimī* merchants set up bases in Cairo, al-Fusṭāṭ, or Aden. From these bases, they expanded their commercial activities to Mecca, ʿAydhāb, Qūṣ, Alexandria, Damascus, Aleppo, Baghdad, and al-Baṣra. Some of them, based in Aden, went further to Calicut in India, Hormuz in Iran, Malacca in Southeast Asia, Guangzhou, Quanzhou, and Yangzhou in China, bringing spices, silk goods, and pottery back to the Islamic world.[33]

27 Al-Ashqar, *Tujjār al-Tawābil*, pp. 105–107, 112–113.

28 Ira. M. Lapidus, *Muslim Cities in the Later Middle Ages*, Cambridge, Mass., 1967, p. 125.

29 Fischel, "Über die Gruppe der Kārimī-Kaufleute," pp. 67–82

30 Ashtor, "The Kārimī Merchants," pp. 51–52.

31 Ibn Ḥajar, *Inbā' al-Ghumr bi-Anbā' al-'Umr*, ed. H. Ḥabashī, 4 vols., Cairo, 1969–98, I, 306; Ibn Ḥajar, *al-Durar al-Kāmina*, I, 482. Zakī al-Dīn was also called "*kabīr al-tujjār*" (al-Maqrīzī, *Kitāb al-Sulūk*, III, 539).

32 Sato, "Slave Traders and Kārimī Merchants," pp. 151–152.

33 *Tujjār al-Tawābil* by al-Ashqar contains a useful list of 201 *Kārimī* merchants with their birth and death years, native countries, official positions, and spheres of their activities. For the *Kārimī* merchants who visited China, see H. Yajima, *A History as Seen from the Sea* (*Kaiiki kara mita rekishi*, in Japanese), Nagoya, 2006, pp. 446–456.

"Merchants of Spices and Perfumes" or "Merchants of Spices and Sugar"

The *Kārimīs* were generally known as "the merchants of spices and perfumes." These spices (*bahār* or *tābil*) included pepper, clove, nutmeg, cumin, ginger, cinnamon, turmeric, cardamom, saffron, and others, from South and Southeast Asia. Meanwhile, the perfumes (*ʿiṭr*) consisted of camphor, sandalwood, ambergris, musk, frankincense, myrrh, and so on, mainly from Arabia, South and Southeast Asia. Yajima, based on the *Nūr al-Maʿārif* compiled in thirteenth-century Yemen, explains that, when trading with India, the *Kārimī* merchants offered copper, tin, ironware, grinding stones, *maḥlab*, cumin, musk, mastic trees, dates and the alcohol produced from them, ivory, silk, gold, silver, cotton, flax, leather, *kuḥl*, sulfur, indigo, and more. While in Egypt, they offered pepper, lac, turmeric, clove, nutmeg, ginger, myrobalan, indigo, myrrh, rice, wheat, and so on.[34]

In addition to the above items, we can confirm that the *Kārimī* merchants also traded timber (*khashab*), horses (*khayl*), sugar (*sukkar*), pottery (*fakhkhār*), and slaves (*raqīq*).[35] As mentioned above, Egyptian sugar and wheat were valuable exports for Italian merchants arriving in Alexandria during the Mamluk period. *Nūr al-Maʿārif* also states that various kinds of sugar, such as refined sugar (*sukkar mukarrar*) and white sugar (*sukkar abyaḍ*), were imported from Egypt to Yemen during the thirteenth century.[36] According to Ashtor, "the *Kārimīs* were active in several branches of trade and industry. They traded in wheat, precious stones and jewels, cloth, and slaves, and they invested great sums of money in the sugar industry."[37]

As we will discuss later, Sultan Barsbāy (reigned 825–841/1422–38) repeatedly implemented price controls and monopolistic policies on pepper and sugar in order to increase the Mamluk state income from the 1420's on. This shows that the amount of business in both pepper and sugar was particularly great compared to other commercial goods. So, perhaps rather than "the merchants of spices and perfumes", the *Kārimīs* could be called "the merchants of spices and sugar."

---

34 Yajima, *A History as Seen from the Sea*, pp. 434–435.

35 Ashtor, "The Kārimī Merchants," pp. 55–56; Lapidus, *Muslim Cities*, p. 125; Sato, *State and Rural Society*, p. 215; al-Ashqar, *Tujjār al-Tawābil*, p. 76.

36 Anon., *Nūr al-Maʿārif*, I, 432; II, 105.

37 E. Ashtor, *Levant Trade in the Later Middle Ages*, Princeton, 1983, p. 273.

The Vicissitudes of the Kharrūbī Family in Mamluk Egypt

From Retailers to Kārimī *Merchants*

During the Mamluk period, various influential families appeared among the *Kārimīs*, including the al-Maḥallīs, the al-Kharrūbīs, the Ibn Kuwayks, and the Ibn Musallams. For example, Nāṣir al-Dīn Muḥammad Ibn Musallam made huge profits by traveling to India, Ethiopia, Yemen, and al-Takrūr for slaves (*ʿabd*), becoming the most influential merchant of his age. It is said that when he died in Cairo in 776/1374, he left a fortune to his sons of 200,000 dinars each.[38] Here, let us look at the al-Kharrūbīs as an example of an ascendant wealthy *Kārimī* merchant family, tracing their rise and fall from the thirteenth to the fifteenth centuries.

Since "*kharrūb*" in Arabic means "carob bean", family ancestor Ṣalāḥ al-Dīn al-Miṣrī al-Kharrūbī might have been a carob retailer. According to Ibn Ḥajar al-ʿAsqalānī, the Kharrūbīs originated from Kharrūb square in al-Fusṭāṭ,[39] where carob was commonly sold.[40] In any case, the family's activities as *Kārimī* merchants lasted for seven generations, from Ṣalāḥ al-Dīn al-Kharrūbī (mid-thirteenth century) to Fakhr al-Dīn Sulaymān (d. 864/1460), who was imprisoned for his large debts.[41] Specific descriptions of the Kharrūbīs first began to appear in Arabic chronicles and biographical dictionaries after the period of the brothers Ṣalāḥ al-Dīn Aḥmad b. Muḥammad (d. 769/1368) and Badr al-Dīn Muḥammad b. Muḥammad (d. 762/1361).

Although he started out as a poor merchant, elder brother Ṣalāḥ al-Dīn Aḥmad attained great wealth through trading and built a large tomb (*turba*) in the al-Qarāfa district, which his grandson, Nūr al-Dīn ʿAlī (d. 802/1400), maintained and later fitted with a fine washroom (*maṭhara*).[42] Ṣalāḥ al-Dīn's son, ʿIzz al-Dīn Muḥammad (d. 776/1374), built a *madrasa* in the suburbs of al-Fusṭāṭ, which was larger than that of his uncle Badr al-Dīn, but ʿIzz al-Dīn died before its completion.[43] Despite achieving considerable success in trading before his brother, Badr al-Dīn seems not to have offered a helping hand to his

---

38 Ibn Ḥajar, *al-Durar al-Kāmina*, V, 26; al-Maqrīzī, *Kitāb al-Muqaffā al-Kabīr*, VII, 257–258; Ibn Taghrībirdī, *al-Manhal al-Ṣāfī*, XI, 122–123.

39 Ibn Ḥajar, *al-Durar al-Kāmina*, I, 481. Brief descriptions of the Kharrūbīs are found in Ashtor, "The Kārimī Merchants," pp. 47–50.

40 Ibn Duqmāq, *Kitāb al-Intiṣār*, I, 35. According to this account, the square was originally called "Raḥbat Dār al-Malik," and later came to be named "Raḥbat Kharrūb" because carob was usually sold there.

41 Al-Sakhāwī, *al-Ḍawʾ al-Lāmiʿ*, III, 267.

42 Al-Maqrīzī, *al-Khiṭaṭ*, II, 369.

43 Al-Maqrīzī, *al-Khiṭaṭ*, II, 370.

poorer elder brother Ṣalāḥ al-Dīn. This also shows that the Kharrūbīs, or the *Kārimī* merchants in general, operated on individual bases, not according to organized systems.

There was also a case wherein the entire Kharrūbī family was ordered by the Mamluk government to provide sugar. In Dhū al-Qaʿda 751/February 1351 the government had neither one dirham of silver nor one *ardabb* of wheat remaining, as the state treasury (*bayt al-māl*) and granary (*ahrāʾ*) had been completely exhausted. Al-Maqrīzī describes the emergency measures taken by the government as follows.

> Fakhr al-Dīn Mājid, who was appointed Chief Secretary (*naẓar al-buyūt*), ordered the Kharrūbī merchants in al-Fusṭāṭ to provide sugar for a sugar allowance (*rātib al-sukkar*) to be given at the beginning of the new year [752]. Fakhr al-Dīn, after being provided with sugar [by the Kharrūbīs], could barely pay the monthly allowance (*jāmakīya*) to the *mamlūk*s in the Sultan's court.[44]

This account clearly shows that the Kharrūbīs were deeply involved in sugar production in the mid-fourteenth century, and had close ties to the Mamluk government.

The Sugar Refinery Merchant

Among the Kharrūbī merchants, the above-mentioned Badr al-Dīn Muḥammad, who was called "the leader of the Kharrūbīs," was particularly well known as a "sugar refinery merchant" (*tājir fī maṭābikh al-sukkar*) in al-Fusṭāṭ.[45] The 751/1351 government order for the Kharrūbīs to provide sugar might have been dealt with under Badr al-Dīn's leadership. He also had a major business rivalry with Nāṣir al-Dīn Muḥammad Ibn Musallam (d. 776/1374). When a dispute arose between them, Ibn Musallam boasted to Badr al-Dīn, "Buy sacks (*shikāra*) for all your money and bring them to me. Then I will fill them for you with my coins."[46] Interestingly enough, however, Ibn Musallam gave his daughter in marriage to Sirāj al-Dīn ʿUmar b. ʿAbd al-ʿAzīz (d. 825/1422), a Kharrūbī merchant, in order to form ties between the two families.[47]

---

44 Al-Maqrīzī, *Kitāb al-Sulūk*, II, 828–829.

45 Al-Maqrīzī, *al-Khiṭaṭ*, II, 369. See also Sato, "Sugar in the Economic Life of Mamluk Egypt," p. 99.

46 Ibn Ḥajar, *Inbāʾ al-Ghumr*, I, 99.

47 Al-Sakhāwī, *Kitāb al-Tibr al-Masbūk fī Dhayl al-Sulūk*, Bulaq, 1896; repr. Cairo, 1974, 107; Ibn Ḥajar, *Inbāʾ al-Ghumr*, III, 289.

As I mentioned in Chapter Three, we find an interesting account in Ibn Duqmāq's *Kitāb al-Intiṣār*, which relates that of the 65 sugar refineries (*maṭbakh al-sukkar*) in al-Fusṭāṭ, 7 were owned by the sultan, 21 by amirs, and 13 by merchants (*tājir*).[48] Among the 13 refineries owned by merchants, 4 were managed by *sukkarī*s (Muslim and Jewish sugar merchants) and another 4 by the *Kārimī* merchants.

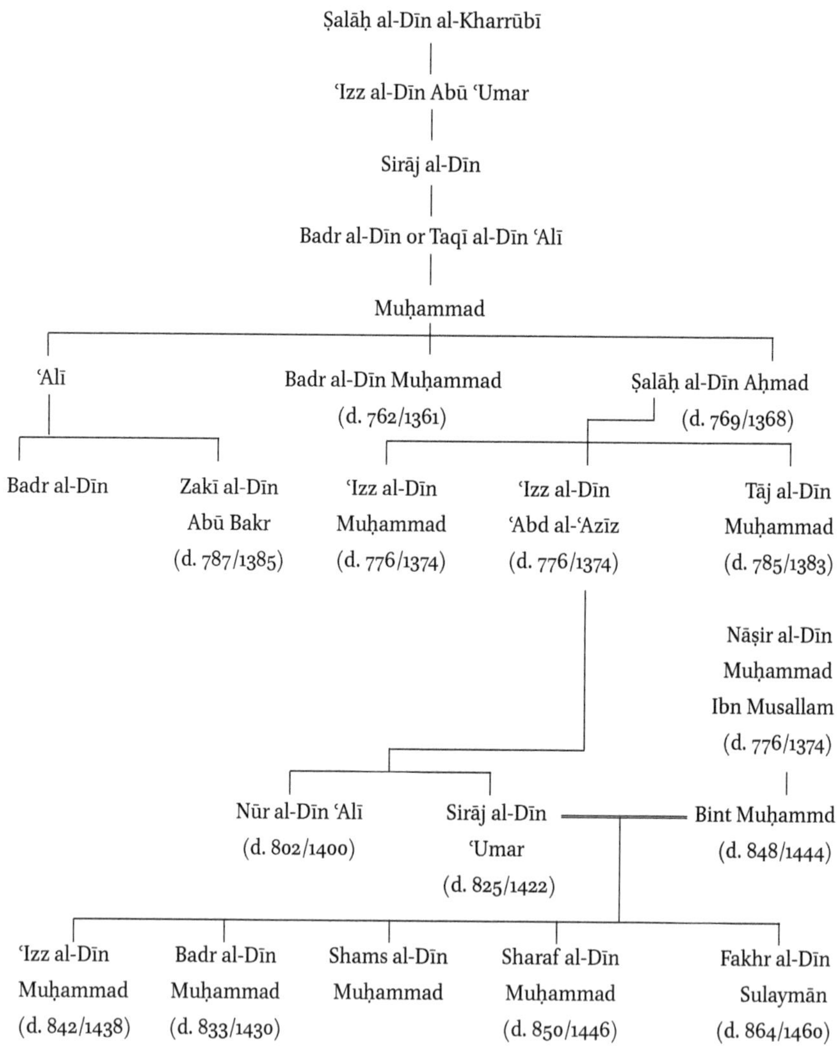

* Revised and enlarged genealogy based on the table by Ashtor, "The Kārimī Merchants."

FIGURE 5 *Genealogical table of the Kharrūbī family*

48 Ibn Duqmāq, *Kitāb al-Intiṣār*, I, 41–46.

Among the four refineries owned by the *Kārimīs*, two were managed by Kharrūbī family members: Maṭbakh Sirāj al-Dīn [ʿUmar] Ibn al-Kharrūbī and Maṭbakh Nūr al-Dīn [ʿAlī] Ibn al-Kharrūbī.[49] Sirāj al-Dīn ʿUmar and Nūr al-Dīn ʿAlī were the sons of ʿIzz al-Dīn ʿAbd al-ʿAzīz, and the grandnephews of the above-mentioned Badr al-Dīn Muḥammad who had already gained a reputation as a "sugar refinery merchant". The rich merchants in the Mamluk period were generally said not to survive for more than two or three generations, due to burdensome property confiscations (*muṣādara*) by the government.[50] Yet, the Kharrūbī merchants were able to manage their sugar refineries for more than three generations and gained immense wealth by trading refined sugar produced in Egypt, and various spices brought in from South and Southeast Asia.

Because of this brisk commerce, both Sirāj al-Dīn and Nūr al-Dīn attained positions as purveyors and were granted the title of *khawājā* by the Mamluk sultans.[51] *Khawājā* (an Arabic corruption of the Turkish term *hoca*) was usually a title (*laqab*) bestowed upon wealthy slave traders (*nakhkhās, jallāb*) from outside the Mamluk domain who served the sultans in an official capacity.[52] However, the above cases of the Kharrūbīs indicate that this title was occasionally granted to a few *Kārimī* merchants as well.

The Position of Chief Merchant (Raʾīs al-Tujjār)

Some Kharrūbī family merchants sought even higher positions or titles from the government. In 781/1379, Kamāl al-Dīn, a grandson of Ṣalāḥ al-Dīn Aḥmad al-Kharrūbī, was arrested and whipped by Amir Barqūq (later reigned

49 Ibn Duqmāq, *Kitāb al-Intiṣār*, I, 46. Regarding the two refineries owned by the Kharrūbīs, there is no detailed description of them in the original text. Ashtor states that three factories were owned by the al-Kharrūbīs: two belonging to brothers Nūr al-Dīn and Sirāj al-Dīn, and another belonging to Zakī al-Dīn al-Kharrūbī ("Levantine Sugar Industry in the Late Middle Ages," p. 101). But, we find no sugar refinery belonging to Zakī al-Dīn in the Arabic sources he refers to.

50 Ashtor, *A Social and Economic History*, p. 301; Goitein, *Studies in Islamic History and Institutions*, p. 351.

51 Al-Sakhāwī, *al-Ḍawʾ al-Lāmiʿ*, III, 267; Ibn Iyās, *Badāʾiʿ al-Zuhūr fī Waqāʾiʿ al-Duhūr*, 3 vols., Bulaq, 1893, I, 340. *Badāʾiʿ al-Zuhūr* edited by M. Muṣṭafā does not have the title *khawājā* for Nūr al-Dīn ʿAlī (I-2, 636).

52 Al-Qalqashandī, *Ṣubḥ al-Aʿshā*, VI, 13. See also D. Ayalon, *L'esclavage du Mamelouk*, Jerusalem, 1951, pp. 3–4; Lapidus, *Muslim Cities*, pp. 122–123, 127–29. Ashtor mistakenly states that the honorific khawaja or khawajaki title bestowed upon them is not mentioned in the great manual of state administration compiled by al-Qalqashandī (*A Social and Economic History*, p. 321).

784–791/1382–89, 792–801/1390–99) for attempting to obtain the rank of vizier with a bribe of 100,000 dinars. Following that incident, Kamāl al-Dīn was exiled to Qūṣ in Upper Egypt, where he was ordered to reside until his death.[53] Fifteen years later, in 796/1394 when Timur attempted to invade Syria, three influential *Kārimī* merchants – Burhān al-Dīn al-Maḥallī, Shihāb al-Dīn Ibn Musallam, and Nūr al-Dīn ʿAlī ibn al-Kharrūbī – supplied Sultan Barqūq with 1,000,000 dirhams for the war against Timur.[54] The three *Kārimī* merchant's share thus amounted to ten percent of the 10,000,000 dirhams spent on Barqūq's royal *mamlūk*s just prior to the war.[55] The exiled Kamāl al-Dīn, of course, had no chance to join in contributing money to the sultan.

Among the Kharrūbīs, Zakī al-Dīn Abū Bakr was the only one granted the title of "chief merchant" (*raʾīs al-tujjār*). Ibn Ḥajar al-ʿAsqalānī states the following in *Inbāʾ al-Ghumr.*

> In 786/1384, when trouble arose between Zakī al-Dīn al-Kharrūbī and Shihāb al-Dīn al-Fāriqī, an influential merchant from Yemen, they were both tried before Sultan Barqūq. In answer to al-Fāriqī's accusations, Zakī al-Dīn quoted a letter written by al-Fāriqī and addressed to the lord of Yemen, which read, "At present Egypt is in a state of corruption (*fasād*). Since there is no credible lord (*ṣāḥib*), you need not send any gifts from here on. The present lord [sultan] is the lowest and the most despicable among the *mamlūks*." After reading this, Barqūq ordered al-Fāriqī seized and his tongue cut out. Then the sultan bestowed on Zakī al-Dīn a fine robe (*khilʿa*) and granted him the title of "great merchant" (*kabīr al-tujjār*).[56]

The account of the Zakī al-Dīn/Shihāb al-Dīn dispute tells us that Zakī al-Dīn was granted the title of "great merchant" (*kabīr al-tujjār*) or "chief merchant" (*raʾīs al-tujjār*) in 786/1384. In *al-Durar al-Kāmina*, Ibn Ḥajar further states, "Zakī al-Dīn approached the state (*dawla*) and gained the title of "leader" (*riʾāsa*), thus surpassing his peers,"[57] showing distinctly that Zakī al-Dīn peti-

---

53 Ibn Ḥajar, *Inbāʾ al-Ghumr*, I, 306.

54 Al-Maqrīzī, *Kitāb al-Sulūk*, III, 811; Ibn al-Furāt, *Taʾrīkh Ibn al-Furāt*, IX, 378–79. Incidentally, Ibn al-Furāt describes each of these three merchants with the title of Qadi. See also W.J. Fischel, "The Spice Trade in Mamluk Egypt," *JESHO*, 1 (1958), p. 171; Ashtor, "The Kārimī Merchants," p. 53.

55 Al-Maqrīzī, *Kitāb al-Sulūk*, III, 803.

56 Ibn Ḥajar, *Inbāʾ al-Ghumr*, I, 288. The account of this dispute between two leading *Kārimī* merchants was previously noted by Labib (*Handelsgeschichte Ägyptens*, p. 228).

57 Ibn Ḥajar, *al-Durar al-Kāmina*, I, 482.

tioned Sultan Barqūq to bestow upon him the title of *riʾāsa*. Zakī al-Dīn held this honorary title for about two years until he died in 787/1385 in al-Fusṭāṭ.[58] According to Ibn Ḥajar, after he gained the title, Zakī al-Dīn's status (*qadr*) in the government rose. He was no longer preoccupied with business, but gradually mellowed, earning the respect of the *Kārimī* merchants.[59]

Religious and Cultural Activities

Though the slave traders of the Mamluk period made their fortunes under the protection of sultans, we find little positive information regarding their work for the public good.[60] We find many more instances of religious and cultural activities among the *Kārimī* merchants than among the slave traders. As mentioned above, Badr al-Dīn Muḥammad al-Kharrūbī (d. 762/1361), who was known primarily as a "sugar refinery merchant," also built a school (*madrasa*, later called "al-Madrasat al-Kharrūbīya") to which he appointed Shaykh Bahāʾ al-Dīn ʿAbd Allāh Ibn ʿUqayl as professor of law (*mudarris al-fiqh*) and Shaykh Sirāj al-Dīn ʿUmar al-Bulqīnī as assistant (*muʿīd*).[61] It is said that Badr al-Dīn set the condition that only Arabs be appointed to its faculty.[62] According to Ibn Ḥajar, ʿIzz al-Dīn ʿAbd al-ʿAzīz b. Aḥmad al-Kharrūbī (d. 776/1374) owned a fine *madrasa* adjacent to his house in al-Fusṭāṭ.[63] His brother, Tāj al-Dīn Muḥammad b. Aḥmad al-Kharrūbī (d. 785/1383), built a large house on a bank of the Nile and converted it into a *madrasa*, to which he donated a *waqf* and appointed a professor of tradition (*mudarris ḥadīth*).[64] ʿIzz al-Dīn ʿAbd al-ʿAzīz's other brother, ʿIzz al-Dīn Muḥammad b. Aḥmad al-Kharrūbī, also built a *madrasa*, larger than that of his uncle Badr al-Dīn, in the suburbs of al-Fusṭāṭ, but died before it was completed.[65] According to Ibn Iyās, Khawājā Nūr al-Dīn ʿAlī al-Kharrūbī was also the owner of a *madrasa* in al-Fusṭāṭ near the Nile.[66]

After he returned from Mecca in 786/1384, Zakī al-Dīn Abū Bakr (*raʾīs al-tujjār*) invited Najm al-Dīn Ibn Razīn to learn *Ṣaḥīḥ al-Bukhārī* from him. Al-

58 Al-Maqrīzī, *Kitāb al-Sulūk*, III, 539; Ibn Taghrībirdī, *al-Nujūm al-Zāhira*, XI, 305; Ibn Ḥajar, *al-Durar al-Kāmina*, I, 482. It is said that Zakī al-Dīn left 30,000 dinars to Sultan Barqūq in his will (Ibn Qāḍī Shuhba, *Taʾrīkh Ibn Qāḍī Shuhba*, ed. A. Darwīsh, 4 vols., Damascus, 1977–97, I/3, 168).

59 Ibn Ḥajar, *Inbāʾ al-Ghumr*, I, 306.

60 Sato, "Slave Traders and Kārimī Merchants," p. 147.

61 Al-Maqrīzī, *al-Khiṭaṭ*, II, 369. Badr al-Dīn also built *rab*ʿs (living quarters) near the school.

62 Al-Maqrīzī, *al-Khiṭaṭ*, II, 369–70.

63 Ibn Ḥajar, *Inbāʾ al-Ghumr*, I, 86–87.

64 Al-Maqrīzī, *al-Khiṭaṭ*, II, 368.

65 Al-Maqrīzī, *al-Khiṭaṭ*, II, 368.

66 Ibn Iyās, *Badāʾiʿ al-Zuhūr*, I/2, 636.

though he had gained the title of *ra'īs al-tujjār* through the entrapment of his rival Shihāb al-Dīn, Ibn Ḥajar praised Zakī al-Dīn as being a person of decency (*ḥishma*), esprit de corps (*ʿaṣabīya*), manliness (*murūwa*), and a generous donor to scholars and poets.[67] His praise of Zakī al-Dīn was probably due to their personal friendship, as Zakī al-Dīn, at the request his father, had taken good care of Ibn Ḥajar when he visited Mecca in his boyhood.[68]

The Beginning of the Downfall

Over time, however, some of the Kharrūbī family merchants devoted themselves to Sufism and other religious activities, neglecting the family business and running up debts. According to al-Sakhāwī, Sirāj al-Dīn ʿUmar b. ʿAbd al-ʿAzīz al-Kharrūbī, who had inherited his uncle's property and expanded his business, wanted nothing more than to hear the Qur'an recited, and died heavily in debt.[69] Nūr al-Dīn ʿAlī, a pious sufi (*mutaṣawwif*), donated 100,000 dirhams to the reconstruction of al-Ḥaram al-Sharīf in Mecca.[70] Although he has been called "the last of the Kharrūbī merchants (*ākhir tujjār Miṣr min al-Kharāriba*)," upon his death at the age of 58, Nūr al-Dīn left behind a huge fortune.[71] However, as he had no children, his four nephews (three Muḥammads and one Sulaymān) likely inherited most of his property.

With this inherited capital, ʿIzz al-Dīn Muḥammad (d. 842/1438), Badr al-Dīn Muḥammad (d. 833/1430), Fakhr al-Dīn Sulaymān, and others continued trading into the early fifteenth century. So, Nūr al-Dīn was actually not the last merchant of the Kharrūbī family. But, Fakhr al-Dīn, for example, had neither the prosperity of the Kharrūbīs, nor their status as notable members (*aʿyān*) of Cairene society.[72] In 826/1423, in response to a deficiency of state revenue, Sultan Barsbāy declared government control (*ṭarḥ*) over sugar refining and trade. According to al-Maqrīzī, the government sealed off the sugar refineries (*khatama ʿalā maṭābikh al-sukkar*) and put them under state control, prohibiting the trade of sugar and sweets not authorized by the sultan.[73] Then, in 832/1429, Barsbāy decreed that the prices of spices traded with Italian merchants in Al-

67 Ibn Ḥajar, *al-Durar al-Kāmina*, I, 482. We also find an account of Zakī al-Dīn constructing al-Khānqāh al-Kharrūbīya (al-Maqrīzī, *al-Khiṭaṭ*, II, 426–427). However, he originally constructed this as a private residence for his family. In 822/1419, the house was converted into a *khānqāh* in accordance with the wishes of Sultan al-Mu'ayyad Shaykh.

68 Ibn Ḥajar, *al-Durar al-Kāmina*, I, 482.

69 Al-Sakhāwī, *al-Ḍaw' al-Lāmiʿ*, VI, 92.

70 Al-Sakhāwī, *al-Ḍaw' al-Lāmiʿ*, V, 240.

71 Al-Sakhāwī, *al-Ḍaw' al-Lāmiʿ*, V, 240.

72 Al-Sakhāwī, *al-Ḍaw' al-Lāmiʿ*, III, 267.

73 Al-Maqrīzī, *Kitāb al-Sulūk*, IV, 647.

exandria would be determined by the government,[74] dealing the *Kārimī* merchants a fatal blow. The above-mentioned Fakhr al-Dīn, who had spent a luxurious life reading the Qur'an, suffered various misfortunes (*nazala bi-hi al-ḥāl*), fell deeply into debt, and was consequently imprisoned,[75] no doubt as a result of the monopolistic spice and sugar policies put in place by Sultan Barsbāy.

The downfall of the Kharrūbī family reflects the fate of all the *Kārimī* merchants, who had uniquely contributed to the prosperity of Ayyubid and Mamluk Egypt. Ibn Taghrībirdī talks about the effects of these monopolistic policies in *Ḥawādith al-Duhūr*.

> As this year (859/1455) comes to an end, firewood (*ḥaṭab*) has already become hard to find. The firewood from tamarisk trees sold at about 120 dirhams per load (*ḥiml*). As for the *Kārimī*s, not a single merchant was to be found [in the market] from the end of Ramaḍān to date, which greatly worsened the situation for the common people.[76]

This account clearly shows that the *Kārimī* merchants had disappeared from the Egyptian markets by the middle of the fifteenth century.

However, the price controls and monopolistic policies on spices and sugar were not always implemented to good effect. As M. Sobernheim has already stated, monopolistic decrees on sugar were repeatedly issued in the 1420s. After the government seized control of sugar refining and sales in 826/1423, it decreed in Shaʿbān 828/July 1425 that the sultan has the exclusive right to buy and sell sugar.[77] Then, in Rabīʿ II 832/March 1429, the government also centralized the production of sugar (*taḥkīr ṣanf al-sukkar*). Al-Maqrīzī criticizes this policy as follows.

---

74 Al-Maqrīzī, *Kitāb al-Sulūk*, IV, 791–792. For the price controls and monopolistic policies under Sultan Barabāy, see the following works. M. Sobernheim, "Das Zuckermonopol unter Sultan Barsbāi," *Zeitschrift für Assyriologie*, 27 (1912), pp. 75–84; A. Darrag, *L'Égypte sous le règne de Barsbāy*, Damascus, 1961; Labib, *Handelsgeschichte Ägyptens*, pp. 94f.; Ashtor, *A Social and Economic History*, p. 321; id., *Levant Trade*, pp. 278f.; al-Ashqar, *Tujjār al-Tawābil*, pp. 439f.: J.L. Meloy, "Imperial Strategy and Political Exigency: The Red Sea Spice Trade and the Mamluk Sultanate in the Fifteenth Century," *JAOS*, 123 (2003), pp. 1–19.

75 Al-Sakhāwī, *al-Ḍaw' al-Lāmiʿ*, III, 267.

76 Ibn Taghrībirdī, *Ḥawādith al-Duhūr fī Madā al-Ayyām wal-Shuhūr*, ed. W. Popper, 4 vols., Berkeley, 1930–42, II, 247.

77 Al-Maqrīzī, *Kitāb al-Sulūk*, IV, 691.

> The order prohibited the operation of waterwheels (*dūlāb*) for sugarcane cultivation and pressing, the refining of sugar from raw sugar (*qand*) to white sugar (*sukkar*), and the sale of sugar, except by the sultan. Moreover, it allotted the supply of another 30,000 dinars to supervisors (*kāshif*) and governors (*wālī*). However, the policy was neglected and never fully implemented. "Praise be to God."[78]

According to J.L. Meloy, Sultan Barsbāy, seeking to expand Mamluk authority into the Ḥijāz, including the sacred cities of Mecca and Medina, carried out a centralization of the economy, through price controls and monopolistic policies on spices and sugar, that consequently brought about the downfall of the *Kārimī* merchants.[79] As we will later see, a new type of Muslim merchant replaced the *Kārimī* merchants from the end of the Mamluk era to the beginning of the Ottoman era.

78 Al-Maqrīzī, *Kitāb al-Sulūk*, IV, 796. See also Ibn Ḥajar, *Inbā' al-Ghumr*, III, 419.

79 Meloy, "Imperial Strategy and Political Exigency," pp. 1–19.

CHAPTER 5

Sugar as Medicine

We have so far discussed sugarcane cultivation, sugar production technologies, sugar as commodity, and the vicissitudes of sugar merchants in medieval Muslim societies. In addition to its roles in sweeteners and as a commodity, sugar was also important as a medicine and for its use in festivals. In this chapter, we will examine how various kinds of sugar were used as medicines by Ibn al-Bayṭār, a famous pharmacologist, and Ibn al-Nafīs, a personal physician of Sultan Baybars. We will also examine the activities of the druggists who sold sugar as a medicine.

A Comprehensive Book of Simple Drugs by Ibn al-Bayṭār

Ibn al-Bayṭār, Pharmacologist

Ibn al-Bayṭār ʿAbd Allāh al-Mālaqī (d. 646/1248) was considered a leading pharmacologist (*ʿashshāb*) of the Islamic world. He was born in Málaga at the end of the twelfth century, and studied botany and pharmacology in Sevilla under Muwaḥḥid Dynasty rule. Arabic biographies tell us that he recorded in great detail the names, shapes, medicinal effects, and native growing areas of numerous herbs while he worked under such masters as Abū al-ʿAbbās al-Nabaṭī, ʿAbd Allāh b. Ṣāliḥ, and Abū al-Ḥajjāj. Around 617/1220, Ibn al-Bayṭār left his homeland for the eastern Islamic world and arrived at the Ayyubid capital city of Cairo via Morocco, Algeria, and Tunisia.[1] Cairo, at that time, was beginning to stand out as a new center of economics and culture in the Islamic world, regardless of ongoing political unrest in Baghdad.

According to his disciple, Ibn Abī Uṣaybiʿa (d. 668/1270), when Ibn al-Bayṭār arrived in Cairo, he was appointed by Sultan al-Kāmil as the "head of all pharmacologists" (*raʾīs ʿalā sāʾir al-ʿashshābīyīn*).[2] While living in Cairo, he conducted new research on herbs, visiting the countries of Agāriqa (Greece) and Rūm.

---

1 For the life of Ibn al-Bayṭār, see the following works. Ibn Abī Uṣaybiʿa, *ʿUyūn al-Anbāʾ fī Ṭabaqāt al-Aṭibbāʾ*, 3 vols., Beirut, 1956–57, III, 220–222; *EI*², s.v. Ibn al-Bayṭār (J. Vernet); C. Brockelmann, *Geschichte der Arabischen Litteratur*, 5 vols., Leiden, 1937–49, I, p. 492; D. Campbell, *Arabian Medicine and its Influence on the Middle Ages*, 2 vols., London, 1926; repr. Amsterdam, 1974, vol. 1, pp. 101–102.

2 Ibn Abī Uṣaybiʿa, *ʿUyūn al-Anbāʾ*, III, 221.

 | DOI 10.1163/9789004281561_007

Even after Sultan al-Kāmil died, Ibn al-Bayṭār was welcomed by his son al-Ṣāliḥ. Not long after, however, he moved to Damascus, where he published an annotated edition (*tafsīr*) of *Materia Medica* by Dioscorides and conducted research in the suburbs with assistants including his disciple, Ibn Abī Uṣaybiʿa. Ibn al-Bayṭār was a strong, respectable, and honest man who wholly devoted himself to the study of pharmacology. He died in Damascus in the winter of 646/1248, shortly before the collapse of the Ayyubid dynasty.[3]

Ibn al-Bayṭār compiled two major works; *al-Mughnī fī al-Adwiyat al-Mufrada* (*A Corpus of Simple Remedies*), and *al-Jāmiʿ li-Mufradāt al-Adwiya wal-Aghdhiya* (*A Comprehensive Book of Simple Drugs and Foods*). Here, we will look at the latter work, *A Comprehensive Book of Simple Drugs*, which is a pharmaceutical encyclopedia listing over 1,400 kinds of simple pharmaceutical substances (*adwiya mufrada*), excluding compound drugs (*adwiya murakkaba*). Each item is explained from Ibn al-Bayṭār's personal observations and quoting from over 260 sources by authors including Dioscorides, Galen, al-Rāzī, Ibn Sīnā, and al-Idrīsī.[4] Ibn Abī Uṣaybiʿa states, "We can not find any book as excellent as the *al-Jāmiʿ li-Mufradāt al-Adwiya*."[5] As Peter E. Pormann and Emilie Savage-Smith state,[6] we can also understand Ibn al-Bayṭār's pharmacopoeia to be the most influential of all Arabic treatises on basic pharmaceutical substances since the mid-thirteenth century.

Sugar in the Comprehensive Book of Simple Drugs

In the *Comprehensive Book of Simple Drugs* entry for "*sukkar*", Ibn al-Bayṭār thoroughly explains the medicinal effects of sugar, quoting the works of physicians and pharmacologists. The following is a full translation of the Arabic text.

> **Dioscorides** [first century] relates: sugar (*sukkar*) is a kind of honey (*ʿasal*), but solid. In fertile lands like al-Hind and Maghrib, it is found on [sugar] cane.[7] It looks like salt, and is similarly brittle when bitten with teeth. And if one drinks it with water, he feels refreshed. It is also effective

3 Ibn Abī Uṣaybiʿa, *ʿUyūn al-Anbāʾ*, III, 220–222.

4 J. Vernet believes that the *al-Jāmiʿ li-Mufradāt* of Ibn al-Bayṭār is merely plagiarized from the pharmacopoeia of al-Ghāfiqī (*EI*², s.v. Ibn al-Bayṭār). But, it should be noted that his account is based on his observations of herbs and drugs over many years.

5 Ibn Abī Uṣaybiʿa, *ʿUyūn al-Anbāʾ*, III, 222.

6 P. Pormann and E. Savage-Smith, *Medieval Islamic Medicine*, Washington, D.C., 2007, pp. 53–54.

7 It is doubtful that the account related by Dioscorides refers to sugar made from sugarcane. Mintz is also skeptical of R.J. Forbes's view that the account by Dioscorides shows that sugar was produced during the first century (*Sweetness and Power*, p. 20).

for stomach (*maʿida*) ailments, as well as against bladder (*mathāna*) and kidney (*kulya*) pain. If one puts it on his eyes, it will heal his weakened eyesight.

Galen [ca. 129-ca. 210] relates in his seventh lecture: it is said that the *sukkar* carried from al-Hind and Maghrib was apparently extracted from cane and had congealed. It looks like honey, but its sweetness is milder than our honey. It is effective for healing weak eyesight, drying affected parts [of the body], and reducing pain. It is neither harmful to the stomach nor causes thirst, unlike our honey. The above are the characteristics of sugar. In his eighth lecture, he also states that sugar cleanses the body of wastes and purges old blood.

Ibn Māsawayh [160–243/775–857] relates: sugar, is "hot" (*ḥārr*) to the first or second degree, and "moist" (*raṭb*) to the middle of the first degree. It is effective for the stomach, in particular for persons suffering from an excess of yellow bile (*mirra ṣafrāʾ*). Persons suffering from hyperacidity are in danger of agitation of yellow bile. Rock sugar (*ṭabarzad*) is not gentle like the white sugar of *sulaymānī* or *fānīdh*. In terms of gentleness (*talyīn*), sugar cane juice (*ʿasal al-qaṣab*) is gentler than *fānīdh* white sugar, and *ṭabarad* is gentler than honey (*ʿasal*), which is not gentle like sugarcane juice.[8]

ʿĪsā al-Baṣrī[9] [3/9 or 4/10 century] relates: new sugar (*ḥadīth*) is 'hot' and "moist", and old sugar (*ʿatīq*) is 'hot' and 'dry' (*yābis*). It is effective against the gas (*rīḥ*) that often rises in the internal organs, like the stomach. If one drinks it with almond powder, it is also effective against colic (*qawlanj*). Old sugar is capable of removing phlegm (*balgham*) from the stomach, but it may make one thirsty and thickens the blood.

Al-Sharīf [al-Idrīsī] [493–560/1100–65] relates: if one drinks sugar with butter, it is effective against retention of urine (*iḥtibās al-bawl*). Its optimal effectiveness has been confirmed through experience. If one drinks one *ūqīya* (37.5 grams)[10] of sugar with two *ūqīyas* of butter, it is effective against stomachache, and it also cleanses placentas. This too has been confirmed through experience. If one drinks sugar with hot water, it soothes sore throat and is effective against cough (*suʿāl*) and asthma (*taḍāyuq*). If one drinks one *ūqīya* of sugar everyday, it is effective. If one puts sugar powder on his eyelids and rubs them until they become red, it

8 For the kinds of sugar, see the entry for *sukkar* in the Glossary.

9 Perhaps ʿĪsā b. Māssa al-Baṣrī (3/9 c.), or ʿĪsā b. Ibrāhīm al-Baṣrī (4/10 c.). See F. Sezgin, *Geschichte des Arabischen Schrifttums*, 13vols., Leiden, 1967–2003, vol. 3, pp.128, 257–258.

10 Hinz, *Islamische Masse und Gewichte*, p. 35.

is effective against their inflammation. This action should be repeated. And if one takes sugar vapor into his nose, it relieves sniffles and sore throat.

The Book of Two Experiences reads: sugar relieves serious cough as it necessitates a rinsing of the throat. Although antimony (*kuḥl*) is an irritant, if one mixes it with sugar, it becomes gentler and will not hurt the eyes.

Al-Rāzī [ca. 250–313 or 323/ca. 854–925 or 935] relates in his book *Kitāb Dafʿ Maḍār al-Aghdhiya* (*Book for the Prevention of Malnutrition*): sugar is a balanced and 'hot' drug that rinses away impurities and relieves chest (*ṣadr*) and lung (*riʾa*) pain. It also relieves bladder disorder, and maintains the patient's balance of 'hot' and 'cold'. But if the 'hot' and 'cold' qualities are well balanced, medical treatment is not needed. If the feces are soft or the bowels are wounded, one should avoid consuming sugar. One afflicted with pulmonary tuberculosis (*maslūl*) should also be careful to avoid sugar. Regarding the types of white sugar (*fānīdh*), *shajarī* sugar is gentle on the stomach, relieves gas, and warms the body. Whereas, *ḥarrānī* sugar also relieves lung pain, but it is less effective than *shajarī*. Regarding sugar's warming effects on the body, this is not a concern as long as one doesn't consume too much white sugar and doesn't consume sugar when he has a fever. If he is concerned, he should eat sour fruits.

Al-Sharīf [**al-Idrīsī**] also relates: *fānīdh* white sugar is gentle on the stomach, clears one's throat of phlegm, and warms the liver (*kulya*).

Another authority states: sugar is quite effective against chest pains that require a poultice (*tarṭīb*).

Al-Rāzī relates: regarding plant-based drinks boiled with sugar (*nabāt al-sukkar*), the effect varies according to the kind of plant used. If sugar is boiled together with rose water (*māʾ al-ward*), it makes the coldest and lightest-colored drink. And if it is boiled together with violet leaves (*waraqat al-banafsaj*), it makes the drink that is gentlest on the body.[11]

The first source quoted, Dioscorides, was a famous Roman botanist in the first century. His major work *Materia Medica* was regarded as the most authoritative work in Europe on botany and pharmacology until the sixteenth century. It was completely translated into Arabic by Ḥunayn b. Isḥāq in Baghdad in the

11 Ibn al-Bayṭār, *al-Jāmiʿ li-Mufradāt al-Adwiya wal-Aghdhiya*, III, 22–23.

third/ninth century,[12] and meticulously annotated by Ibn al-Bayṭār.[13] However, it is curious that this first account states that sugar was produced in the fertile lands of al-Hind and Maghrib, since sugar production didn't expand to the Maghrib countries until the tenth century, as mentioned in Chapter One. When we examine the original text by Dioscorides, we do find the following passage: "And there is a kind of 'concreted' honey, called saccharin, found in reeds in India and Arabia Felix."[14] Which is to say, Dioscorides originally states not that sugar is found in reeds in India and Maghrib, but in India and Arabia Felix. This shows that some translator after Dioscorides or some pharmacologist, possibly even Ibn al-Bayṭār, changed the text from "Arabia Felix" to "Maghrib."

Next comes Galen, a Greek physician and philosopher born in Pergamon in the first half of the second century. He studied medicine in Alexandria, and then lived in the capital city of Rome at the invitation of Imperator Marcus Aurelius (reigned 161–180). He was respected as the first authority on pharmacology in the Arab world, and the work cited here might be an Arabic translation of his treatise *On the Powers of Simple Drugs*.[15] At the beginning of the paragraph, Galen relates that "the *sukkar* carried from al-Hind and Maghrib was apparently extracted from cane and had congealed," which is probably an alteration to make it coincide with the description of Dioscorides. Galen's account is unique in that it explains sugar as having various medicinal effects, rather than simply being honey.

Thirdly, Yuḥannā Ibn Māsawayh is well known as the physician who, in addition to serving ʿAbbasid caliphs such as Hārūn al-Rashīd and al-Maʾmūn, translated Greek medical books into Arabic at the famous "House of Wisdom" (Bayt al-Ḥikma). The book cited here is probably *Kitāb al-Adwiyat al-Munaqqīya*, which explains the medicinal effects of herbs.[16] Ibn Māsawayh relates that sugar is "hot" (*ḥārr*) to the first or second degree, and "moist" (*raṭb*) to the middle of the first degree. Arabic medicine, which was handed down from the Greeks, explains that the body is made up of four humors (*khilṭ*, pl. *akhlāṭ*): blood, phlegm, yellow bile, and black bile. And each humor is associated with two of the four fundamental qualities: hot or cold, and dry or moist. When a person has a good balance of the four humors, he is thought to be healthy. But,

12 Diyusquridīs, *Hayūlā ʿIlāj al-Ṭibb*, or *Kitāb al-Adwiyat al-Mufrada*. See EI[2], s.v. Diyusḳuridīs (C.E. Dubler); Pormann and Savage-Smith, *Medieval Islamic Medicine*, p. 51.

13 *Tafsīr Kitāb Diyusḳuridīs*.

14 Translated by R.T. Gunther, *The Greek Herbal of Dioscorides*, p. 125.

15 Pormann and Savage-Smith, *Medieval Islamic Medicine*, p. 51.

16 EI[2], s.v. Ibn Māsawayh (J.C. Vadet).

when a person has an imbalance, his condition is believed detrimental and needs to be counter-balanced through nutrients with the appropriate of the four fundamental qualities.[17] Ibn Māsawayh, therefore, explains the various effects of sugar in terms of this medical tradition inherited from the Greeks.

Next is ʿĪsā al-Baṣrī, whose exact life is not known, just that he lived during the tenth century. He is unique in contrasting the "hot" and "moist" qualities of new sugar (*ḥadīth*) with the "hot" and "dry" qualities of old sugar (*ʿatīq*). He explains that old sugar is capable of removing phlegm (*balgham*) from the stomach, but may make one thirsty and thicken one's blood.

The fifth citation is that of Abū ʿAbd Allāh Muḥammad al-Idrīsī, a well-known Arabic geographer of the twelfth century, who was also known as al-Sharīf. The title of "al-Sharīf" came from the fact that al-Idrīsī was a descendant of the Prophet Muḥammad. He completed his book on geography, *Kitāb Nuzhat al-Mushtāq fī Ikhtirāq al-Āfāq*, in 548/1154, and dedicated it to Roger II (reigned 1130–54), the Norman king of Sicily. He wrote another book, entitled *Kitāb al-Adwiyat al-Mufrada* (*The Book of Simple Drugs*), which is likely the source that Ibn al-Bayṭār quoted from.[18] Al-Idrīsī states that if one takes sugar with butter, it is effective against urinary dysfunction and stomachaches, and cleanses placentas. He is unique in affirming that its optimal effectiveness has been confirmed through experience.

The author of the following work, *The Book of Two Experiences*, is not identified.

And finally, al-Rāzī, who was born in Rayy in the mid-ninth century, published an annotated edition (*tafsīr*) of the Qur'an, and studied Ashʿarite theology in Baghdad and Rayy. As Ibn al-Bayṭār relates in the above text, he was also known as the author of the *Book for the Prevention of Malnutrition*.[19] A lack of detailed information prevents us from distinguishing between *shajarī* and *ḥarrānī* white sugar.

As seen above, in medieval Arabic medicine, which had inherited the four humors theory of the Greeks, it was generally thought that sugar was hot and moist, and old sugar was hot and dry. Based on extensive experience, it was widely believed that the various kinds of sugar were particularly effective against colic, eye disease, cough, asthma, and urinary dysfunction, were gentle on the kidneys and liver, and did not cause thirst, as did honey.

---

17 For humorism theory, see the following works. Pormann and Savage-Smith, *Medieval Islamic Medicine*, pp. 43–44; M. Levey, *Early Arabic Pharmacology*, Leiden, 1973, pp. 33–35.

18 *EI*², s.v. al-Idrīsī (G. Oman).

19 Sezgin, *Geschichte des Arabischen Schrifttums*, vol. 3, p. 286.

Ibn al-Nafīs, the Personal Physician of Sultan Baybars I

The Second Ibn Sīnā

Ibn al-Nafīs 'Alā' al-Dīn 'Alī b. Abī al-Ḥaram al-Qurashī al-Dimashqī (d. 687/1288), who was born in or near Damascus, studied medicine, grammar, logic, and Islamic religious sciences there. He later moved to Egypt at an unknown date. After settling in Cairo, Ibn al-Nafīs was appointed as a chief physician of Egypt (*ra'īs al-aṭibbā'* or *shaykh al-ṭibb bil-Diyār al-Miṣrīya*),[20] and also became the personal physician of Sultan Baybars I. He was quite distinguished in clinical medicine and thereby came to be called "the second Ibn Sīnā." What's more, his reputation for medical treatments (*'ilāj*) sometimes exceeded that of Ibn Sīnā.[21] While he devoted himself to advancing Arabic medicine, Ibn al-Nafīs also lectured at Madrasat al-Masrūrīya on Shāfi'ite law. Thus, Ibn al-Nafīs lived his life under quite favorable circumstances. When he died in Cairo in Dhū al-Qa'da 687/December 1288, his entire estate (*milk*), including his extensive library, was donated to Manṣūrī Hospital as *waqf*.[22]

While his research activities encompassed fields as varied as medicine, logic, and law, his main work was *al-Shāmil fī al-Ṣinā'at al-Ṭibbīya* (*An Encyclopedia of Medicine*). Spanning eighty volumes, the encyclopedia still fell short of his original plan for three hundred volumes. The ninth lecture in the fifteenth volume, entitled "The Principles of Sugar (*aḥkām al-sukkar*)," explains the various kinds, qualities, and effects of sugar. In addition to this work, Ibn al-Nafīs also produced a new explanation of pulmonary bloodflow that challenged Galen's theories, and published an annotated edition of Ibn Sīnā's *Canon of Medicine* (*Sharḥ Tashrīḥ al-Qānūn*).[23] As he was well known for not consulting books while writing, Ibn al-Nafīs was likely a learned man with a keen memory.[24]

---

20 The Arabic sources refer to him variedly as "*ra'īs al-aṭibbā'*" (al-Maqrīzī, *Kitāb al-Sulūk*, I, 746), "*al-ḥakīm al-ra'īs*" (Ibn Kathīr, *al-Bidāya wal-Nihāya*, 14 vols., Beirut, 1966, XIII, 313), and "*shaykh al-ṭibb bil-Diyār al-Miṣrīya*" (al-Subkī, *Ṭabaqāt al-Shāfi'īyat al-Kubrā*, ed. M.M. al-Ṭanāḥī and A.M. Ḥulw, 8 vols., Cairo, 1964, VIII, 305; Ibn 'Imād al-Ḥanbalī, *Shadharāt al-Dhahab fī Akhbār Man Dhahaba*, 8 vols., Beirut, n. d., V, 401). See also D. Behrens-Abouseif, *Fatḥ Allāh and Abū Zakariyya: Physicians under the Mamluks*, Cairo, 1987, pp. 5–6.

21 Al-Subkī, *Ṭabaqāt al-Shāfi'īyat al-Kubrā*, VIII, 305.

22 Al-Subkī, *Ṭabaqāt al-Shāfi'īyat al-Kubrā*, VIII, 306; Ibn al-Ṣuqā'ī, *Tālī Kitāb Wafayāt al-A'yān*, ed. J. Sublet, Damascus, 1974, 114–115; Ibn Taghrībirdī, *al-Manhal al-Ṣāfī*, VIII, 32–33; Ibn 'Imād al-Ḥanbalī, *Shadharāt al-Dhahab*, V, 402.

23 Pormann and Savage-Smith, *Medieval Islamic Medicine*, p. 47.

24 Ibn Taghrībirdī, *al-Manhal al-Ṣāfī*, VIII, 32.

The Principles of Sugar as Described by Ibn al-Nafīs

The first section of the ninth lecture in the fifteenth volume of *al-Shāmil* relates the following:

> Sugar (*sukkar*), which is extracted from cane and congeals, has a moist quality. Externally, it looks like Persian cane (*al-qaṣab al-fārisī*). Internally, it differs in that it is stuffed rather than hollow, and its interior shows a pale coloration. Since the pressed juice is a sweet liquid, it becomes dry and congeals hard like a stone when it is boiled down.
>
> When one wants to melt sugar, he adds water to it or puts it over fire. When one adds water to it, it slowly becomes dry. When he puts it on fire, its water content exudes from within. The cane's leaves and joints resemble those of Persian cane.
>
> There are various kinds of sugar. Among these, *ṭabarzad* sugar[25] is the most popular in Egypt and Syria. It is also called "*sukkar ublūj*," formed in a cone shape. The *mukarrar* (repeatedly refined sugar) is dissolved in water, refined with an *ublūj*, and then refined once again. As it is repeatedly refined, it becomes whiter and purer, but both the sweetness and taste suffer. It has the properties of the earth (*arḍīya*) element, and its impurities are further eliminated with each successive boiling.
>
> The *sukkar al-nabāt* is another kind of sugar that is boiled repeatedly. After the boiled juice is solidified with an *ublūj*, it is dissolved in water, and left in a vessel (*qidr*). When the twigs from a date palm (*qaḍīb min al-nakhl*) are thrown in the vessel, small rock sugar (*ḥajar ṣaghīr*) crystallizes on them. What is left remains in the pot as liquid.
>
> *Sukkar ḥawzī* is another kind of sugar, also known as *sukkar sīnatāb*.[26] The *fānīdh* sugar, forming small sticks and rings, has a reddish color because its impurities have not been completely removed.
>
> The sugar with the most reddish color is called *sukkar aḥmar*, which is [raw sugar] made from boiled cane juice. What remains in the pot is molasses (*ʿasal*) or high-quality molasses (*quṭāra*) [after repeated refinements].

25 *Ṭabarzad* sometimes refers to a rock sugar, but here, based on the explanation in the following paragraph, it seems to be used in reference to solid white sugar.

26 *Ḥawz* in Arabic means "to collect" or "to drive camels," and *sīnatāb* in Persian denotes "to heat the breast." As we do not have another example usage to compare with, it is difficult to know what kinds of sugar *sukkar ḥawzī* and *sukkar sīnatāb* are.

> Yet another kind of sugar product is a natural one, rather than a processed one. This is the salt-like lump that congeals on the cane, like a sort of cane resin.[27]

Although Ibn al-Nafīs differentiates Persian cane from sugarcane, these are generally understood to have been the same thing.[28] Nevertheless, this paragraph provides us with the most detailed information on the various kinds of sugar and their qualities. According to this, there are two kinds of rock sugar: one is *sukkar ṭabarzad*, also known by the name *sukkar ublūj*, which is a cone-shaped piece of sugar (*ublūj*). And the other one is *sukkar al-nabāt*, rock sugar made with date twigs through repeated boilings. However, as previously noted, rather than rock sugar, Ibn al-Nafīs might have used the term *sukkar ṭabarzad* to refer to white sugar, which was commonly known as *ṭabarzad* in the medieval Islamic world.[29] As mentioned in Chapter Two, al-Nuwayrī explained that as one repeatedly boils pressed juice, it becomes pure white sugar, and the molasses becomes like rock sugar (*sukkar al-nabāt*). The above account by Ibn al-Nafīs is invaluable in that it provides the details of the production process for *sukkar al-nabāt*. As previously explained, the white sugar obtained from repeated refinements was called *sukkar mukarrar* or *sukkar fānīdh*. However, this account by Ibn al-Nafīs shows that the *sukkar fānīdh*, forming small sticks and rings, has a reddish color due to remaining impurities.

The second section describes the properties and medicinal effects of sugar.

> An atom of sugar (*jawhar al-sukkar*) is comprised of elements of water (*mā'īya*), gentle hot earth (*al-arḍīyat al-laṭīfat al-ḥārra*), and air (*hawā'īya*). Sugar's predominant quality is its "hot" quality, due to its water element. Even if the water element is dominant, the heat properties of the earth and air elements overcome the cold property of the water element. This is because when the water element's properties arise, but there is little water present, the properties of the air element overtake those of the water element. When boiled sugar congeals, its water element properties naturally recede.

27 Ibn al-Nafīs, *al-Shāmil*, XV, 115–116.

28 For example, see Al-Muqaddasī, *Aḥsan al-Taqāsīm*, 188; Ibn Ḥawqal, *Kitāb Ṣūrat al-Arḍ*, 122; Ibn Mammātī, *Kitāb Qawānīn al-Dawāwīn*, 204.

29 Solid white sugar (*ṭabarzad* or *thalij*) was regarded as the highest-quality sugar in the medieval Islamic world. See al-Thaʿālibī, *Laṭā'if al-Maʿārif*, 82–83; Lippmann, *Geschichte des Zuckers*, pp. 98–102; Ahsan, *Social Life under the Abbasids*, p. 102.

> So, when pressed juice is repeatedly refined without boiling, the "hot" quality decreases relative to that of congealed sugar. This is due to the increase of the water element's properties. But boiling is ultimately required, because an excess of water element properties causes rotting.
>
> The "hot" quality of sugar is not dominant because sugar's water element properties overcome its earth element properties. Sugar's combination of different atoms has a "moist" quality (*ruṭūba*) because it has the properties of its water and air elements.
>
> This combination, that is to say, sugar, is effective on the human body. It has only a slight "moist" quality, because only its water element properties add to its moistness. As repeatedly explained, the air element properties do not increase moistness. Accordingly, sugar as medicine has only a slight "moist" quality, which decreases as the water element's properties diminish. Old sugar, therefore, is dry due to its greatly reduced water element properties. And yet, sugar that has congealed after a first boiling still has some moistness to it.[30]

This second section, based on the theories of Hippocrates (BC. ca. 460-BC. ca. 375), explains that sugar consists of three elements: water, earth, and air.[31] The qualities and degrees of these three elements produce the sugar's qualities of heat/cold and dryness/moistness. Applying this theory to medicine, various kinds of sugar were given to patients in order to regain the body's lost balance of humors.

Sugar as Medicine

Ibn al-Nafīs shows the various medicinal effects of sugar in the following passages from the third to the sixth sections. The third section explains the effects of sugar on the organs in the head (*aʿḍāʾ al-raʾs*).

> If the qualities of its earth element properties are "hot" and "gentle", sugar tends to ascend mostly to the brain (*dimāgh*), which helps the patient maintain a balance [of humors]. If sugar is hindered from ascending to the brain, the brain loses its balance of qualities and starts to go bad. If the sugar does not ascend to the brain, it takes on the "hot" quality, which is an unfavorable condition.

30 Ibn al-Nafīs, *al-Shāmil*, XV, 118–120.

31 Hippocrates explained that the human body was comprised of atoms of the four elements; water, fire, earth, and air. This theory was incorporated into Arabic medicine. See Pormann and Savage-Smith, *Medieval Islamic Medicine*, pp. 44–45.

> Since the earth element has a "gentle" quality, the brain's state takes on this gentleness as the sugar ascends to it. That is, the sugar that reaches the brain brings with it a considerable gentle quality. Even if one consumes sugar repeatedly, it will not become excessive or do harm to the brain. However, too much sugar intake may cause headaches.
>
> As sugar has both cleansing and drying effects due to its earth element properties, it is effective on the eyes (*ʿayn*), cleansing them and drying their wetness (*ruṭūba*). From sugar is made powdered medicine that cures trachoma (*jarab*) of the eyelids. If one mixes sugar with antimony (*kuḥl*), it is more effective in curing inflammation of the eyes. So, *kuḥl* mixed with sugar is given to patients as a powdered medicine to combat inflammation of the eyes.
>
> Similar in appearance to salt, the sugar crystals that accumulate on sugarcane are extremely effective against eye disease. Vapor medicines, when mixed with these sugar crystals, are also quickly and remarkably effective against colds (*zukām*).[32]

The third section describes the medicinal effects of sugar on both the brain and the eyes. Above, Ibn al-Bayṭār explained the effects of sugar when used against eye disease, but did not mention its effect on the brain. Nor did he explain that the sugar crystals appearing on sugarcane were a particular remedy aginst eye disease and colds.

The fourth section describes the medicinal effects of sugar on the organs in the chest (*aʿḍāʾ al-ṣadr*).

> Sugar contains atoms with a "gentle" quality, and as it dissolves easily in liquids, it moves easily into the organs of the chest and is highly effective on them. Since sugar has a "gentle" quality and a cleansing effect, it is no doubt effective on the organs of the chest.
>
> Accordingly, if one repeatedly drinks sugar with hot water, it is effective against hoarseness of the throat (*buḥḥat al-ṣawt*). If one drinks sugar with borage (*lisān al-thawr*) juice, it is particularly effective against cough (*suʿāl*). Sugar is also effective if one drinks it with barley water (*māʾ al-shaʿīr*) or hot water.
>
> Sugar reduces hemoptysis (*nafth*, the coughing up of blood, etc.), regulates breathing (*nafas*), and is effective against breathing difficulties (*ʿusr al-nafas*), asthma (*rabw*), and shortness of breath (*nafas al-intiṣāb*). It is also effective against pleurisy (*dhāt al-janb*) and pneumonia (*dhāt al-riʾa*),

32 Ibn al-Nafīs, *al-Shāmil*, XV, 121–122.

> expels pus from the chest (*ṣadr*), and reduces inflammations in the chest and lungs (*ri'a*). It is also effective against chest ailments and hoarseness of voice (*ṣawt*).[33]

Here, Ibn al-Nafīs gives a more detailed explanation than Ibn al-Bayṭār, stating that sugar is effective against hoarse throat, hemoptysis, asthma, pleurisy, pneumonia, etc. As I will explain later, for example, when fierce disease or epidemic ravaged the people, they rushed to the druggists (*ʿaṭṭār*) to buy sugar as a medicine for chest and joint pains.

The fifth section describes the medicinal effects of sugar on the digestive organs (*aʿḍāʾ al-ghidhāʾ*).

> As sugar has gentle and cleansing qualities, it is mild on the stomach (*maʿida*) and cleanses away phlegm (*balgham*). When bile (*mirra*) increases in the stomach, sugar present in the stomach may cause harmful bitterness. This is due to the gentle and warm sweetness (*ḥalāwa*) of sugar. Since sugar does not assimilate into the blood much, it is somewhat absorbed by the digestive organs. However, because sugar has strong air and mild earth qualities, the spirit (*rūḥ*) of the sugar can be transferred to the body of the person consuming it. The spirit becomes like an atom of spirit (*jawhar al-arwāḥ*), and it therefore strengthens the body. Sugar – Allāh knows best – opens obstructions in the liver (*sadad al-kibd*) and cleanses them. However, sugar may also damage the liver with its "hot" quality because sugar, as mentioned above, can take on a bitter quality. When consuming sugar, one feels less thirsty than when consuming honey because sugar reduces the thirst caused by phlegm (*al-ʿaṭsh al-balghamī*). Also, old sugar cleanses the stomach and cleanses away phlegm, but it also causes strong thirst and leads to impure blood.[34]

Ibn al-Nafīs describes the same things as Ibn al-Bayṭār in stating that sugar is gentle on the stomach and cleanses away phlegm, and that old sugar causes strong thirst and leads to impure blood. While Ibn al-Bayṭār further states that sugar is effective against urinary retention and is gentle on the kidneys and liver, Ibn al-Nafīs explains that by consuming sugar, one can obtain the sugar's spirit (*rūḥ*), which strengthens one's body.

The sixth and final section discusses the urinary organs (*aʿḍāʾ al-nafḍ*).

---

33 Ibn al-Nafīs, *al-Shāmil*, xv, 123.

34 Ibn al-Nafīs, *al-Shāmil*, xv, 124–125.

> Since sugar has a gentle and cleansing quality, it is effective for causing urination (*idrār*). If one consumes sugar with butter, it is quite effective against the retention of urine (*iḥtibās al-bawl*). Sugar relieves the stomach, without forming lumps in it. If one consumes sugar with fresh butter (*zubd*), his stomach feels relieved. *Fānīdh* white sugar in particular has this remarkable effect.
>
> Red sugar (*sukkar aḥmar*) [that is, raw sugar] is most gentle and effective for the body whether it is drunk or used for enema (*iḥtiqān*). This is due to its strong cleansing quality. Rock sugar (*sukkar al-nabāt*) is also effective because it has this same quality. Sugar crystals accumulated on sugarcane are quite effective on the stomach because they have the strongest cleansing quality.
>
> If one consumes too much sugarcane, his stomach swells, due to the sugarcane's excessive water. However, the sugar itself reduces flatulence (*nafakh*). So, if one drinks sugar with almond oil, it is effective against flatulence and colic (*qawlanj*).[35]

What Ibn al-Nafīs explains in the above paragraphs may be summarized as follows: (1) When sugar ascends to brain, it helps the patient maintain balance of humors, but if one takes too much sugar, it may cause headaches. Sugar is also used to make powdered medicine to treat trachoma. (2) Regarding its medicinal effects on the organs of the chest, if one drinks sugar with hot water, it is effective against hoarse throat. And if one drinks sugar with borage herbs, it reduces cough. It is also effective against hemoptysis, asthma, pleurisy, pneumonia, and other ailments. (3) If one drinks sugar with butter, it is quite effective against urinary retention. Red sugar (raw sugar) is most gentle and effective, whether it is drunk or used for enema. However, sugar crystals accumulated on sugarcane are among the most effective for cleansing the stomach.

---

35 Ibn al-Nafīs, *al-Shāmil*, xv, 126. For the medical and pharmacological terms, see the following works. H. Kamal, *Encyclopaedia of Islamic Medicine*, Cairo, 1975; Academy of Arabic Language ed., *Modern Dictionary of Chemical and Pharmaceutical Terms*, Cairo, 2004; Ibn Buṭlān, tr. by H. Elkhadem, *Le Taqwīm al-Ṣiḥḥa*; Pormann and Savage-Smith, *Medieval Islamic Medicine*.

ʿAṭṭārs: Merchants who Profited from Sugar

Who were the ʿAṭṭārs?

Even today, when walking around the markets of the Islamic world, one can find *ʿaṭṭār* shops that sell various spices, like pepper, clove, nutmeg, coriander, cumin, ginger, cinnamon, turmeric, cardamom, and saffron, as well as perfumes, like camphor, sandalwood, ambergris, musk, frankincense, and myrrh. We also see that they sell pomegranate rinds and roots, various kinds of herbs, dried fruits, rose water, soap, candles, white sugar, and rock sugar. The *ʿaṭṭārs* sell several kinds of sugar particularly because, as described above, sugar has been regarded as a precious medicine with remarkable medicinal effects.[36] Regarding the *ʿaṭṭārs* of medieval history, however, we have no comprehensive study of their activities. ʿAbd al-Wahhāb al-Subkī (d. 771/1370) lists, in his *Kitāb Muʿīd al-Niʿam* (*The Restorer of Favours*),[37] 110 different kinds of occupation, including sultan, wazir, amir, judge (*qāḍī*), public notary (*shāhid*), storyteller (*qāṣṣ*), tailor (*khayyāṭ*), money changer (*ṣayrafī*), washer of dead bodies (*ghāṣil al-mawtā*), gatekeeper (*bawwāb*), and even street beggar (*shaḥḥādh fī al-ṭurqāt*), but alas, he makes no mention of the *ʿaṭṭārs*. So, we must seek out the actual activities of the *ʿaṭṭārs* in other Arabic source materials.

First, let me quote an account from *Kitāb al-Ishāra ilā Maḥāsin al-Tijāra* by al-Dimashqī (eleventh century), which reads:

> The *ʿaṭṭār* should have knowledge of drugs (*ʿaqqār*), medicine (*dawāʾ*), drinks (*sharāb*), and flavors (*ṭīb*). Furthermore, he should be able to distinguish good from bad, [genuine from] fakes, perishables, unperishables, and keepables. He should also have the ability to mix ointments, internal medicines, and powdered medicines.[38]

36 Regarding the *ʿaṭṭārs*, we find brief accounts in the following works. *EI*², s.v. ʿAṭṭār (A. Dietrich); A. Raymond, *Artisans et commerçants au Caire au XIIIᵉ siècle*, 2 vols., Damascus, 1973–74, pp. 334–335; E.W. Lane, *An Account of the Manners and Customs of the Modern Egyptians*, repr. Cairo, 2003, p. 318; Sato, *State and Rural Society*, pp. 182, 215; Chipman, *The World of Pharmacy and Pharmacists in Mamlūk Cairo*, p. 172. Chipman states that the *ʿaṭṭārs* of Ibn Taghrībirdī's day were regarded first and foremost as providers of medicines, rather than purveyors of perfumes.

37 Al-Subkī, *Kitāb Muʿīd al-Niʿam wa-Mubīd al-Niqam*, ed. D.W. Myhrman, London, 1908; repr. New York, 1978.

38 Al-Dimashqī, *Kitāb al-Ishāra*, 40. We have no detailed information on the author Abū al-Faḍl Jaʿfar b. ʿAlī al-Dimashqī.

This account shows that the *ʿaṭṭārs* were required to mix ointments, and internal and powdered medicines, in addition to being knowledgeable about drugs, medicines, drinks, and flavors. Whereas Ibn al-Ḥājj, a Mālikī jurist in Cairo, describes the *ʿaṭṭār* in his *al-Madkhal* as follows.

> Some *ʿaṭṭārs*, when selling goods, don't tell their customers when the goods are spoiled. At present, an *ʿaṭṭār* must acquire his goods from one of two sources. That is, he must obtain his commercial goods either from the *Kārimī* merchants or from the [major] *ʿaṭṭārs*. In the former case, the *ʿaṭṭār* is first requested to declare his intention (*nīya*) of purchase and sale as God wishes. However, in reality, Muslim brothers[39] rarely have the opportunity to carry out this, because the "weak [minor] *ʿaṭṭārs* (*ʿaṭṭār ḍaʿīf*)," even if they wish to purchase a full *ūqīya* (37.4 grams) of civet (*zabād*) or musk (*misk*) from the *Kārimī* merchants, could never get such a small quantity of the commodity from them.
>
> In the latter case, the [minor] *ʿaṭṭār* obtains his goods from a [major] *ʿaṭṭār*. In such case, he is also required to declare his intention of purchase and sale for his Master Allāh. As mentioned above, he (the minor *ʿaṭṭār*) provides a local place for his Muslim brothers to obtain what they need. That is, when it is difficult for them to visit the remote shops of the major *ʿaṭṭārs* (*ʿaṭṭār kabīr*), the nearby minor *ʿaṭṭārs* can accommodate them instead. Also, if a common person wants to buy just one, or one-half, quarter, or eighth *ūqīya* of a valuable drug, the major *ʿaṭṭārs* take no notice of it, leaving dealings with the Muslim brothers to the minor *ʿaṭṭār*. Moreover, if the local shop is far from the major *ʿaṭṭārs*, the minor *ʿaṭṭārs* can provide various advantages. For example, if women can get drugs nearby, they do not need to go out to remote drug stores.[40]

Ibn al-Ḥājj stresses that the *ʿaṭṭārs* are at first requested to express their intent (*nīya*) of purchase and sale in accordance with the wishes of God. The *nīya* indicates the clear expression of the merchant's will to conduct business according to the wishes of God. For example, when he performs his five daily salats, he is expected to express his will each time, "I perform my salat for God." Next, Ibn al-Ḥājj explains that there were actually two classes of *ʿaṭṭārs* in Muslim society in Egypt: the major *ʿaṭṭārs* who stocked drugs from the *Kārimī* merchants, and the minor *ʿaṭṭārs* who stocked from the major *ʿaṭṭārs*. As discussed

39 Ibn al-Ḥājj uses the term "Muslim brothers", referring to the "weak *ʿaṭṭārs*" in the following sentence.

40 Ibn al-Ḥājj, *al-Madkhal*, IV, 71, 74–75.

previously, the *Kārimīs* were Muslim merchant groups[41] who traded along the East-West routes connecting the Red Sea and the Mediterranean Sea from the twelfth to the fifteenth centuries. They dealt in spices, perfumes, and drugs (including sugar) and sold them wholesale to the major *ʿaṭṭārs*. The minor *ʿaṭṭārs*, however, weren't able to purchase drugs from the *Kārimī* merchants in small quantities. Interestingly enough, Ibn al-Ḥājj presumes that the minor *ʿaṭṭārs* were better suited to serving the common people than were the major *ʿaṭṭārs*.

Al-Maqrīzī's View of the Troubles in Egypt

Taqī al-Dīn Aḥmad al-Maqrīzī, who was born in Cairo under the Mamluks, compiled a historical geography of Egypt entitled *al-Khiṭaṭ* and a voluminous chronicle of Egypt and Syria entitled *Kitāb al-Sulūk*. Over the course of his lifetime, Egyptian society faced political, economic, and social difficulties following the prosperous age of Sultan Malik al-Nāṣir Muḥammad (third reign 709–741/1310–41). Al-Maqrīzī sought ways of overcoming these difficulties by writing a booklet entitled *Kitāb Ighāthat al-Umma bi-Kashf al-Ghumma* (*Book to Help the Community by Eliminating Grief*). The term "*al-Umma*" generally means "the Islamic Community," but is used here to mean "Egyptian society."

Al-Maqrīzī, who was raised in the Barjawān quarter of old Cairo, saw the drastic changes that followed the great plague (*ṭāʿūn*) in Egypt in the years 748–749/1347–48. According to the account in his chronicle, in 776/1374, when al-Maqrīzī was about ten years old, an epidemic (*wabāʾ*) once again spread across Egypt.

> In the middle of Jumādā II/September, an epidemic began to spread among the people in Cairo and al-Fusṭāṭ, and the number of poor (*faqīr*) and beggars (*miskīn*) who died of starvation increased. I heard a poor man crying out until his death, "Give me even just an earlobe of bread, or at least let me smell it."[42]

In 806/1403, another disaster was brought about by insufficient water levels on the Nile and the spread of plague following the seasonal hot winds (*khamsīn*) and drought. Al-Maqrīzī further relates.

---

41 Although some Christian or Jewish merchants were occasionally found among the *Kārimī* merchants, most of them were Muslims. See Ashtor, "The Kārimī Merchants," p. 55.

42 Al-Maqrīzī, *Kitāb al-Sulūk*, III, 233–234.

> The year (807/1404) did not pass before disaster prevailed in Egypt, destroying even Upper Egypt. Many towns and villages were abandoned, and most of the lands were left uncultivated. The people dispersed (*tamazzaqa ahluh aydī Sabā*)[43] and countless children were sold.[44]

During these years, as discussed in Chapter Three, the Bedouins (*ʿUrbān*) repeatedly attacked sugar pressing factories and sugar refineries in Upper Egypt to plunder raw sugar, white sugar, and the oxen that drove the waterwheels. Moreover, al-Maqrīzī lost his daughter to an epidemic in 807/1404, which may have prompted him to write this book.[45] In 808/1405, he completed *Kitāb Ighāthat al-Umma*, a book that sought to elucidate the true causes of these hardships.

The book consists of seven chapters, after the Preface: (1) A Logical Premise, (2) The Price Increases (*ghalāʾ*) in Egypt from Ancient to Contemporary Times, (3) The Causes and Endurance of Our Tragedy, (4) The Current Conditions of the Seven Classes of Population, (5) Supplementary Account of Current Prices and Present Difficulties, (6) Eliminating Disease from the Muslims and Recovery from Illness, and (7) The Advantages for the People of this Proposal. In Chapter Three especially, al-Maqrīzī aims to identify the causes of the hardships (*miḥna*) that the Egyptian people were suffering. Let me summarize what he explains.

> Among the causes of price increases that have beset the people since ancient times, the shortfall of Nile flooding and damage from droughts, hot winds (*khamsīn*), and locusts are the so-called "natural disasters (*āfāt samāwīya*)," that are usually acts of God. However, in Egypt the situation is a little more complicated. A shortfall of Nile flooding leads to abandoned cultivation, which in turn leads to abandonment again the following year because of a shortage of crops for seeds. That is, a famine in Egypt continues for at least two years.
>
> Now, we can identify the three causes of the famine and price increases of 806/1403. The first is political corruption. It should be noted that this was the principal cause of the disaster (*aṣl hādhā al-fasād*). Political posts such as minister (*wazīr*), judge (*qāḍī*), and local governor (*wālī*) could not be obtained without paying bribes (*rishwa*), which resulted in a

43 "*Tamazzaqa ahluh aydī Sabā*" or "*tafarraqū aydī Sabā*" means "the people dispersed" (Ibn Manẓūr, *Lisān al-ʿArab*, 15 vols., Beirut, 1955–56, I, 94).

44 Al-Maqrīzī, *Kitāb al-Sulūk*, III, 1167.

45 M.M. Ziyāda, "Taʾrīkh Ḥayāt al-Maqrīzī," *Dirāsāt ʿan al-Maqrīzī*, Cairo, 1971, p. 16.

> weakening of the government. Particularly, after the death of Sultan Barqūq, a power struggle between the Mamluk amirs ensued, and because of such ineptitude, peasant revolts (*thawrat ahl al-rīf*) increased, as did offences committed by miscreants (*zu''ār*) in urban areas, and highway bandits (*quṭṭā' al-ṭarīq*) in the outlying areas.
>
> The second cause was the land tax increases (*ghalā' al-aṭyān*) that took place. The managers of *iqṭā'* watched over cultivated fields, and brought in tenant farmers (*musta'jir min al-fallāḥīn*) to increase the land tax (*ujra*) every year. It is said that during these two years, the land tax increased almost ten-fold. This inflated the price of wheat, and the costs of plowing, seeding, and harvesting. Moreover, the monopoly of crops held by high officials and soldiers was a major cause of the high prices of commodities and the devastation of villages (*qarya*).
>
> The third and final cause was the circulation of copper coins (*rawāj al-fulūs*). The first ruler who issued copper coins (*fals*) in Egypt was the Ayyubid Sultan al-Kāmil Muḥammad.[46] The devaluation of copper coins in the early Mamluk period put great pressure on the lives of common people, but, as "the sons of tradition (*abnā' al-'awā'id*)," they managed to adapt to these severe changes. During the reign of Barqūq, dinars and dirhams disappeared from the market place, and all transactions came to be done with copper coins.[47]

Al-Maqrīzī believed that the corruption of the Mamluk rulers, the exploitation of peasants by *iqṭā'* holders, and the disruption of the monetary system were more important factors in triggering the hardships than were natural disasters, such as epidemics, seasonal hot winds, and droughts. Ibn Khalīl al-Asadī (9/15 century), in his booklet *al-Taysīr wal-I'tibār wal-Taḥrīr wal-Ikhtibār fī mā yajibu min Ḥusn al-Tadbīr wal-Taṣarruf wal-Ikhtiyār* (*Facilitation, Consideration, Liberation, and Examination Concerning What is Needed in Just Administration*) written in 854/1450, similarly attributes the corruption (*fasād*) in Egypt to the following four causes: (1) the failure of the *'imāra* to cultivate lands and open new canals (*ḥafr al-khalīj wal-tur'a*) to foster prosperity, (2) the increase of rebellious *'Urbān* forcing the peasantry to abandon cultivation (*zirā'a*), (3) the exploitation of peasants (*fallāḥ*) by officials and those who held the right to

46 The earliest *fals* is of the year 87/705–6 struck at Damascus, somewhat later than the gold and silver coins that resulted from 'Abd al-Malik's reform (ca. 77/696). See *EI*², s.v. Fals (A.L. Udovitch).

47 Al-Maqrīzī, *Kitāb Ighāthat al-Umma*, 43–47.

levy taxes (*aṣḥāb al-jibāya*), and (4) the appointment of governors through bribery (*badhl*) and the extension of this custom to *iqṭāʿ* allocations.[48]

In these assessments by al-Maqrīzī and al-Asadī, we find mostly the same causes; that is, both authors attribute the difficulties in Egypt to the corruption of the central and provincial governments, and the exploitation of peasants, regardless of the farming conditions. The natural disasters of course inflicted severe damage, but both historians regarded political corruption and the lack of justice as the real causes of the calamities that devastated Egyptian societies in the later Mamluk period.

The Prosperous ʿAṭṭārs

As mentioned above, al-Maqrīzī was appointed to the office of *ḥisba* in Cairo three times, in 801/1399, 802/1400, and 807/1404. Based on these experiences, he would have had access to accurate information about the market traders in Cairo from the late fourteenth to early fifteenth centuries. In Chapter Four of *Kitāb Ighāthat al-Umma*, he acknowledges the strong position of the market traders (*bāʿa* or *sūqa*), that is, the middle class of merchants (*mutawassiṭū al-ḥāl min al-tujjār*) including *ʿaṭṭār*s, noting that they could live on their own income (*ribḥ*) even in times of hardship.[49] Thus, we will examine how these *ʿaṭṭār*s in Cairo profited from sugar while the plague raged. Al-Maqrīzī gives the following account of the famine and disease that prevailed in Egypt in 695/1296.

> In 695/1296, when the prices increased and the provisional supplies from local countries decreased, people had no choice but to await the next crops. However, in the harvest season the black wind blew from Barqa [in Libya], carrying yellow sand to the crops in the districts of al-Buḥayra, al-Gharbīya, al-Sharqīya, and Upper Egypt. Summer crops, which were cultivated with waterwheels (*sāqiya*), such as rice (*aruzz*), sesame (*simsim*), taro (*qulqās*), sugarcane (*qaṣab al-sukkar*), and others, were damaged, and the prices therefore increased. Also, since the wind spread disease and fever among the people, the prices of goods for sick people,

48 Ibn Khalīl al-Asadī, *al-Taysīr wal-Iʿtibār wal-Taḥrīr wal-Ikhtiyār fī Mā Yajibu min Ḥusn al-Tadbīr wal-Taṣarruf wal-Ikhtiyār*, ed. A.A. Ṭulaymāt, Cairo, 1968, 92–96. Al-Asadī also relates that the *iqṭāʿ* holders exploited peasants under the pretext of protection (*ḥimāya*) in order to recover the amounts they had paid as bribes (*ibid.* 135–136).

49 Al-Maqrīzī, *Kitāb Ighāthat al-Umma*, 74. For a comparison of *tujjār* and *sūqa*, see also al-Thaʿālibī, *al-Tamthīl wal-Muḥāḍara*, ed. A.M. Ḥulw, Riyad, 1983, 196–199.

> like sugar (*sukkar*) and molasses (*ʿasal*) increased, and the stocks of fruits (*fākiha*) were exhausted.[50]

When young Sultan al-Nāṣir (first reign 693–694/1293–94) was dethroned in 694/1294, amir Zayn al-Dīn Kitbughā al-Manṣūrī proclaimed himself sultan (694–696/1294–96) and gave himself the royal name al-Malik al-ʿĀdil. However, as he ascended the throne in a year when famine was beginning to spread across Egypt, he was regarded as a "bad-omen sultan (*sulṭān ẓālim*)."[51] Moreover, this famine occurred in the wake of crop price increases by cunning merchants who, after seeing the insufficient flooding of the Nile, concealed crops, hoping to make big profits the following year. Sultan Kitbughā assigned each of his amirs a certain number of poor (*faqīr*) and needy (*dhū al-ḥājāt*) people to assist; an *amīr miʾa* (amir of hundred) had one hundred poor people, an *amīr ṭablkhāna* (amir of forty) had forty, and an *amīr ʿashara* (amir of ten) had ten. The amirs provided relief to their assigned poor in the form of loafs of bread (*raghīf*) or cakes (*kaʿk*). Nevertheless, an epidemic (*wabāʾ*) raged forth into the outlying areas.[52] Al-Maqrīzī gives the following account in *Kitāb Ighāthat al-Umma*.

> The disease (*maraḍ*) also spread across Cairo and al-Fusṭāṭ, claiming many lives. So many sick people needed drugs (*dawāʾ*) that one *ʿaṭṭār* in the Daylam quarter in Cairo was earning 32,000 dirhams a month. Another shop, one at Suyūfiyīn market named Sharīf ʿAṭūf, and other shops at al-Wazīrīya and outside of Zuwayla gate, each earned the same amount. Since the number of wealthy individuals seeking physicians (*ṭabīb*) increased, some physicians earned as much as 100 dirhams a day. But the people were growing tired of the ever-increasing death toll. Every day, the names of over 3,000 dead were crossed off government administrative ledgers (*dīwān sulṭānī*).[53]

As previously explained, the *ʿaṭṭārs* sold several different kinds of sugar, because they were regarded as precious medicines with various remarkable medicinal effects. Now, let us estimate the value of the above-mentioned 32,000

50 Al-Maqrīzī, *Kitāb Ighāthat al-Umma*, 33–34.

51 Ibn Aybak al-Dawādārī, *Kanz al-Durar*, VIII, 356–357; Ibn al-Ṣuqāʿī, *Tālī Kitāb Wafayāt al-Aʿyān*, 132; M. Chapoutot-Remadi, "Une grande crise à la fin du XIIIe siècle en Égypte," *JESHO*, 26 (1983), pp. 227–229.

52 Al-Maqrīzī, *Kitāb Ighāthat al-Umma*, 35.

53 Al-Maqrīzī, *Kitāb Ighāthat al-Umma*, 35–36.

dirhams per month under the *iqṭāʿ* system of the early Mamluk period. Since one dinar was equal to 20 dirhams in Egypt at that time,[54] 32,000 dirhams corresponded to about 1,600 dinars. After the cadastral survey (*al-Rawk al-Ḥusāmī*)[55] of Sultan Ḥusām al-Dīn Lājīn (reigned 696–698/1296–99) in 697/1298, the *iqṭāʿ* revenue of a *ḥalqa* cavalryman[56] was 250–1,000 dinars.[57] So, in one month during the famine, an *ʿaṭṭār* earned more than the annual income of a *ḥalqa* cavalryman. Looking at wheat for comparison, since one *ardabb* (90 liters) of wheat (*qamḥ*) cost one dinar (20 dirhams),[58] one could purchase about 1,600 *ardabb*s of wheat for 32,000 dirhams. This would have been enough to feed more than 1,000 people for a year.

Again in 709/1309, an epidemic (*wabāʾ*) spread over Cairo, as al-Maqrīzī relates.

> In this year, a severe disease spread among the people, becoming an epidemic. The demand for drugs and physicians increased, and the price of medical attention rose to the extent that one *raṭl* (967 grams) of sugar (*sukkar*) and chicken (*farrūj*) sold for five dirhams, and melon (*baṭṭīkh*) for one dirham. Consequently, one of the *ʿaṭṭār*s in Cairo earned 200–300 dirhams a day.[59]

According to al-ʿUmarī, one *raṭl* of regular sugar (*sukkar*) sold for 1.5 dirhams, and repeatedly refined sugar (*mukarrar*) for 2.5 dirhams.[60] This shows that the price of regular sugar increased more than three-fold (around 3.3-fold), and refined sugar two-fold. Sales of 200–300 dirhams per day equates to nearly 6,000–9,000 dirhams per month, which is less than the above 32,000 dirhams, but still a considerable income.

---

54 Rabie, *The Financial System of Egypt*, p. 180.

55 In 697/1298, Sultan Ḥusām al-Dīn Lājīn conducted a cadastral survey of Egypt to ascertain the *iqṭāʿ* holdings by amirs, *mamlūk*s, and the *ḥalqa* cavalrymen. In 698/1299, the sultan was assasinated by soldiers who were dissatisfied with the resulting reassignment of *iqṭāʿ*s. See Sato, *State and Rural Society*, pp. 124–134.

56 During the Ayyubid and Mamluk periods, the term *ḥalqa* denoted a free-born cavalryman, such as a Kurd, an Arab, or the child of a *mamlūk* (*awlād al-nās*). Regarding the *ḥalqa* cavalrymen, see R.S. Humphreys, "The Emergence of the Mamluk Army," *SI*, 45 (1977), pp. 67–99; D. Ayalon, "From Ayyubids to Mamluks," *REI*, 49 (1981), pp. 43–58.

57 Sato, *State and Rural Society*, p. 133.

58 Ashtor, *Histoire des prix et des salaires*, p. 293.

59 Al-Maqrīzī, *Kitāb al-Sulūk*, II, 55.

60 Al-ʿUmarī, *Masālik al-Abṣār fī Mamālik al-Amṣār: Dawlat al-Mamālīk al-Ūlā*, 84.

Then, during the end of land allocation (*taḥḍīr*)[61] in autumn 748/1347, the plague (*ṭāʿūn*) spread from Syria to Egypt, sweeping from Lower into Upper Egypt the next year. Al-Maqrīzī says the epidemic was more severe than any in Islamic history.[62] His disciple Ibn Taghrībirdī relates that the plague started at the beginning of land allocation in 748/1347, and most of the peasants (*fallāḥūn*) had died off by the time the harvest season came.[63] The *ṭāʿūn* (the Black Death), with symptoms of both bubonic and pneumonic plagues, raged among the merchant fleets of the eastern Mediterranean and spread into Egypt, Sicily, and Italy almost simultaneously.[64] In 749/1348, the daily mortality rate in Cairo rapidly increased from 300 to 2,000, devastating the Barjawān quarter[65] where al-Maqrīzī was born and raised, and leaving 42 houses vacant.[66] During this time, the price of medicinal sugar increased to 23–27 dinars per *qinṭār* (96.7 kilograms) in the transactions of Italian merchants in Alexandria,[67] equivalent to 4.6–5.4 dirhams per *raṭl* (967 grams). The skyrocketing price of sugar might have provided the *ʿaṭṭār*s with another chance for big money. However, as al-Maqrīzī relates, the quickness of death after onset of the disease denied victims even the time to order drinks and drugs or to invite physicians.[68]

In 806/1403, as mentioned above, a great famine occurred due to insufficient water levels on the Nile and the spread of plague following the seasonal hot winds and drought. Al-Maqrīzī relates.

> As the disease raged and the demand for drugs increased, the price of the drugs rose even more. The price of one *qidḥ* (about 0.1 liter) of gourd

---

61 The *taḥḍīr* was an annual allocation of land for lease to peasants with *qabāla* contracts, after the flood of the Nile in autumn. The land to be cultivated was registered by the officials (*mubāshir*) in a document called a *sijill*. See Sato, *State and Rural Society*, pp. 192–197.

62 Al-Maqrīzī, *Kitāb al-Sulūk*, II, 772.

63 Ibn Taghrībirdī, *al-Nujūm al-Zāhira*, X, 209. While al-Maqrīzī states that the plague began at the end of land allocation, Ibn Taghrībirdī believes it came at the beginning of land allocation.

64 M.W. Dols, *The Black Death in the Middle East*, Princeton, 1977, pp. 53–67; Borsch, *The Black Death*, pp. 1–23.

65 The Barjawān quarter (Ḥārat Barjawān) still exists in northern Old Cairo. Al-Maqrīzī says, "At the south end of the quarter was a market (*sūq*) which, I think, was the largest in Cairo. We youth (*shabāb*) were proud of it, stating that there were such public baths as Ḥammām Rūmī and Ḥammām Suwayd, and inside the quarter two ovens (*furn*) and enough various markets to meet the demands of the residents" (*al-Khiṭaṭ*, II, 95–96).

66 Al-Maqrīzī, *Kitāb al-Sulūk*, II, 780, 782.

67 Dols, *The Black Death*, p. 258.

68 Al-Maqrīzī, *Kitāb al-Sulūk*, II, 781.

> kernels (*lubb al-qarʿ*) rose to 100 dirhams, one *wayba* (15 liters) of purslane seed (*badhr al-rijla*) from 2 to 70 dirhams, one *raṭl* (450 grams) of manna (*shīr khushk*) to 130 dirhams, one *ūqīya* (37.4 grams) of rock sugar (*sukkar al-nabāt*) to 8 dirhams, white sugar (*sukkar bayāḍ*) to 4 dirhams, and then to 80 dirhams, one *raṭl* of melon (*baṭīkh*) to 8 dirhams and Syrian pears (*kummathrā shāmī*) to 55 dirhams, one *raṭl* of congealed milk (*ʿaqīd*) to 60 dirhams, a cooked foreshank of lamb (*ʿaḍud al-kharūf al-ḍaʾn al-masmūṭ*) to 4 dirhams, one white water lily (*līnūfar*)[69] to 1 dirham, and one cucumber (*khiyāra*) to 1.5 dirhams.[70]

According to R. Dozy, *shīr khushk* is a kind of *manna*,[71] perhaps similar to the thin bread-like food provided by God to the Israelites wandering the desert after the Exodus described in the Bible. Here, however, it denotes a sweet pasty sap obtained from manna ash, which was commonly used as a laxative.[72] The account by al-Maqrīzī indicates that the *ʿaṭṭār*s handled numerous kinds of drugs, like gourd kernels, purslane seeds, manna, rock sugar, white sugar, congealed milk, cooked lamb, and water lilies. His account also indicates that the spread of epidemics drove up the prices of medicinal products in Mamluk Cairo.

As shown in the above examination, we know that in medieval times, unlike today, sugar was regarded as a medicine effective against diseases of throat, lungs, and stomach. The *ʿaṭṭār*s profited greatly during the epidemics and plagues because sugar was particularly believed to relieve pains of the throat, lungs, and joints.

---

69 *Līnūfar* is called also *nīlūfar*, denoting nenuphar, that is, white water lily.

70 Al-Maqrīzī, *Kitāb al-Sulūk*, III, 1125.

71 Dozy, *Supplément aux dictionnaires arabes*, vol. 1, p. 810.

72 Academy of Arabic Language ed., *Modern Dictionary of Chemical and Pharmaceutical Terms*, s.v. Manna, p. 361. Ibn al-Quff relates that the *manna* is a sap obtained from oak (*ballūṭ*) and oleander (*diflā*) trees, and from the leaves of the marsh mallow plant (*khiṭmī*) in Sinjār, Naṣībīn, and Diyār Bakr (*Jāmiʿ al-Gharaḍ*, 316).

CHAPTER 6

Sugar and Power: Festivals and Gifts from Royalty

In addition to its roles as a commodity and medicine, during the Fatimid period precious and expensive sugar also came to be used at festivals. Moreover, caliphs and sultans often used sugar and sweets for political means and to demonstrate their authority. In this chapter, we will first examine the management of the storehouse where raw sugar was kept (the *Dār al-Qand*), a topic that has not been fully studied to date. Then, we will look at political authority as it relates to sugar in the month of Ramaḍān, and the role of sweets in pilgrimages to Mecca.

The Storehouse for Raw Sugar (*Dār al-Qand*)

The Repeal of Miscellaneous Taxes by Sultan Ṣalāḥ al-Dīn

As mentioned in Chapter Three, many sugar refineries (*maṭbakh al-sukkar*) were set up in al-Fusṭāṭ during the Ayyubid and Mamluk periods. Sultan Ṣalāḥ al-Dīn al-Ayyūbī, who came to power in Cairo in 564/1169, conducted a tax survey in Egypt in 567/1171–2 to ascertain *iqṭāʿ* revenues and repeal miscellaneous taxes (*maks*) levied in and around Cairo and al-Fusṭāṭ. This series of measures is called the Ṣalāḥī cadastral survey (*al-Rawk al-Ṣalāḥī*).[1] At the final stage of this cadastral survey, miscellaneous taxes amounting to 100,000 dinars annually were abolished, including the following.

The tax on spices (*maks al-bahār*)	33,364 dinars
The tax on commodities and caravansaries (*maks al-baḍāʾiʿ wal-qawāfil*)	9,350 dinars
The tax on the storehouse for raw sugar (*rusūm dār al-qand*)	3,108 dinars
The tax on the storehouse for cotton ([*rusūm*] *funduq al-quṭn*)	2,000 dinars
The tax on sheep markets ([*rusūm*] *sūq al-ghanam*)[2]	3,311 dinars

1 For the Ṣalāḥī cadastral survey, see Sato, *State and Rural Society*, pp. 60–63; Rabie, *The Financial System of Egypt*, p. 51.

2 The markets were located at Cairo and al-Fusṭāṭ (*al-Khiṭaṭ*, I, 104).

 | DOI 10.1163/9789004281561_008

The tax on crops (*rusūm wājib al-ghallāt*)[3] .... 6,000 dinars
The tax on the storehouse for apples and dates
([*rusūm*] *dār al-tuffāḥ wal-rutab*)[4] ....1,700 dinars
The tax on the storehouse for flax
(*rusūm dār al-kattān*) .... 60 dinars
The tax on the public bath at the Cereals Bank
(*rusūm al-ḥammām bi-Sāḥil al-Ghalla*) .... 534 dinars
The tax on the sugar merchants market
([*rusūm*] *sūq al-sukkarīyīn*) .... 50 dinars
The half raṭl tax on sugar refineries
(*niṣf al-raṭl min maṭābikh al-sukkar*) ....135 dinars[5]

The first two taxes, the tax on spices and the tax on commodities and caravansaries, were miscellaneous taxes, separate from the ordinary taxes on commercial goods (*ʿushr*).[6] Among the other taxes repealed, we find three items closely related to sugar and sugar refineries. The first, *rusūm dār al-qand,* was levied on the storehouse for raw sugar in al-Fusṭāṭ. The raw sugar stored at this facility was likely refined at the adjacent sugar refinery, but there remains no Arabic source to tell us when the *Dār al-Qand* was established or how it was managed. Nevertheless, since the tax on it was abolished in the early Ayyubid era, we can safely conclude that its construction dates back to the preceding Fatimid period.

Regarding the next tax [*rusūm*] *sūq al-sukkarīyīn,* Ibn Duqmāq states that *Sūq al-Sukkarīyīn* was home to the al-Muʿallaq mosque, at which the *imām* was named Ibn al-Muḥtasib al-Sukkarī.[7] However, we find several mosques named al-Muʿallaq in al-Fusṭāṭ,[8] so it is still difficult for us to identify the exact location of Sūq al-Sukkarīyīn. Regardless, the sugar refineries (*maṭābikh*) were often written about along with al-Sukkarīyīn in the Arabic sources,[9] which indicates that both were probably located in nearby al-Fusṭāṭ.

So then, what is the third *niṣf al-raṭl min maṭābikh al-sukkar*? In medieval Egypt, one *raṭl* of sugar was equal to 1/100 *qinṭār jarwī,* around 967 grams, which means that 1/2 *raṭl* was equal to 484 grams. According to the above

3 The tax was levied on cereals arriving at ports on the Nile bank, such as al-Ṣināʿa, al-Maqs, al-Minya, and al-Jisr etc. (*al-Khiṭaṭ*, I, 104).
4 This storehouse was located at al-Fusṭāṭ (*al-Khiṭaṭ*, I, 104).
5 Al-Maqrīzī, *al-Khiṭaṭ*, I, 104–105.
6 *EI*², s.v. ʿUshr (T. Sato).
7 Ibn Duqmāq, *Kitāb al-Intiṣār*, I, 85.
8 A.A. Harīdī, *Fihrist Khiṭaṭ Miṣr*, vol. 3, pp. 342–343.
9 For example, Ibn Duqmāq, *Kitāb al-Intiṣār*, I, 26.

account by al-Maqrīzī, 1/2 *raṭl* per one *qinṭār jarwī* means that a tax rate of 1/200 was levied on the sugar produced at the sugar refineries in al-Fusṭāṭ during the Fatimid period.[10] The total amount of this tax abolished by Ṣalāḥ al-Dīn was estimated as 135 dinars, so the total sugar production was presumably 200 times that, 27,000 dinars or 540,000 dirhams. Since one *raṭl* of refined sugar, as mentioned above, sold for 2.5 dirhams, 27,000 dinars would have bought 216,000 kilograms of sugar. We may, therefore, presume that over 200,000 kilograms of refined sugar were produced annually at the sugar refineries in al-Fusṭāṭ from the Fatimid to the Ayyubid periods.

Al-Nashw Enacts Attachment on Raw Sugar

Al-Qāḍī Sharaf al-Dīn ʿAbd al-Wahhāb b. Tāj Faḍl Allāh al-Nashw al-Kātib (d. 740/1339), who was born into a Coptic family in Cairo, served several amirs and then Sultan al-Malik al-Nāṣir Muḥammad as a high official chosen from among the Coptic Muslims (*Muslimānī al-Qibṭ*).[11] Since the Coptic officials had inherited several generations' worth of family knowledge on local government, the Muslim rulers were dependant on their expertise to manage the state effectively, in particular, in levying taxes on Egyptian peasants. This state of affairs often led to a cozy relationship between the sultans and the Coptic-Muslim officials. The common Muslims greatly envied this relationship, which sometimes exacerbated religious confrontations and conflicts.

According to al-Ṣafadī's biographical dictionary, al-Nashw was a clerk (*kātib*) in his youth, first serving amir Sayf al-Dīn Baktamur al-Ḥājib, and then amir ʿAlāʾ al-Dīn Aydaghmish. One day, Sultan al-Malik al-Nāṣir Muḥammad chose the handsome al-Nashw from among the amir's clerks and appointed him as state treasurer (*mustawfī al-dawla*), stationed in al-Jīza. Next, he was made superintendent of the royal treasury (*nāẓir al-khāṣṣ*), and accompanied Sultan al-Nāṣir's pilgrimage to Mecca in 732/1332. Al-Nashw was known for his amiable personality and his face was "shining brightly". People were also appreciative of al-Nashw's prompt responses to their requests. However, upon being appointed superintendent of the royal treasury, al-Nashw ingratiated himself with Sultan al-Nāṣir by enforcing the sultan's self-interested proclamations

10 Rabie says rather vaguely that 135 dinars [were] derived from a tax of half a pound on sugar products (*The Financial System of Egypt*, p. 81).

11 For the subject of Coptic conversion to Islam, see the following works. Donald P. Little, "Coptic Converts to Islam during the Baḥrī Mamluk Period," M. Gervers and R.J. Bikhazi ed., *Conversion and Continuity: Indigenous Christian Communities in Islamic Lands, Eighth to Eighteenth Centuries*, Toronto, 1990, pp. 263–288; T. Sato, "The Proposers and Supervisors of *al-Rawk al-Nāṣirī* in Mamluk Egypt," *Mamlūk Studies Review*, 2 (1998), pp. 74–77.

and was repeatedly rewarded with favoritism. Al-Nashw, subsequently had to "open the gates" of confiscating the property (*abwāb al-muṣādara*) of amirs and clerks in order to comply with the sultan's unreasonable requests. The unfairness of these actions brought al-Nashw into public disfavor, as people thought he had lost his mind.[12]

In Jumādā II 733/February 1333, al-Nashw put the confiscation policy into practice, as al-Maqrīzī relates in *Kitāb al-Sulūk.*

> In this month, al-Nashw gathered the merchants of Cairo and al-Fusṭāṭ, and put commercial goods like timber (*khashab*), broadcloth (*jūkh*), and cloth (*qumāsh*) under government control, fixing each price at a threefold increase. He rode to the Dār al-Qand to inspect the amount of raw sugar (*qand*) that the amirs received from their sugarcane pressing factories (*maʿṣara* [*li-qaṣab al-sukkar*]). It was a great quantity. Until then, the sultan had exempted the amirs from state taxes levied on raw sugar. But, al-Nashw repealed the sultan's exemption (*musāmaḥa*), and forced the amirs' officials (*mubāshir*) to pay. He then rode back to the sultan to report that the taxes levied on raw sugar [at the Dār al-Qand] had increased to 6,000 dinars in a single day.[13]

We find nearly the same account in al-Yūsufī's biography of Sultan al-Malik al-Nāṣir, *Nuzhat al-Nāẓir.*[14] Both accounts clearly show that the raw sugar produced at the amirs' sugar factories was brought to the Dār al-Qand in al-Fusṭāṭ, where it was taxed; after which, as mentioned above, the amirs would refine the raw sugar at their private refineries (*maṭbakh al-sukkar*). This is crucial to our understanding of the mechanisms for sugarcane cultivation, sugar production, and sugar refinement by the amirs, who were the *iqṭāʿ* holders of the Mamluk period.

Then in 737/1336–7, al-Nashw imposed attachment (*ḥawṭa*) on the property of local governors and officials in Upper Egypt. Al-Yūsufī describes this in *Nuzhat al-Nāẓir.*

---

12 Al-Ṣafadī, *Kitāb al-Wāfī bil-Wafayāt*, XIX, 324–325; Ibn Ḥajar, *al-Durar al-Kāmina*, III, 42–44.

13 Al-Maqrīzī, *Kitāb al-Sulūk*, II, 360. According to Mūsā al-Yūsufī, al-Nashw went to the Dār al-Qand to impose the attachment of property (*ḥawṭa*) on the sugar merchants (*sukkarī*) and druggists (*ʿaṭṭār*) also in the following year, 734/1334 (*Nuzhat al-Nāẓir*, 186).

14 Al-Yūsufī, *Nuzhat al-Nāẓir*, 127.

> Al-Nashw imposed an attachment of property on the governor (*wālī*) of Ushmūnayn, the upper management of sugar factories and waterwheels (*mubāshirū al-ma'āṣir wal-dūlāb*), and all the other clerks (*kātib*) and officials (*shādd*) in the provinces of Upper Egypt and al-Fayyūm. He then informed the sultan that a group of [general] merchants (*tājir*) and sugar merchants (*sukkarī*) had sought the protection of [amirs] Qawṣūn, Bashtak, Āqubughā, and others. Among those seeking protection was a sugar merchant in al-Fusṭāṭ who headed several sugar refineries (*maṭbakh sukkar*) that falsely produced sugar and molasses, insisting that those sugar refineries belong to amir Qawṣūn. Upon hearing this, Sultan al-Nāṣir ordered the sugar merchant to surrender his estate and appear before him. Al-Nashw carried out the sultan's wishes, ordering the sugar merchant to appear and imposing on him a fine of 100,000 dirhams.[15]

According to *al-Khiṭaṭ* by al-Maqrīzī, the Mallawī district in Ushmūnayn was famous for sugarcane cultivation. It had many stone mills (*ḥajar*) managed by the descendants of the Fuḍayl family.[16] In 738/1338, this fertile district for sugar production in Upper Egypt caught the attention of al-Nashw.

> This year, al-Nashw sent an inspector to the owners of the waterwheels used to produce raw sugar (*arbāb dawālīb al-qand*). He found a great deal of raw sugar belonging to the descendants of the Fuḍayl family, specifically, 14,000 *qinṭār*s [*jarwī*] (1,260,000 kilograms) of raw sugar produced this year. The land area they were using for sugarcane crops had already grown to 1,500 *faddān*s (about 955 hectares) annually. However, their agreement with the governmental officials (*mubāshir*) was that only 1,000 *qinṭār*s of raw sugar were to be paid as tax to the government. When al-Nashw found out about this, he imposed an attachment (*ḥawṭa*) on their products, and brought their raw sugar to the Dār al-Qand. He issued them documents (*ḥujja*) declaring that 8,000 *qinṭār*s (720,000 kilograms) of raw sugar belonged to the sultan. After this was taken, they were found to still have another 10,000 *qinṭār*s (967,000 kilograms) of raw sugar that al-Nashw had missed. He also confiscated the property of the officials

15 Al-Yūsufī, *Nuzhat al-Nāẓir*, 370.

16 Al-Maqrīzī, *al-Khiṭaṭ*, I, 204. For the genealogy of the Fuḍayl family, see also Labib, *Handelsgeschichte Ägyptens*, pp. 186–187; Ashtor, "Levantine Sugar Industry in the Late Middle Ages," p. 101.

overseeing the royal waterwheels (*shādd dawālīb al-khāṣṣ*) in Upper Egypt, carrying another 160,000 dirhams back to the sultan.[17]

This account shows that the descendants of the Fuḍayl family in Mallawī used waterwheels (*dūlāb*) to produce 14,000 *qinṭārs jarwī* (1,260,000 kilograms) of *qand* annually. As al-Muqaddasī (4/10 century) states, there were many *dūlāb*s on the banks of the Nile to irrigate orchards (*bustān*) when the water level was low.[18] Judging from the use of the expression "*arbāb dawālīb al-qand*" in the above account by al-Maqrīzī, we can take this to mean that the *dūlāb*s were used not only for irrigating the sugarcane fields but also for compressing the harvested sugarcane to produce raw sugar (*qand*). Al-Maqrīzī further relates that after the death of Sultan al-Nāṣir in 741/1341, the price of sugar rose due to the destruction of both the waterwheels in Upper Egypt and the sugar refineries (*maṭbakh al-sukkar*) in the town of al-Fusṭāṭ.[19] This suggests that the maintenance of both the *dūlāb*s in Upper Egypt and the *maṭbakh al-sukkar*s in al-Fusṭāṭ were vital to successful sugar production and trade in medieval Egypt.

Ibn Baṭṭūṭa, who visited Mallawī at the beginning of the fourteenth century, gives us a vivid account of the booming sugar production in that district. According to his description, the town had 11 *maṭbakh al-sukkar*s where even beggars or sufi mendicants (*faqīr*) could freely come to the factories with warm bread, put it into pots boiling pressed juice, and leave with sugar-soaked bread.[20] The *ḥawṭa* in the account denotes that the government sealed off property belonging to major merchants and high officials to impose an attachment on their movable and immovable assets. The actual confiscation of property after the *ḥawṭa* was called *muṣādara*. From the ʿAbbasid period onward, confiscation of property was often used to compensate for fiscal deficits.[21] The raw sugar confiscated from the Fuḍayl family was transferred to the Dār al-Qand, which indicates that both Sultan al-Nāṣir and al-Nashw as his superintendent had deep ties to the management of the Dār al-Qand.

At any rate, Sultan al-Nāṣir seems to have been firmly committed to supporting al-Nashw's authority. And yet, two years after the confiscation at al-Mallawī,

17 Al-Maqrīzī, *Kitāb al-Sulūk*, II, 431. We find almost the same account in al-Maqrīzī, *al-Khiṭaṭ*, I, 204. According to *al-Khiṭaṭ*, a total amount of 14,000 *qinṭārs* of raw sugar was transferred to the Dār al-Qand in al-Fusṭāṭ. See also Levanoni, *A Turning Point in Mamluk History*, p. 150.

18 Al-Muqaddasī, *Aḥsan al-Taqāsīm*, 208.

19 Al-Maqrīzī, *al-Khiṭaṭ*, II, 99.

20 Ibn Baṭṭūṭa, *Tuḥfat al-Nuẓẓār*, I, 100–101.

21 For the *ḥawṭa* and *muṣādara*, see *EI*², s.v. Ḥawṭa (J. Chelhod), Muṣādara (C.E. Bosworth); Ashtor, *A Social and Economic History*, p. 324; Sato, *State and Rural Society*, pp. 20, 252.

confronted by amirs harshly criticizing al-Nashw, al-Nāṣir eventually decided in 740/1339 to arrest him and confiscate his property. Al-Maqrīzī describes the attachment (*ḥawṭa*) of al-Nashw's property and the people's reaction as follows.

> When the amirs set out to confiscate the property of those arrested, they got the news that the females of al-Nashw's household were staying in a garden on al-Fīl Island [in the Nile]. They hurried to the island. There they found sixty female slaves (*jāriya*), al-Nashw's mother, wife, sister, two sons, and all the other family members. They had two hundred leather bags of grapes (*ʿinab*), abundant raw sugar (*qand*), and grape juice. The amirs sealed off the residences (*dār*) and revenues (*ḥāṣil*), commanding that none of them be removed.
>
> The markets (*sūq*) of Cairo and al-Fusṭāṭ were closed, and people, women and children included, gathered at al-Rumayla beneath the Citadel. They lit candles, held up Qur'ans above their heads, and hoisted flags, shouting and crying out with delight at the news of al-Nashw's arrest. The amirs encouraged them to continue the spectacle for three nights.[22]

Al-Maqrīzī does not state the amount of raw sugar confiscated at that time, but the amirs concerned carried out thorough ongoing investigations into al-Nashw's properties. Consequently, they seized a great number of pearls, emeralds, crystals; a golden cross (*ṣalīb dhahab*); various kinds of cloth and clothes; pork (*laḥm al-khanzīr*), and wine (*khamr*), in addition to 15,000 dinars of cash.[23] Al-Nashw and his family were executed and buried in a Jewish cemetery (*maqābir al-Yahūd*) rather than a Christian one. It is said that his term of office was seven years and seven months.[24]

We have looked at various issues concerning the Dār al-Qand in al-Fusṭāṭ which show that those in power during the Mamluk period were keenly intent on profiting from the control of this storehouse for raw sugar. It is very interesting to learn that the raw sugar produced at the amirs' sugar factories in their respective *iqṭāʿ*s was brought to the Dār al-Qand in al-Fusṭāṭ, where it was

---

22 Al-Maqrīzī, *Kitāb al-Sulūk*, II, 478–479.

23 Al-Maqrīzī, *Kitāb al-Sulūk*, II, 481–482. For the career and works of al-Nashw, see the following works. H.N. al-Ḥajjī, *Aḥwāl al-ʿĀmma fī Ḥukm al-Mamālīk, 678–784/1279–1382: Dirāsa fī al-Jawānib al-Siyāsīya wal-Iqtiṣādīya wal-Ijtimāʿīya*, Kuwait, 1994, pp. 370–380; A. Levanoni, "The al-Nashw Episode: A Case Study of 'Moral Economy.'" *Mamlūk Studies Review*, 9-1 (2005), pp. 207–220. But note that these works, while referring to the Dār al-Qand, are not detailed investigations of it.

24 Al-Maqrīzī, *Kitāb al-Sulūk*, II, 486.

taxed. The amirs then refined that raw sugar at their own sugar refineries (*maṭbakh al-sukkar*) before selling it. Next, we will discus how the rulers demonstrated their authority through social customs, such as through gifts of sugar in the month of Ramaḍān, and serving sugar candy to pilgrims travelling to Mecca.

Sugar in the Month of Ramaḍān

Fasting and Sweets

The Prophet Muḥammad, just after he made the *hijra* to Medina, declared the 10th of Muḥarram to be a day of fasting in the custom of the Jews. However, after his great victory over the Meccans in Baḍr in Ramaḍān 2/ March 624, Muḥammad declared Ramaḍān to be a sacred month of fasting. The Qur'an reads.

> In the month of Ramaḍān the Qur'an was revealed, a book of guidance with proofs of guidance distinguishing right from wrong. Therefore whoever of you is present in that month let him fast. But he who is ill or on a journey shall [instead] fast a similar number of days later on.
>
> God desires your well-being, not your discomfort. He desires you to fast the whole month so that you may magnify God and render thanks to Him for giving you His guidance. ....
>
> Eat and drink until you can tell a white thread from a black one in the light of the coming dawn. Then resume the fast till nightfall and do not approach your wives, but stay at your prayers in the mosques.[25]

According to hadith, the night of power and excellence (*laylat al-qadr*) when Muḥammad received the first revelation of the Qur'an falls on an odd night in the last ten days in Ramaḍān, commonly accepted to be the 27th night. Based on the sacred hadith, the fast of Ramaḍān was incorporated into the five pillars of Islam (*arkān al-Islām*): (1) Witnessing the oneness of God and the prophethood of Muḥammad (*shahāda*), (2) The five daily prayers (*ṣalāt*), (3) The giving of alms (*zakāt*), (4) Fasting (*ṣawm*), and (5) The pilgrimage to Mecca (*ḥajj*). With the exceptions of children, sick and weak persons, pregnant or nursing mothers, travelers, and soldiers on the battlefield, all Muslims are required to abstain from eating, drinking, and sexual activity during daylight hours for one month. Those who observe this daily fast, particularly during the longer

25 *Al-Qur'ān*, II/185–187.

daylight hours of summer, are quite debilitated by the experience. The Muslims of the world, therefore, have held on to a long-established custom of having sweets just after sunset during Ramaḍān to quickly recover their strength.

As previously mentioned, in *The Thousand and One Nights* we find a dialogue between Ibrāhīm al-Naẓẓām, a poet of the ʿAbbasid court, and Tawaddud, a wise female slave: al-Naẓẓām asked, "We often chew on it after sunset during Ramaḍān." She answered, "It is sugarcane (*qaṣab al-sukkar*)." Although manufactured sugar had already spread into Iraq during the ʿAbbasid period, most people continued the custom of biting or sucking sugarcane. Moreover, we may regard this story as one of the earliest accounts describing the close relationship between the month of Ramaḍān and the consumption of things sweet. Ibn al-Jazarī also mentions this in his chronicle.

> It is said that Ibn al-Salʿūs Shams al-Dīn Muḥammad al-Tanūkhī (d. 693/1294),[26] who was trusted with market inspection (*ḥisba*) in Damascus, rode around the city at night during the month of Ramaḍān. He did this to inspect those who produced *kunāfa* (vermicelli baked in sugar, melted butter, and honey), *qaṭāʾif* (a doughnut mixed with walnuts, rock sugar, rose water, and almonds), *ḥalāwa* (sweets), and other foods. He inspected the small-scale bazaar merchants (*bāʿa*), protecting the poor (*mutaʿayyishūn*), and correcting measures and weights.[27]

This account shows that various kinds of sweets like *kunāfa* and *qaṭāʾif*, were produced and sold in the month of Ramaḍān in Damascus also during the Mamluk period.

Even in contemporary Cairo, *kunāfa*, *qaṭāʾif*, and *luqmat al-qāḍī* are widely known as "sweets for Ramaḍān (*ḥalwayāt Ramaḍān*)." Egyptian Muslims, when they have their first meals after sunset (*ifṭār*) during Ramaḍān, begin by eating dates, in accordance with the *Sunna* of the Prophet, then drinking fruit juice, followed by main courses and sweets. In the Maghrib countries, Muslims also break fast with a communal *ifṭār* meal after the post-sunset signal has been given. First, they have dates and drink fruit juice or milk, then they slowly bring out the main dishes. Around ten o'clock at night, they have tea or coffee with sweets. They await daybreak after a final pre-dawn meal (*saḥūr*) of couscous (*kuskus*), yogurt (*laban*), boiled eggs, dried meats, bread, and so on.[28] Tunisian

---

26 For the career of Ibn al-Salʿūs, see al-Ṣuqāʿī, *Tālī Kitāb Wafayāt al-Aʿyān*, 152–153.

27 Ibn al-Jazarī, *Taʾrīkh Ḥawādith al-Zamān*, I, 212.

28 K. Ohtsuka ed., *Food Culture in the World* (*Sekai no shokubunka*, in Japanese), vol. 10, *Arab*, Tokyo, 2007, pp. 223–229, 274–275.

Muslims, in particular, are fond of having "sweets for Ramaḍān" like *dibla* (ring-shaped pancakes fried and topped with sugar and honey), *maqrūd* (semolina cakes, filled with date paste, fried and dipped in syrup), and *samosa* (triangle-shaped pastries, filled with almonds, pistachio, and sugar paste, and fried).[29] When I visited a Shanghai mosque during Ramaḍān in 1990, I was served a round fried cake with sugar, called "*you xiang*" (油香), meaning literally "flavored fried cake."

The Royal Custom of Giving Sugar

As explained in Chapter Three, on Friday at the end of Ramaḍān in 415/1024, under the reign of Fatimid Caliph al-Ẓāhir, a diorama, made of sugar candy and depicting a banquet (*simāṭ*) with 152 figurines, and 7 castles was paraded the streets of Cairo. Nāṣir Khusraw, who visited Cairo in 439/1047, describes the following in his travel journal *Safar Nāma*.

> A gift of 50,000 *mans* (41,650 kilograms) of sugar (*shakar*) was granted by the sultan (the Fatimid caliph) in the month of Ramaḍān. I saw a citron tree (*turanj*) with 1,000 branches, leaves, and fruits, all made of sugar.[30]

Nāṣir Khusraw arrived in Cairo in 439/1047, the early days of Caliph al-Mustanṣir, who later ruled during the Seven-year Famine (459–464/1067–72).[31] Al-Mustanṣir demonstrated his authority by continuing the Ramaḍān policy of his predecessor, Caliph al-Ẓāhir, allocating a large quantity of sugar and producing a citron tree made of sugar.

The Ayyubid and Mamluk sultans followed the Fatimid caliphs in this tradition of giving sugar during Ramaḍān. Al-Maqrīzī describes the custom as practiced by Sultan al-Nāṣir as follows.

> During the reign of [Sultan] al-Nāṣir Muḥammad b. Qalāwūn, the allowance of sugar (*rātib al-sukkar*) given by the sultan every Ramaḍān amounted to 1,000 *qinṭār*s [*jarwī*] (96,700 kilograms). Then, in 745/1344–5 [during the reign of Sultan Ṣāliḥ Ismāʿīl b. Muḥammad al-Nāṣir], it

---

29 F. Béllahsen and D. Rouche, *Cuisine Tunisienne*, Barcelona, 2003; L. Zaouali, *Medieval Cuisine of the Islamic World*, English tr. by M.B. DeBevoise, Berkeley and Los Angeles, 2007, p. 197.

30 Nāṣir Khusraw, *Safar Nāma*, 79.

31 *EI*^{2}, s.v. al-Mustanṣir (H.A.R. Gibb and P. Kraus); C. Petry ed., *The Cambridge History of Egypt*, vol. 1, *Islamic Egypt, 640–1517*, Cambridge, 1998, pp. 152–153.

> increased to 3,000 *qinṭārs* [*jarwī*] (290,000 kilograms), equivalent to 600,000 dirhams, or 30,000 Egyptian dinars.[32]

The *rātib* of the Mamluk period denotes a "stipend in kind" paid to the royal *mamlūk*s and state officials. The sultans occasionally granted the *mamlūk* cavalrymen, whose main income was from *iqṭāʿ* revenues, supplementary stipends in cash or in kind. Ibn Faḍl Allāh al-ʿUmarī also states that the Mamluk sultans gave sugar (*sukkar*) and sweets (*ḥalwāʾ*) to the amirs during Ramaḍān.[33] According to David Ayalon, the royal *mamlūk*s, particularly during the Circassian period, were given monthly payments (*jāmakīya*), as well as allowances (*nafaqa*) upon the accession of a new sultan to the throne, or on the eve of a military campaign. There were also special allowances for Ramaḍān clothing expenses (*kiswa*), and daily meat (*laḥm*) rations.[34] However, during the reign of Sultan Ṣāliḥ Ismāʿīl the government came under financial hardship as al-Maqrīzī plainly states in his *Kitāb al-Sulūk*.

> In the month of Ramaḍān [745/1344–5], state affairs (*aḥwāl al-dawla*) came to a dead end in all aspects. The minister (*wazīr*) could not afford the meat rations for the court laborers (*muʿāmil*), the monthly payments to the *mamlūk* slaves, or the sugar customarily given during Ramaḍān. The sugar grant, which was 1,000 *qinṭārs* [*jarwī*] under Sultan al-Nāṣir Muḥammad, had increased to over 3,000 *qinṭārs* [*jarwī*] this Ramaḍān. However, the state treasury (*bayt al-māl*) had been depleted through increased payment of stipends (*rātib*), and it was difficult [for the government] to get sugar because the previous year's sugarcane crops had suffered [significant] damage. Accordingly, sugar was given only to the females of the court, and the stipends for amirs, *mamlūk*s, and state officials were reduced.[35]

Even under Sultan al-Nāṣir Muḥammad the state treasury was already struggling because of both the increasing number of *mamlūk* slaves purchased by the sultan, and the inflating stipends paid by the government. Amaria

32 Al-Maqrīzī, *al-Khiṭaṭ*, II, 231. See also A. Sabra, *Poverty and Charity in Medieval Islam: Mamluk Egypt, 1250–1517*, Cambridge, 2000, p. 135.

33 Al-ʿUmarī, *Masālik al-Abṣār fī Mamālik al-Amṣār: Mamālik Miṣr wal-Shām wal-Ḥijāz wal-Yaman*, 30.

34 D. Ayalon, "The System of Payment in Mamluk Military Society," *Studies on the Mamlūks of Egypt (1250–1517)*, Variorum reprints, London, 1977, pp. 37–65, 257–296.

35 Al-Maqrīzī, *Kitāb al-Sulūk*, II, 671.

Levanoni notes that historians in the later Mamluk period, like al-Maqrīzī, who had overestimated the reign of al-Nāṣir, couldn't fathom the harshness of the realities or the changes wrought by the Mamluk system during the third reign of al-Nāṣir Muḥammad Ibn Qalāwūn.[36] As mentioned in Chapter Five, in 748/1347, just three years after this economic collapse, the plague (*ṭāʿūn*) swept across Syria and Egypt, decimating sugar and textile production by killing off most of the artisans and laborers.

Sweets for Banquets and Charities

Sugar Candies for Banquets (Simāṭ)

In Shaʿbān 732/May 1332, a reception was held at the Cairo citadel for the wedding of Sultan al-Nāṣir's son, amir Ānūk, to the daughter of amir Sayf al-Dīn Baktamur al-Sāqī, with attendees including chief amirs and their wives. The amirs, each carrying a candle (*shamʿ*), entered the Castle one after another and walked to the sultan and his son Ānūk. There were 3,300 candles used that evening. According to Ibn al-Jazarī, Sultan al-Nāṣir held the following luxurious feast.

> Over 20,000 horses (*khayl*), camels (*jamal*), oxen (*baqar*), sheep (*ghanam*), geese (*wazz*), and chickens (*dajāj*) were slaughtered. The candles brought in for the reception weighed a total of 760 *qinṭārs* (34,200 kilograms), and 18,000 *qinṭārs* [*jarwī*] (about 1,740,600 kilograms) of sugar were used for sweets (*ḥalāwa*) and other things. Shaykh Abū Bakr al-Raḥbī wrote me the above account.[37]

One ʿulama, named Shihāb al-Dīn al-Dimyāṭī, criticized the wedding reception, held in the evening of Friday 11 Shaʿbān, for using so much money for the banquet.[38] Elsewhere, a wedding reception was held in Damascus on 7 Muḥarram 891/13 January 1486 for Muḥammad Ibn Sayyidī al-Shaykh[39] and

36 Levanoni, *A Turning Point in Mamluk History*.

37 Ibn al-Jazarī, *Taʾrīkh Ḥawādith al-Zamān*, II, 525. Al-Maqrīzī gives a slightly different account: "Over 20,000 sheep, oxen, horses, geese, and chickens were slaughtered, and 18,000 *qinṭārs* [*jarwī*] of sugar were used for sweets (*ḥalwā*) and drinks (*mashrūb*)" (*Kitāb al-Sulūk*, II, 346). See also Abū al-Fidāʾ, *al-Mukhtaṣar fī Akhbār al-Bashar*, 4 vols., Cairo, 1325H., IV, 106.

38 Ibn al-Jazarī, *Taʾrīkh Ḥawādith al-Zamān*, II, 525.

39 Sayyidī al-Shaykh denotes Taqī al-Dīn Ibn Qāḍī ʿAjlūn, a prominent Shāfiʿite jurist of Damascus from the late fifteenth to early sixteenth centuries.

Fāṭima, daughter of *qāḍī* Zayn al-Dīn ʿAbd al-Raḥmān. Eight grilled sheep, Māmūnīya cakes covered with sugar (*māmūnīya sukkarīya*), yogurt, breads, and drinks were served at the reception banquet.[40] No account of the banquet itself survives, but it is impressive that even though sugar production was on the decline, cakes of *māmūnīya* covered with sugar were served at a reception held by a prominent ʿulama in Damascus.

Moreover, we find yet another example. This time involving a hadith scholar, Sharaf al-Dīn ʿUmar b. Muḥammad al-Fārisī.

> In 702/1302–3, Sharaf al-Dīn ʿUmar b. Muḥammad al-Fārisī, professor of hadith at Dār al-Ḥadīth al-Ẓāhirīya, died at nearly ninety years of age. Prior to his death, he left a will instructing his family to purchase 500 dirhams worth of *ṣābūnīya* cakes with sugar (*ḥalāwa ṣābūnīya*), and serve them to people attending his funeral.[41]

500 dirhams would have bought over 320 kilograms of regular sugar.[42] It is said that his family complied with his wishes, and the attendants ate sweet cakes and spoke reverently of him.[43] Also, in Ramaḍān 726/August 1326, when al-Malik al-Ṣāliḥ Ṣalāḥ al-Dīn Yūsuf, lord of Ḥiṣn al-Kayfā on the Upper Tigris, visited Cairo, Sultan al-Nāṣir Muḥammad greeted him warmly, presenting meat, chickens, sugar, and sweets exceeding the 10,000 dirhams worth appropriate to his status.[44]

Also of note, al-Maqrīzī mentions that, in addition to buying Turkic, Slavic, and Circassian *mamlūk* slaves, Sultan al-Nāṣir was quite eager to purchase horses for his military.

> When the news that Sultan al-Nāṣir was firmly intent on getting excellent horses reached the ʿArabs, they brought him horses from the countries of Iraq, al-Baḥrayn, al-Ḥasā, and al-Ḥijāz. When the horses arrived, he inspected them and paid as much as 10,000, 20,000 or even 30,000 dirhams for a single horse, in addition to compensating the owner of the horse. As the Sultan's demand for horses increased, the horse owners

40 Ibn Ṭawq, *al-Taʿlīq: Yawmīyāt Shihāb al-Dīn Aḥmad b. Ṭawq*, ed. J. al-Muhājir, 3 vols., Damascus, 2000–04, II, 581.

41 Al-ʿAynī, *ʿIqd al-Jumān*, IV, 289–290.

42 According to al-ʿUmarī, one *raṭl* (967 grams) of regular sugar cost 1.5 dirhams, and one *raṭl* of refined sugar cost 2.5 dirhams (*Masālik al-Abṣār fī Mamālik al-Amṣār: Dawlat al-Mamālīk al-Ūlā*, 84).

43 Al-ʿAynī, *ʿIqd al-Jumān*, IV, 290.

44 Al-Maqrīzī, *Kitāb al-Sulūk*, II, 276.

> (*ṣāḥib al-faras*) rose to meet it. When the ʿArabs returned home after being paid for their horses, the Sultan gave them clothes for themselves and their families, as well as sugar and other gifts.[45]

Here we see that sugar was one of the gifts given by the sultan to the ʿArabs who had provided him with excellent horses. Regarding al-Nāṣir's intention to purchase *mamlūk* slaves, al-Maqrīzī says the following.

> Sultan al-Nāṣir increased the number of *mamlūk*s and *jāriya*s (female slaves) he purchased. He ordered the merchants (*tājir*) to appear before him and bestowed them with money, describing to them the desirable qualities in *mamlūk*s and *jāriya*s. He sent the merchants to Uzbek, Tabriz, al-Rūm, Baghdad, and other countries. When they returned with the *mamlūk*s, the Sultan rewarded the merchants handsomely, giving them splendid clothes (*al-malābis al-fākhira*), golden girth-straps (*ḥawāʾiṣ al-dhahab*), and horses, and giving gifts to the *mamlūk*s that would have amazed them. The previous kings did not behave so [extravagantly].[46]

The newly conscripted young *mamlūk*s were enrolled at military school (*ṭibāq*)[47] at the citadel, where they underwent the education (*adab*) required by the Muslim rulers and mastered the arts of war, including training in Arab horsemanship (*furūsīya*) through playing polo (*kura*). Upon the completion of training, as we will see later, the sultans often held luxurious banquets in celebration. Al-Maqrīzī further expounds upon what was taught to the *mamlūk*s at military school.

> The *mamlūk*s enrolled at the school were taught according to a well-ordered system. When the merchants brought the *mamlūk*s to Cairo, they were introduced to the sultan and grouped by ethnicity (*jins*). Eunuchs (*ṭawāshī*) were appointed to teach each group the art of Arabic writing (*kitāba*). Qur'an was the first item to be learned, and each group of *mamlūk*s studied it everyday under [Islamic] jurisprudents (*faqīh*). They

45 Al-Maqrīzī, *Kitāb al-Sulūk*, II, 526. Al-Maqrīzī also states that horses were brought to Sultan al-Nāṣir by ʿArabs, in particular by Āl Muhannā and Āl Faḍl (*Kitāb al-Sulūk*, II, 525).

46 Al-Maqrīzī, *Kitāb al-Sulūk*, II, 524.

47 The *ṭibāq* (pl. of *ṭabaqa*) denotes classes composed of the various *mamlūk* ethnicities like Turks, Slavs, Kurds, Greeks, Armenians, Georgians, Circassians, and so on. For more on the *ṭibāq*, see Ayalon, *L'esclavage du Mamelouk*, pp. 4–6; A. Mājid, *Nuẓum Dawlat Salāṭīn al-Mamālīk wa-Rusūmhum fī Miṣr*, 2 vols., Cairo, 1964–67, I, p. 15. According to Mājid, Cairo during the Mamluk period had several *ṭibāq*s managed by the sultans and amirs.

> also received instruction and training in Arabic calligraphy (*khaṭṭ*), Islamic law (*adab al-sharīʿa*), and the way of prayer (*ṣalāt*) and invocation of God (*dhikr*). However, these were merely elementary courses for the child *mamlūk*s brought by merchants. If they were already adolescents (*shabb*), the instructor would teach them something about jurisprudence (*fiqh*).
>
> When the *mamlūk*s attained manhood (*sinn al-bulūgh*)[48], they trained in arts of war including archery (*ramy al-sahm*) and spear fighting (*laʿb al-rumḥ*), and came to completely master the required arts and crafts under the instructor (*muʿallim*) of each group.[49]

Learning Qur'an, Arabic language, Islamic law, and the way of prayer and invocation of God was regarded as the core of proper conduct (*adab*) and decency (*ḥishma*) commonly required of all Muslims. Al-Maqrīzī says in *Kitāb al-Sulūk*, "When a *mamlūk* attains manhood, he is usually appointed to an appropriate position (*waẓīfa*), which he manages based on the proper conduct (*adab*) he learned in his youth."[50] This clearly shows that full-fledged *mamlūk*s could not properly perform their duties if they lacked *adab*, even if they held high positions in the government.

The subsequent training in war arts, such as archery, spear fighting, and horsemanship, was principally a means of learning the *furūsīya* (Islamic martial arts and equestrianism) particular to Arab society. According to Ibn Qayyim al-Jawzīya (691–751/1292–1350), the *furūsīya* is classified into two categories: one being knowledge (*ʿilm*) and distinction (*bayān*), and the other being shooting spears (*ramy*) and charging with lances (*ṭaʿn*). Those who master both categories completely are said to be able to conquer their opponents' hearts with arguments (*ḥujja*) and proof (*burhān*), and their countries with swords (*sayf*) and spearheads (*sinān*).[51] That is, the *furūsīya* was regarded as a form of horsemanship that required more than simple bravery or boldness. Ibn Taghrībirdī, a great authority on the *furūsīya* practices of the *mamlūk*s, also writes that *furūsīya* was something other than bravery (*shujāʿa*) and boldness (*iqdām*), for

48 Abū ʿAbd Allāh Muḥammad al-Shāfiʿī (150–204/767–820) gives the following legal explanation of puberty and manhood in Muslim society: "a youth (*ṣabī*) has no duty of *ḥajj* until he attains puberty (*ḥulum*) or she experiences her first menstruation, irrespective of his/her age. However, if he/she reaches fifteen years old, or he/she attains puberty, in either case they are obligated to perform the *ḥajj*." (Al-Shāfiʿī, *Kitāb al-Umm*, 8 vols., Beirut, n. d., II, 110–111).

49 Al-Maqrīzī, *al-Khiṭaṭ*, II, 213.

50 Al-Maqrīzī, *Kitāb al-Sulūk*, II, 521–522.

51 Ibn al-Qayyim al-Jawzīya, *al-Furūsīya*, Cairo, n. d., 27.

a brave man could topple his opponent with sheer strength, but a horseman is one who handles his horse well when charging forward in attack.[52]

As mentioned above, the *mamlūk*s, even after graduating from military school and being assigned *iqṭā*'s appropriate to their ranks, continued to train themselves toward a mastery of Arab horsemanship (*furūsīya*) by playing polo (*kura*). D. Ayalon informs us that the Mamluk sultans, particularly those of the Baḥrī period, constructed a considerable number of hippodromes (*maydān*) in and around Cairo.[53] Let me cite the example of a polo game played between Sultan Barqūq and amir al-Atābak Aytamish in Cairo on 12 Dhū al-Qaʿda 800/27 July 1398. Ibn Ḥajar al-ʿAsqalānī documents it in his chronicle *Inbāʾ al-Ghumr* as follows.

> 12 Dhū al-Qaʿda was a memorable day for the royal stable (*iṣṭabl al-sulṭān*), because on that day the sultan [Barqūq] played polo with amir al-Atābak Aytamish and won. Barqūq entrusted Aytamish with 200,000 dirhams with which to hold a banquet (*simāṭ*). Wazīr Ibn al-Ṭawkhī and Ustādār Yalbughā were ordered to carry out the preparations for the important event. They pitched tents (*khayma*) at the hippodrome (*maydān*) and prepared 20,000 *raṭl*s (about 9,000 kilograms) of meats (*laḥm*), 200 pairs of geese (*iwazza*), 1,000 birds (*ṭayr*) and chickens (*dajāj*), 20 horses (*faras*) – elsewhere said to be 30 horses – 50 *qinṭār*s [*jarwī*](4,800 kilograms) of sugar (*sukkar*), and 70 *ardabb*s (6,300 liters) of flour (*daqīq*) for making sweets (*būza*). Water was poured into 100 *ardabb*s (9,000 liters) earthen jars (*dann*), to which herbs (*ḥashīsh*) were added, boiled, and mixed. Additionally, 60 *qinṭār*s (2,700 kilograms) of wine (*nabīdh*) were produced from dried grapes (*zabīb*). When the sultan descended from the citadel, the table cloths (*simāṭ*) were unfurled and the common people (*ʿāmma*) hungrily devoured the food and drinks provided. Meanwhile, a sufi mendicant (*faqīr*) beneath the citadel vociferously decried such a luxurious banquet.[54]

52 Ibn Taghrībirdī, *al-Nujūm al-Zāhira*, XIV, 131. See also D. Ayalon, "Notes on the *Furūsiyya* Exercises and Games in the Mamluk Sultanate," U. Heyd ed., *Studies in Islamic History and Civilization*, Jerusalem, 1961, p. 34.

53 Ayalon, "Notes on the *Furūsiyya* Exercises," pp. 38–46.

54 Ibn Ḥajar, *Inbāʾ al-Ghumr*, II, 15. According to al-Maqrīzī, two kinds of *simāṭ* were known during the Mamluk period, one was "banquets of food" (*simāṭ al-ṭaʿām*) and the other was "banquets of sweets" (*simāṭ al-ḥalwā*). Al-Maqrīzī, *Kitāb al-Sulūk*, IV, 738.

That the sultan descended from the citadel to the *maydān* shows that the hippodrome was located beneath the western wall of the citadel, called *Maydān bil-Qalʿa*.[55] That is, Sultan Barqūq, who won the polo game with amir Aytamish, allotted 200,000 dirhams for the staging of the opulent banquet beneath the citadel. However, a sufi mendicant familiar with honest poverty loudly criticized the indulgent feast, which consumed large quantities of sugar, wine, and other comestibles. The account also notes that, in addition to amirs and soldiers, commoners were, as a matter of course, present at the banquet. Inviting them might have been an opportunity for the sultan to publicly demonstrate his generosity.

On the other hand, we find accounts of a reverse custom wherein amirs presented the sultan with offerings of sugarcane, sugar, and sweets. Let me take one example, quoting from an account by Ibn Faḍl Allāh al-ʿUmarī.

> The sultan [of the Mamluk period] has the following customary right: when the sultan passes through a great amir's *iqṭāʿ* [in Egypt] while hunting (*mutaṣayyida*), the amir presents him with sheep (*ghanam*), geese (*iwazz*), chickens (*dajāj*), sugarcane (*qaṣab al-sukkar*), and barley (*shaʿīr*) as the entitlements of a sultan. Upon receiving these, the sultan presents the amir with an ornate robe (*khilʿa*) in return.[56]

The Mamluk sultans traditionally hunted (*ṣayd*) in parts of Egypt with small groups of amirs and *mamlūks*.[57] As the above account indicates, when the sultan passed through a great amir's *iqṭāʿ* while hunting, the amir had a customary obligation to present the sultan with things like sheep, geese, chickens, sugarcane, and barley. Similarly, we can infer that such tributary goods (*ḍiyāfa*) would have at times been given to the *iqṭāʿ* holders (*muqṭaʿ*) by the peasants of medieval Egypt.[58] As I noted in the account of *al-Rawk al-Nāṣirī* in 715/1315, the *ḍiyāfa* consisted of produce (*ghalla*), chickens (*dajāj*), lamb (*kharūf*), clover

---

55 Ayalon does not refer to a hippodrome at *Maydān bil-Qalʿa* ("Notes on the *Furūsiyya* Exercises," pp. 38–44). However, we do find a detailed account of *Maydān bil-Qalʿa* in *al-Khiṭaṭ* by al-Maqrīzī, according to which the *Maydān* originated from the Ayyubid period and continued to be used for polo games and congregational prayers, throughout repairs by Sultan al-Nāṣir Muḥammad, until the reign of Sultan Barqūq in 800/1397–8 (al-Maqrīzī, *al-Khiṭaṭ*, II, 228–229). See also N.O. Rabbat, *The Citadel of Cairo: A New Interpretation of Royal Mamluk Architecture*, Leiden, New York, and Köln, 1995, pp. 104–105, 194–195.

56 Al-ʿUmarī, *Masālik al-Abṣār: Mamālik Miṣr wal-Shām wal-Ḥijāz wal-Yaman*, 31.

57 Sato, *State and Rural Society*, pp. 90, 149 n. 3, 166, 188.

58 Sato, *State and Rural Society*, p. 141.

(*birsīm*), dough (*kishk*), cakes (*ka'k*) and so on.[59] The last 'cake' (*ka'k*) was of course a kind of baked sweet made of flour, eggs, and sugar.

Sweets for Charities

Authorities also donated sugar and sweets to mosques, *khānqāh*s, and *zāwiya*s, and to their staffs. As cited above, Ibn al-Ma'mūn al-Baṭā'iḥī, the son of the Fatimid wazir, gives the following account.

> On Thursday 12 Muḥarram 516/1122, the birthday of Caliph al-ʿĀmir bi-Aḥkām Allāh (reigned 495–524/1101–30), an order was given to prepare forty trays (*ṣīnīya*) of round cakes (*khushkanānij*), sweets (*ḥalwā*), and another kind of cakes (*ka'k*). In addition, sugar (*sukkar*), honey (*'asal*), almonds (*lawz*), wheat flour (*daqīq*), and sesame oil (*sīraj*) were, by order of the caliph, delivered to the tombs of prominent persons. Specifically, 500 *raṭl*s (484 kilograms) of sweets were distributed to mosque leaders (*mutaṣaddir*), Qur'an readers (*qāri'*), and sufi mendicants (*faqīr*).[60]

Ṣīnīya literally meant "Chinese goods", but was used to indicate the round brass trays made in medieval Egypt. And *khushkanānij* was a kind of round cake with almond and pistachio in its hollowed center.[61] The following year also, from the beginning of Shaʿbān to the end of Ramaḍān, on the four bonfire nights (*arbaʿ layālī al-waqūd*),[62] [four times over two months], two kinds of sweets, *khushkanānij* and *basandūd*, were donated. They were made daily using one *qinṭār* (96.7 kilograms) of sugar, two *mithqāl*s (9.4 grams) of musk, and two dinars (about 8 grams) of *mu'na* (a mixture of butter and olive oil) and donated to mausoleums (*mashhad*), and to mosques including al-Azhar, al-Aqmar, al-Anwar in Cairo, al-Ṭūlūnī and al-ʿAtīq ('Amr) in al-Fusṭāṭ, and al-Qarāfa. These

59 Al-Maqrīzī, *al-Khiṭaṭ*, 88. See also al-Maqrīzī, *Kitāb al-Sulūk*, II, 149; Ibn Taghrībirdī, *al-Nujūm al-Zāhira*, IX, 43.

60 Ibn al-Ma'mūn, *Nuṣūṣ min Akhbār Miṣr*, 35–36.

61 Ibn al-Ma'mūn, *Nuṣūṣ min Akhbār Miṣr*, 35. See also note 5 by the editor, Aymān Fu'ād Sayyid.

62 Since the Fatimid period, the mosques in Cairo had had a custom of making bonfires for celebrations like the birthdays of the Prophet Muḥammad, al-Ḥusayn, and others. These were generally called "the four bonfire nights" (*layālī al-waqūd al-arbaʿ*) from the beginning of Shaʿbān to the end of Ramaḍān every year (Al-Maqrīzī, *al-Khiṭaṭ*, 491; al-Qalqashandī, *Ṣubḥ al-Aʿshā*, IV, 497–498). See also M.Q. al-Baqlī, *al-Taʿrīf bi-Muṣṭalaḥāt Ṣubḥ al-Aʿshā*, Cairo, 1984, p. 293.

six mosques were widely known as sacred buildings of noble births in early Islamic Egypt.[63]

In 624/1227, the Ayyubid Sultan Muḥammad al-Malik al-Kāmil (reigned 615–635/1218–38), who was to be blamed for delivering Jerusalem to Friedrich II in 626/1229, gave bread (*khubz*), meat (*laḥm*), sweets (*ḥalwā*), and sugar (*sukkar*) to every jurist (*faqīh*) in all the *madrasas*, *ribāṭ*s, and *khānqāh*s, and held banquets (*simāṭ*) in Cairo.[64] We can not with certainty say the exact reason for this generous royal grant, but the more pious sovereigns of that era had already established a tradition of protecting the sufi scholars and mendicants under their rule. For example, Nūr al-Dīn Maḥmūd b. Zangī (reigned 541–569/1147–74) constructed *khānqāh*s for the sufis in Damascus.[65]

To take some examples from the Mamluk period, in 811/1408 amir Jamāl al-Dīn Yūsuf al-Bīrī, the sultan's chief secretary (*ustādār al-sulṭān*), built a *madrasa* in the old city area of Cairo. Ibn Ḥajar al-ʿAsqalānī gives an account of its opening ceremony.

> On 3 Rajab 811/22 November 1408 amir Jamāl al-Dīn Yūsuf al-Bīrī al-Bajāsī, the sultan's chief secretary, finished the construction of a *madrasa* at al-ʿĪd square in Cairo. He appointed the professors (*mudarris*) of four schools for Islamic law, Qur'an interpretation (*tafsīr*), and Prophetic tradition (*ḥadīth*). ... On the opening day, he held an amazing banquet (*simāṭ hāʾil*), filling a large basin (*fasqīya*) with refined sugar (*sukkar mukarrar*). One professor gave continuous lectures for a full week. When he finished, he was bestowed with a robe of honor (*khilʿa*). The next week began with another lecture on Qur'an interpretation by professor and chief judge (*qāḍī al-quḍāt*) Jalāl al-Dīn al-Balqīnī. He sat down and recited this verse of the Qur'an (IX/18), "The mosques of Allah shall be visited and maintained by such as believe in Allah."[66]

This account notes that amir Jamāl al-Dīn held an amazing banquet (*simāṭ hāʾil*) with large quantities of white sugar for the opening ceremony for his *madrasa*. Ibn Ḥajar also states that Ṣarghitmish al-Nāṣirī, a handsome young boy purchased by Sultan al-Malik al-Nāṣir for the expensive price of 80,000 dirhams (about 4,000 dinars), was eventually promoted to amir of one hun-

63 Ibn al-Ma'mūn, *Nuṣūṣ min Akhbār Miṣr*, 63–64.

64 Ibn Aybak al-Dawādārī, *al-Durr al-Maṭlūb fī Akhbār Mulūk Banī Ayyūb*, ed. S.A. ʿĀshūr, Cairo, 1972, 283.

65 Ibn Jubayr, *Riḥlat Ibn Jubayr*, 279–281.

66 Ibn Ḥajar, *Inbāʾ al-Ghumr*, II, 399.

dred, and later built the Madrasa Ṣarghitmish adjacent to Ibn Ṭūlūn mosque in Cairo.[67] When the *madrasa* was completed in 757/1356, Ṣarghitmish appointed Qawām al-Dīn Abū Ḥanīfa Amīr Kātib al-Fārābī as a professor of the Hanafi school of Islamic law.[68] According to al-Maqrīzī, Ṣarghitmish also held a sumptuous feast to celebrate the opening of his *madrasa*.

> On Tuesday 9 Jumādā I 757/11 May 1356, when Ṣarghitmish visited the *madrasa* accompanied by amirs, judges (*qāḍī*), and other notables (*shaykh*), Qawām al-Dīn gave [the first] lecture there. Afterwards, a lavish banquet (*simāṭ jalīl*) was held, featuring a pond (*birka*) filled with melted sugar (*sukkar mudhāb*). People ate, drank, and left.[69]

It is interesting to read that both amirs held extravagant banquets as opening ceremonies for their *madrasa*s in Cairo, and both with large quantities of sugar. So, we can see that there was an established social custom in the Ayyubid and Mamluk periods of sultans and amirs sometimes giving gifts of sugar to sufi mendicants and using sugar in ceremonies to celebrate cultural enterprises.

Sugar Candies in Sultans' Pilgrimages to Mecca

Amīr al-Ḥājj – *The Official Guard of Pilgrims to Mecca*

In Jumādā I 834/January 1431, al-Maqrīzī, an Egyptian historian approximately sixty-eight years of age, departed Cairo with his family to make the *ḥajj* pilgrimage to Mecca. Let me summarize his personal account of the journey.

> Al-Maqrīzī and his family joined in a caravan (*rakb*) of about 1,500 camels, commanded by amir Saʿd al-Dīn Ibrāhīm b. al-Marra, governor of Judda (*nāẓir Judda*). Not long after the caravan had departed from Birkat al-Ḥājj, about 1,000 men and women died of thirst. Forty days into the journey, Zubaydī Bedouins assaulted the caravan, violating a peace treaty (*ṣulḥ*) that had been agreed to in exchange for 100 dinars. Two pilgrims and about ten ʿArabs died in the battle between one hundred guards and the Bedouins. The treaty was renewed for over 10,000 dinars, which were levied on the pilgrims according to the amount of money they had with

---

67 Ibn Ḥajar, *al-Durar al-Kāmina*, II, 305–306.

68 Al-Maqrīzī, *Kitāb al-Sulūk*, III, 28.

69 Al-Maqrīzī, *Kitāb al-Sulūk*, III, 28; Ibn Qāḍī Shuhba, *Taʾrīkh Ibn Qāḍī Shuhba*, III, 100.

> them. On 28 Jumādā II/13 March, forty-six days after departure, they arrived at the sacred city of Mecca. After performing the rites of the *ḥajj*, the caravan, with al-Maqrīzī and his family, left Mecca under the command of *amīr al-ḥājj* Qarāsunqur, and returning safely to Cairo on 23 Muḥarram 835/1 October 1431. The long journey took 200 days. Al-Maqrīzī criticized amir Qarāsunqur's merciless treatment of pilgrims suffering from thirst.[70]

Since, as the above account vividly shows, a *ḥajj* pilgrimage meant risking one's life, the caliphs and sultans needed a way to maintain public order for the pilgrimage. The Muslim rulers of the medieval ages, therefore, appointed an *amīr al-ḥājj* to command the army protecting the pilgrim caravans (*rakb*) against Bedouin assaults.

There were three main pilgrimage routes arriving at Mecca: the first was the Kufa route for Muslims from Central Asia, Iran, and Iraq. The second was the Damascus route for pilgrims from Anatolia and Syria, and the third was the Cairo route for those from Africa, al-Andalus, Maghrib, and Egypt.[71] The exact date when an *amīr al-ḥājj* was first appointed remains unknown. Let us examine the subject based on Arabic source materials. In 367/978 amir Bādīs b. Zīrī was appointed by the Fatimid Caliph al-ʿAzīz as the *amīr al-ḥājj* for the Egyptian caravan.[72] He was most likely the first *amīr al-ḥājj* in Islamic history. For the Damascus route, in 583/1187 when Ṣalāḥ al-Dīn regained Jerusalem, Ṭāshtigīn was appointed as the *amīr al-ḥājj* for the Syrian caravan.[73] As for the Kufa route, Qāymāz, a Turkish amir, was probably first selected by Seljuqid Sultan Muḥammad II for the role of *amīr al-ḥājj* for the Iraqi caravan in 552/1157.[74]

Generally speaking, the military rank of *amir* was held for several years, sometimes lifelong, but the honorary rank of *amīr al-ḥājj* was usually reassigned each year. During the Mamluk period, an amir of one hundred, which was the highest amir rank attainable, was often selected as the *amīr al-ḥājj* in the month of Rajab. Then, in the month of Shawwāl, the Egyptian caravan

---

70 Al-Maqrīzī, *Kitāb al-Sulūk*, IV, 854–855, 858, 863.

71 F.E. Peters, *The Hajj: The Muslim Pilgrimage to Mecca and the Holy Places*, Princeton, 1994, pp. 71–96.

72 Al-Suyūṭī, *Ḥusn al-Muḥāḍara fī Taʾrīkh Miṣr wal-Qāhira*, ed. M.A. Ibrāhīm, 2 vols., Cairo, 1967–68, II, 280–281.

73 ʿImād al-Dīn al-Iṣfahānī, *al-Fatḥ al-Qussī fī al-Fatḥ al-Qudsī*, ed. M.M. Ṣubḥ, Cairo, 1965, 188–189.

74 Ibn al-Jawzī, *al-Muntaẓam fī Taʾrīkh al-Mulūk wal-Umam*, vols. 5–10, Hyderabad, 1357–58H., X, 170.

departed from Cairo led by him and the palanquin (*maḥmil*). The *amīr al-ḥājj* was fully authorized by the sultan to manage matters like the supply of provisions to the pilgrims, the organization of the caravan, the protection of accompanying merchants, the distribution of drinking water, the assistance of the sick and the poor, and the punishment of criminals.[75] In reality, however, the *amīr al-ḥājj* was often less than fair to the pilgrims, which caused complaints.[76] As F.E. Peters believes, the *amīr al-ḥājj* was likely a crucial figure in the success or failure of a *ḥajj* pilgrimage caravan.[77]

The Maḥmil *and* Kiswa

Abū Muḥammad al-Qāsim al-Ḥarīrī al-Baṣrī's (446–516/1054–1122) illustrated *Maqāmāt* text, the manuscript of which is preserved at the Bibliotèque Nationale, contains a depiction of a pilgrim caravan led by an *amīr al-ḥājj*. This is believed show the party accompanying a palanquin (*maḥmil al-ḥājj*) leading a pilgrimage to Mecca from Baghdad in the early thirteenth century.[78] According to Edward W. Lane, the *maḥmal* (or *maḥmil*) is empty except for two *muṣḥafs* (copies of the Qur'an), one on a scroll, and the other in the more common form of a small book.[79] It is uncertain whether the *maḥmil* of the Mamluk period were empty or, as Lane says, held two different forms of the Qur'an.[80]

Al-Qalqashandī, an encyclopedist in the Mamluk period, explains that two rounds of practice journeys of the caravan (*dawarān al-maḥmil*) were held in Cairo before the departure for Mecca. The first round, in the month of Rajab, was led by four qadis and the *muḥtasib*. It went from Naṣr Gate to Zuwayla Gate, up to the Citadel, descended south to al-Fusṭāṭ, and then returned to Cairo. After this first procession, the sultan publicly selected an amir and a qadi as the *amīr al-ḥājj* and the *qāḍī al-rakb* (judge of the Meccan pilgrimage) respectively. The second round was in the month of Shawwāl. It went to the Citadel, soon returned north to Naṣr Gate, and went further to al-Raydānīya, bound for the holy city of Mecca.[81] Since the Cairene people so eagerly awaited

75 *EI*², s.v. Amīr al-Ḥādjdj (J. Jomier); Holt, *The Age of the Crusades: The Near East from the Eleventh Century to 1517*, London, 1986, p. 81; Grunebaum, *Muhammadan Festivals*, p. 37.

76 We find many other examples in Arabic chronicles in addition to the above account given by al-Maqrīzī.

77 Peters, *The Hajj*, p. 162.

78 R. Ettinghausen, *Arab Painting*, Cleveland, 1962, p. 119.

79 Lane, *An Account of the Manners and Customs of the Modern Egyptians*, pp. 438–439. See also Grunebaum, *Muhammadan Festivals*, p. 37.

80 Fr. Buhl and J. Jomier believe that in medieval times the *maḥmil* was usually empty (*EI*², s.v. Maḥmal).

81 Al-Qalqashandī, *Ṣubḥ al-Aʿshā*, IV, 57–58.

the *dawarān al-maḥmil*, it was not even unusual for women to stake out good positions the day before, and spend the night in the company of men to see the *dawarān* the following day.[82]

The Egyptian *ḥajj* pilgrimage caravan annually brought a new silk drape (*kiswa*) to cover the Kaʿba. The dedication of this silk drape was a privilege held by the Mamluk sultans who had proclaimed themselves the protectors of the two holy cities of Islam (*al-Ḥaramayn*). The Arabic verses of witness (*shahāda*) were embroidered onto the *kiswa*, which was replaced each year. The old *kiswa* was cut into small pieces and sold to pilgrims who wanted them as souvenirs.[83] It is said that the dedication of the *kiswa* had been the exclusive privilege of the Mamluk sultans since Shajar al-Durr (reigned 648/1250). However, the Arabic sources of the era provide no proof to support the claim that this tradition began with the first Mamluk sultan is a historical fact. As J. Jomier supposes, Sultan Baybars (reigned 658–676/1260–77) seems to have initiated the *maḥmil* and *kiswa* traditions when he first sent them in 664/1266.[84] In the Circassian period, Shāh Rukh (reigned 811–850/1409–47), son of Timur, repeatedly sent envoys to Cairo requesting approval to make and present *kiswa* from Samarqand as well. But in 838/1434, Sultan Barsbāy, after asking the opinions of the four chief judges, gave the following reply to Tāj al-Dīn ʿAlī, an envoy sent again from Shāh Rukh.

> The custom (*ʿāda*) stipulates that no one is permitted to bestow the *kiswa* except the Egyptian kings (*mulūk Miṣr*). This custom has been acknowledged legitimate by divine law (*al-sharʿ*) in Islamic countries.[85]

Even after the Egyptian sultan refused his request, Shāh Rukh nevertheless continued to claim the right to present the *kiswa*, but never achieved this goal. When the Mamluk sultanate collapsed in the early sixteenth century, the right to present the *kiswa* went to the Ottoman sultans who had assumed protection of the two holy cities. In the international politics of the Islamic world, the problem of which sovereigns had rights regarding the *kiswa* continued to be a crucial point in the legitimization of authority.

---

82 Al-Maqrīzī, *Kitāb al-Sulūk*, IV, 614. See also *EI²*, s.v. Maḥmal (Fr. Buhl and J. Jomier).

83 Grunebaum, *Muhammadan Festivals*, p. 24.

84 *EI²*, s.v. Maḥmal (Fr. Buhl and J. Jomier), citing al-Maqrīzī, *Kitāb al-Sulūk*, I, 544. See also, Peters, *The Hajj*, p. 165.

85 Al-Maqrīzī, *Kitāb al-Sulūk*, IV, 932.

The Mamluk Sultans' Pilgrimages to Mecca

Many caliphs and sultans throughout Islamic history made the *ḥajj* pilgrimage to Mecca, often with political significance. For example, in 187/803 when Hārūn al-Rashīd (reigned 170–193/786–809), the fifth 'Abbasid caliph, returned from Mecca, he unexpectedly imprisoned the Barmakid wazir Yaḥyā and killed his capable son Ja'far.[86] This was not a capricious punishment, but a prudent decision to prevent a Barmakid influence on his policies, while using the opportunity to frame it as a religious act. Ayyubid Sultan Ṣalāḥ al-Dīn was firmly intent on performing his religious duties, but ultimately was unable to visit the holy cities of Islam because of the severity of his political circumstances.[87] The Mamluk Sultan Baybars, in 667/1269, went to al-Karak with a few of his amirs, *mamlūks*, and *ajnād al-ḥalqa*, concealing his true intention of visiting Mecca. When he arrived in Mecca, Baybars behaved not as a sovereign, but as a pious Muslim, praying alone, washing the Ka'ba (Bayt Allāh) with his hands, and helping, along with his followers, to hang the Egyptian-made *kiswa*.[88] Prior to this, in 659/1261, he had publicly claimed to be a serious protector of Islam through his establishment of the 'Abbasid caliphate in Cairo. Moreover, having completed the pilgrimage, in 667/1269 as mentioned, Baybars was well-positioned to consolidate his sovereignty over the holy cities of Mecca and Medina.[89]

Sultan al-Malik al-Nāṣir Muḥammad visited Mecca three times, in 712/1313, 719/1320, and 732/1332. The second of these *ḥajj* pilgrimages is the best documented.

> In Jumādā II 719/July-August 1319, the sultan began to arrange for the journey to Mecca, sending [Coptic official] Karīm al-Dīn [Akram] al-Kabīr to Alexandria to prepare the *kiswat al-Ka'ba*, and ordering Karīm al-Dīn Akram al-Ṣaghīr and other officials (*mubāshir*) to arrange for provisions

---

86 Al-Ṭabarī, *Ta'rīkh al-Rusul wal-Mulūk*, II, 667f. See also H. Kennedy, *The Prophet and the Age of the Caliphates: The Islamic Near East from the Sixth to the Eleventh Century*, London and New York, 1986, pp. 142–144.

87 Abū Shāma, *Kitāb al-Rawḍatayn*, Beirut ed., II, 205. Abū Shāma says, quoting Qāḍī al-Fāḍil, "The Franks still remain in Syria and do not forget Jerusalem. It is uncertain whether they keep the peace treaty or not. We should therefore take full precautions against their surprise attack on Jerusalem in the absence of the sultan."

88 Ibn 'Abd al-Ẓāhir, *al-Rawḍ al-Zāhir fī Sīrat al-Malik al-Ẓāhir*, ed. A. al-Khuwaytir, Riyad, 1976, 354–355; al-Maqrīzī, *Kitāb al-Sulūk*, I, 580–581. Peters states that Baybars led his own "private pilgrimage" in 1268 (*The Hajj*, p. 110), but the correct year is 667/1269.

89 R. Irwin, *The Middle East in the Middle Ages: The Early Mamluk Sultanate 1250–1382*, London, 1986, p. 56; Holt, *The Age of the Crusades*, p. 186.

> (*iqāma*), feed for the animals (*ʿulūfa*), and other necessities. Then, a constant stream of gifts (*taqādim*) arrived from amirs and governors (*nāʾib*) from all the provinces of Syria. The first gifts, from amir Tankiz, governor of Syria (*nāʾib al-Shām*), included horses with golden saddles, golden and silver chains, and silk leading ropes. Next were gifts from al-Malik al-Muʾayyad, lord of Ḥamā. And then, Karīm al-Dīn [al-Ṣaghīr] personally arranged for what was needed, providing cooking pots (*qidr*) of gold, silver, and copper to be carried on camels. Moreover, he called upon the gardeners (*khawlī*) to grow herbs (*mabqala*) and aromatic plants (*rayḥān*) in camel-mounted planters that allowed plants to be grown, watered, and harvested whenever needed. These included many kinds of aromatic plants like herbs (*baqal*), leeks (*karrāth*), coriander (*kuzbara*), mint (*naʿnaʿ*), and the like. ... Then 500 loads (*ḥiml*) of sweets (*ḥalwā*), sugar boxes (*sukkardān*), and fruits were brought from Damascus in addition to 180 loads of pomegranates (*rummān*), almonds (*lawz*), and other ingredients necessary for cooking. Karīm al-Dīn [al-Ṣaghīr] also supplied 1,000 geese (*iwazz*) and 3,000 chickens (*dajāj*).[90]

It is noteworthy that such a large quantity of sugar, sweets, and fruits were brought to Cairo from Damascus, amounting to 500 *ḥiml* camel-loads (about 125,000 kilograms). These were to hold the sugar and sweets to be granted to Meccan residents and pilgrims that year. Sultan al-Malik al-Nāṣir eagerly anticipated arriving in the holy city. When he did, he refrained from *ṭawāf* on camelback, as the Prophet had done, and walked instead on foot, together with the commoners. Moreover, al-Maqrīzī tells us that al-Nāṣir washed the Kaʿba with his hands[91] in the same way Baybars had done in his *ḥajj* journey.

In the later Mamluk period, several sultans performed more extravagant pilgrimages as a way of demonstrating their importance. Let me describe the journey of Sultan al-Malik al-Ashraf Shaʿbān (reigned 764–778/1363–77), grandson of al-Malik al-Nāṣir Muḥammad, in 778/1377.

> Innumerable dishes (*maṭbakh*), drinks (*mashrab*), and various kinds of foods were prepared [for the sultan's pilgrimage]. Among them were 30,000 boxes (*ʿulba*) of sweets (*ḥalwā*), 5 *raṭl*s (about 4.8 kilograms) per box, and 180,000 *raṭl*s (actually 150,000 *raṭl*s, that is 145,050 kilograms) in

---

90 Al-Maqrīzī, *Kitāb al-Sulūk*, II, 195–196; al-Maqrīzī, *al-Dhahab al-Masbūk fī Dhikr Man Ḥajja min al-Khulafāʾ wal-Mulūk*, ed. J. al-Shayyāl, Cairo, 1955, 102. See also Ibn Aybak al-Dawādārī, *al-Durr al-Fākhir fī Sīrat al-Malik al-Nāṣir*, ed. H.R. Roemer, Cairo, 1960, 295.

91 Al-Maqrīzī, *Kitāb al-Sulūk*, II, 197.

> total. All the sweets were made of pure sugar (*sukkar naqī*), and were flavored with 100 *mithqāls* (468 grams) of musk (*misk*), and also sandalwood (*ṣandal*) and aloe (*ʿūd*). Amirs arranged the same quantity of sweets. *Ḥalqa* cavalrymen and other notables (*aʿyān*) also prepared an immeasurable amount of sweets. Witness the grandeur of a country where 360,000 *raṭls* (1,728,000 kilograms) of sugar were cooked for the sultan and amirs within a month.[92]

3,000 boxes of sweets were to be given to the pilgrims to demonstrate the sultan's piety and generosity. But, the people regarded this as an extravagance unsuitable for the pilgrimage. Al-Maqrīzī also criticized the sultan for disrupting the happiness of the state (*saʿādat al-dawla*) with his silly conduct.[93] Along with this negative public sentiment, when Sultan al-Ashraf visited ʿAqaba in Dhū al-Qaʿda 778/March 1377, news of a coup d'état by the amirs and *mamlūks* spread through the capital city of Cairo. The sultan promptly returned to Cairo with his followers, but was arrested by the *mamlūks* and put to death. He was twenty-four years old, having reigned fourteen years and two months.[94]

As shown above, caliphs and sultans throughout history granted large quantities of sugar to their subjects each year as a part of Ramaḍān, and provided the ʿulama and sufis with sweets and sugar on special occasions. A great deal of sugar was consumed at the sultan's banquets, and some sultans arranged indulgent gifts of sweets to those making the pilgrimage to Mecca. Figurines and castles made of sugar were paraded through the streets for the enjoyment of the Cairene spectators. On the other hand, the rulers were often criticized for extravagance inappropriate for a religious obligation.

---

92 Al-Maqrīzī, *Kitāb al-Sulūk*, III, 273; al-Maqrīzī, *al-Dhahab al-Masbūk*, 118–121.

93 Al-Maqrīzī, *Kitāb al-Sulūk*, III, 273.

94 Al-Maqrīzī, *Kitāb al-Sulūk*, III, 281–283.

CHAPTER 7

Cooking Innovations in Medieval Islam

Cooking in the ʿAbbasid Caliph Courts

In this chapter, we will discuss the cooking innovations that took place in Muslim societies as sugar production increased during the early Islamic period. First, let us examine the changes in the diets of the ʿAbbasid court, based on Arabic language cookbooks (*kitāb al-ṭabīkh*) and nutrition books (*kitāb al-ghidhāʾ*) from the tenth century and after.

The ʿAbbasid Caliph Courts

We will begin by describing conditions in the ʿAbbasid caliph courts in the early eleventh century. As previously discussed in Chapter Three, Baghdad (aka Madīnat al-Salām), the capital of the new Islamic state, was established in 146/766 on the west bank of the Tigris River. At the center of the round wall-enclosed city was Golden Gate Palace, a residence for the caliph that was capped with an enormous green dome symbolizing the unity and authority of the state.[1] But shortly after, in 157/773, al-Manṣūr constructed a new palace called al-Khuld (eternity) along a bank of the Tigris where Hārūn al-Rashīd later resided.[2] At the time, Baghdad extended across the west bank to the east bank, where the quarters of al-Shammāsīya and al-Ruṣāfa emerged as the new city centers of the capital. Then, in 280/893, Caliph al-Muʿtaḍid (reigned 279–289/892–902) rebuilt the old palace on the east bank, expanding its area and adding new buildings. That last palace came to be called Dār al-Khilāfa in the later ʿAbbasid period. As previously mentioned, *ʿayyārūn* bandits appeared in Baghdad in the tenth and eleventh centuries, attacking the caliphal courts and the homes of the rich, often setting fires and killing people. In Jumādā II 334/ January 946 the Shiʿite army of the Buwayhids entered Baghdad and put the Sunnite ʿAbbasid caliphs under its protection.[3]

---

1 Lassner relates that the architectural features of the walled area, and in particular the green dome of al-Manṣūr's palace, reflected the imperial style of the Caliph and served as a visual symbol of the unity and authority of the state (*The Topography of Baghdad*, p. 169).

2 Lassner, *The Topography of Baghdad*, p. 55; *EI*[2], s.v. Baghdād (A.A. al-Duri).

3 Sato, *State and Rural Society*, p. 18; M. Kabir, *The Buwayhid Dynasty of Baghdad*, Calcutta, 1964, p. 6.

 | DOI 10.1163/9789004281561_009

Hilāl al-Ṣābī (359–448/970–1056), a member of Ṣābians who pray toward the stars, was born to a distinguished family of scientists and bureaucrats in Baghdad in a period of decline that restrained the lifestyles of the caliphs of the ʿAbbasid court. After converting to Islam in his early forties, Hilāl served the caliph's court as a secretary (*kātib*) under the Buwayhid sovereignty. Toward the end of his life, he published *Rusūm Dār al-Khilāfa* (*The Rules and Regulations of the ʿAbbasid Court*), which was dedicated to Caliph al-Qāʾim (reigned 422–467/1031–75). Based on this book, I will give an overview of the caliph's court, focusing on the conduct and responsibilities of the positions of wazir, amir, and *ḥājib* (chamberlain), the caliph's meetings with his subjects, the granting of robes (*khilʿa*) and descriptive nicknames (*laqab*), the drums at the five prayers, and so on.

First, an overview of Dār al-Khilāfa in the eleventh century. The court area had already been significantly reduced with the destruction of a considerable number of palaces and residences during contestations and riots over the legitimacy of the caliph. The preceding Caliph, al-Muktafī (reigned 289–295/902–908), employed 20,000 court *ghulāms* and 10,000 black and Slav eunuchs (*khādim*) for whom 400 baths (*ḥammām*) were furnished. According to the budget for 306/918–9, the total income was 14,829,834 dinars, while the annual expenses for the caliph's kitchens (*maṭābikh khāṣṣa*), Turkish soldiers' kitchens, and other costs were 528,840 dinars.[4]

When an amir, a wazir, or a high dignitary saw the caliph, the previous custom had been that they addressed him saying: "Peace be upon you, O Commander of the Faithful, and may the mercy and blessings of Allāh be upon you." However, this practice was replaced by kissing the ground, a rule with which everyone now complied.[5] Hilāl also relates that it is most appropriate for a wazir, or anyone of a similar rank, to enter the presence of the caliph cleanly dressed, groomed, reverent in his stride, and perfumed with aromatic scents emanating from his body and clothes.[6] When a wazir or someone else converses with the caliph, he must keep his voice low and not raise it, except as necessary to prevent repetition or for clarification.[7] The caliph, when receiving his subjects, sat on a throne behind a curtain (*sidillā*) and had ʿUthmān's copy of the Qurʾan in front of him. On his shoulder was the garment (*burda*) [of the Prophet]; and in his hand, the stick (*qaḍīb*) [of the Prophet]. He was girded

4 Hilāl al-Ṣābī, *Rusūm Dār al-Khilāfa*, ed. M. ʿAwwād, Baghdad, 1964, 7–8, 21–22.

5 Hilāl al-Ṣābī, *Rusūm Dār al-Khilāfa*, 31; English tr. by E. Salem, *The Rules and Regulations of the ʿAbbasid Court*, Beirut, 1977, p. 29.

6 Hilāl al-Ṣābī, *Rusūm Dār al-Khilāfa*, 32; Salem tr., *The Rules and Regulations*, p. 30.

7 Hilāl al-Ṣābī, *Rusūm Dār al-Khilāfa*, 33; Salem tr., *The Rules and Regulations*, p. 31.

with the sword of the Apostle of Allah (*sayf Rasūl Allāh*).[8] He was dressed in black, and on his head he wore a *ruṣāfīya*.[9] Regarding the gifts conferred by the caliph, the robes of honor at banquets (*khilaʿ al-munādama*) were: A gilded and embroidered turban (*ʿimāma*), a garment worn under chainmail coats, a lined garment, and a *dabīqī* mantle. The person being honored was given precious gifts, rare ornaments, and perfumes.[10]

That is an overview of the manners and customs of the ʿAbbasid court as described in *Rusūm Dār al-Khilāfa* by Hilāl al-Ṣābī. Unfortunately, we find no reference there to the meals in the caliph's court. But the following two cookbooks (*Kitāb al-Ṭabīkh*) provide us with ample information on the caliph's kitchens in ʿAbbasid Baghdad. So, let's look at these two works written in the tenth and the thirteenth centuries, focusing on dishes cooked with various kinds of sugar.

Ibn Sayyār's Kitāb al-Ṭabīkh

Ibn Sayyār al-Muẓaffar al-Warrāq was an Arab intellectual who lived in Baghdad in the latter half of the tenth century. His name "al-Warrāq" may indicate that he was a specialist of paper (*waraqa*) or the owner of a bookshop. L. Zaouali states: A gifted compiler, trained in medical and dietary matters, he wrote a cookbook (*Kitāb al-Ṭabīkh*) that gave an inventory of food products, as well as all the relevant rules and prescriptions for the proper maintenance of kitchen equipment and cooking utensils.[11] This is regarded as the oldest existing Arabic language cookbook, the Introduction of which provides us with the principal aim of its writing.

> Your Majesty (the exalted caliph) asked of me, may God bestow longevity upon you, to write a book on dishes (*ṭaʿām*) cooked for kings (*malik*),

8 This account shows that the sword (*sayf*), garment (*burda*), and stick (*qaḍīb*) of the Prophet were the symbols of the ʿAbbasid caliphate. According to T.W. Arnold, "Whereas the symbols of Umayyad rule had been the sceptre and the seal, under the Abbasids increased emphasis was laid on the religious character of their dignity, and the mark of their exalted office became the mantle of the Prophet" (*The Caliphate*, Oxford, 1924, p. 27).

9 Hilāl al-Ṣābī, *Rusūm Dār al-Khilāfa*, 81; Salem tr., *The Rules and Regulations*, p. 65. *Al-Ruṣāfīya* denoted a tall headpiece (*qalanswa*) worn by the ʿAbbasid caliphs. See R. Dozy, *Dictionnaire détaillé des Noms des vêtements chez les Arabes*, Amsterdam, 1845; repr. Beirut, n.d., pp. 188–189.

10 Hilāl al-Ṣābī, *Rusūm Dār al-Khilāfa*, 96; Salem tr., *The Rules and Regulations*, p. 77.

11 Lilia Zaouali, *Medieval Cuisine*, pp. 10–11. Regarding Arab cook books, see K. Suzuki, "On the Importance of the Arab Cookery Books in Medieval Islamic Period (Chusei Arabu ryorisho no keito to tokucho nitsuite, in Japanese)," *Oriento*, 37–2 (1994), pp. 88–107.

> caliphs (*khalīfa*), lords (*sayyid*), and dignitaries (*ra'īs*), and here it is, may God bestow longevity upon you, an illustrious and fine collection of whatever benefits the body and fends off any harm that foods might induce.[12]

This account clearly shows that it was a court cookbook, created for kings, caliphs, lords, and dignitaries gathering in the ʿAbbasid court. We can also make inferences about the social background of its writing through the following anecdote included in the book.

> So, Ibrāhīm [Ibn al-Mahdī] went home and ordered the slave girl be brought to him. Her name was Bidʿa. He said to her, "Bidʿa, your master al-Amīn, Amīr al-Muʾminīn (Commander of the Faithful) wants me to serve him *sikbāj*. He said you cooked it once for Caliph al-Rashīd and that he had it with him and liked it a lot. It was made with different kinds of meat." She replied, "I hear and obey the commands of Amīr al-Muʾminīn." Ibrāhīm ordered the kitchen manager (*wakīl al-maṭbakh*) to make available whatever Bidʿa asked for and needed to make the dish.[13]

M.M. Ahsan explains that *sikbāj*, a word indicative of a Persian origin, was made with fatty meat, carrots or eggplants, almonds, currants, dried figs, a mixture of date juice (*dibs*) and vinegar, and the usual spices.[14] According to Ibn Sayyār, the ingredients of *sikbāj*, whether prepared in a caliph's kitchen or a commoner's kitchen, are precisely the same: vinegar, meat, vegetables, eggplant, gourd, saffron, and everything else that is necessary.[15] L. Zaouali mistakenly translated *qarʿ* (gourd) as "sugar"[16]; but in another section Ibn Sayyār says that honey (*ʿasal al-naḥl*) or sugar syrup (*ʿasal al-sukkar*), rather than date juice (*dibs*), should be added to the *sikbāj* cooking pot as a sweetener.[17]

Ibrāhīm, the son of Caliph al-Mahdī (reigned 158–169/775–785), was well-rounded with talents for music, poetry, and cooking. Meals of his own creation

---

12 Ibn Sayyār, *Kitāb al-Ṭabīkh*, ed. K. Öhrnberg and S. Mroueh, Helsinki, 1987, 1; Nasrallah tr., *Annals of the Caliphs' Kitchens*, p. 67. Ouerfelli laments that both editors of the Arabic text (K. Öhrnberg and S. Mroueh) were unfortunately content not to supplement the interesting text with critical comments (*Le sucre*, p. 599, note 8). The English translation by N. Nasrallah is fully annotated based on the Istanbul manuscript.

13 Ibn Sayyār, *Kitāb al-Ṭabīkh*, 133; Nasrallah tr., *Annals of the Caliphs' Kitchens*, p. 250.

14 Ahsan, *Social Life under the Abbasids*, p. 83.

15 Ibn Sayyār, *Kitāb al-Ṭabīkh*, 9; Nasrallah tr., *Annals of the Caliphs' Kitchens*, p. 81.

16 Zaouali, *Medieval Cuisine*, p. 3.

17 Ibn Sayyār, *Kitāb al-Ṭabīkh*, 132; Nasrallah tr., *Annals of the Caliphs' Kitchens*, p.249.

were particularly well known in the ʿAbbasid court by the name "*Ibrāhīmīya*". According to Ibn al-Nadīm (d. 385/995), the owner of a bookshop (*warrāq*) in Baghdad, Ibrāhīm wrote what was probably the first Arabic language cookbook (*Kitāb al-Ṭabīkh*) in Islamic history,[18] but unfortunately it was misplaced and lost to us.

Ibn Sayyār's *Kitāb al-Ṭabīkh* is comprised of 132 chapters, presenting over 200 recipes. Let us look at some recipes that show the variety of meals served in the ʿAbbasid caliph court. In interpreting the Arabic text, I am quoting from Nasrallah's new English translation, entitled *Annals of the Caliph's Kitchens*, with my own revisions and added Arabic terms.

(1) *Tharīd* (Chickpea Broth) for Caliph al-Maʾmūn
Take 1/2 *raṭl* (150 grams) chickpeas (*ḥimmiṣ*) and soak them in water until they puff. Put in a clean pot, 2 disjointed plump pullets (*farrūj samīn*), and 3 dirhams (9 grams) whole cumin seeds tied in a piece of linen cloth, and enough salt. Pour on these the chickpeas liquid and add half the amount of the soaked chickpeas.

Set the pot on the fire and let it cook until the meat is half done. Add 1 *raṭl* (300 grams) of whole onions (*baṣal*) and 7 pieces of aged sharp cheese (*jubn*), each piece weighs 1 dirham (3 grams). When the two pullets and the onions are done, add to the pot 1 dirham black pepper. Break on them 7 eggs so that they look like cows' eyes (*ʿuyūn al-baqar*). Put the pot away from the heat.

Break semolina bread (*khubz samīdh*) into pieces and pour broth (*maraq*) all over the bread. Distribute the pullet pieces and onions over the sopped bread, but do not put any of the chickpeas.[19] Pour about 1/2 *raṭl* sweet olive oil (*zayt ʿadhb*) all over the dish and serve it, God willing.[20]

(2) *Samak Maḥshū* (Stuffed Fish)
Choose what you like of big fish (*samak*). Cut open it starting with the back but do not slit the belly open. The head, fins, tail, and skin should stay in one whole piece. Now, take the meat, discard the gallbladder (*marāra*) and set aside the entrails (*buṭūn*). Take additional meat from

18 Ibn al-Nadīm, *Kitāb al-Fihrist*, ed. G. Flügel, Leipzig, 1867; repr. Beirut, 1964, 116; English tr. by B. Dodge, *The Fihrist of al-Nadīm*, 2 vols., New York, 1970, vol. 1, p. 254.

19 Nasrallah notes that chickpea broth was deemed more nourishing than the chickpeas themselves (*Annals of the Caliphs' Kitchens*, p. 288, note 4).

20 Ibn Sayyār, *Kitāb al-Ṭabīkh*, 162; Nasrallah tr., *Annals of the Caliphs' Kitchens*, pp. 287–288.

other fish until you have enough to stuff the prepared fish skin (*jild*). Discard all bones.

Put the fish meat on a board and pound it very well with a knife. Sprinkle a little salt, and continue pounding until it has the consistency of the brain. Crack some eggs on it and continue pounding. Add a little sugar (*sukkar*) or honey (*ʿasal*) and ground spices (*afāwīh*) as needed such as spikenard, cloves, cassia, ginger, black pepper, cumin, and caraway seeds. Also add fermented sauce (*mā' kāmakh*) and olive oil. Chop fresh rue (*sadhāb*) and coriander leaves and add them to the fish. Add as well skinned almonds and sesame seeds. Mix all.

Stuff the mixture into the fish skin with the head, fins, and tail intact. Let the stuffing be tight no matter how big the fish is. Arrange split canes (*qaṣab*) lengthwise around the filled fish and tie it with the canes using threads at two or three places.

Line the bottom of the oven (*tannūr*) with flat tiles, enough to accommodate the length of the fish, press them onto the fire. Place the fish on the bricks and let it bake slowly.[21]

(3) *Jūdhāba* (Meat baked with Bread Pudding) for Caliph al-Muʿtamid
Take a whole semolina bread (*raghīf samīdh*) made with the finest flour, let its weight be 1 *raṭl* (300 grams). Cut it into morsel-size pieces, which you then soak in water in a green-glazed bowl (*ghaḍāra*) for about an hour. When bread pieces are saturated and puffed, put them in a big baking pan (*jūdhābadān*). Pour on them 1 *raṭl* honey, 2 *raṭl*s [pounded] rock sugar (*sukkar ṭabarzad*),[22] and 1 *raṭl* water. Mix in aromatic spices and saffron, too. Put a plump chicken (*dajāja samīna*) over the saturated and puffed bread in the pan, [and let it roast until done,] God willing.[23]

(4) *Harīsa* (Porridge) by [Ibrāhīm] Ibn al-Mahdī
Wash and scald the tripe (*kirsha*), cut it into pieces, and wash it repeatedly until it is very clean. Beat it the way you beat the meat then shred it into thin threads, the thinnest you can get them. Put the shredded tripe in the pot and pour enough fresh milk (*laban ḥalīb*) to cover it. Add cassia (*dār ṣīnī*) and galangal (*khūlanjān*), a piece each. Add as well melted

21 Ibn Sayyār, *Kitāb al-Ṭabīkh*, 78; Nasrallah tr., *Annals of the Caliphs' Kitchens*, p. 176.

22 Nasrallah notes that *ṭabarzad* was "pure and white cane sugar" (*Annals of the Caliphs' Kitchens*, p. 374, note 20), but *ṭabarzad* indicated the same rock sugar as *sukkar al-nabāt*. See Chapter Two.

23 Ibn Sayyār, *Kitāb al-Ṭabīkh*, 236; Nasrallah tr., *Annals of the Caliphs' Kitchens*, p.374.

chicken fat and ground rice (*aruzz maṭḥūn*). Stir the porridge [on the fire] until it thickens. Season it with enough salt and moisten it with kidney tallow (*shaḥm kulya*), which has been rendered in a frying pan. Ladle the porridge into a big serving bowl (*ṭayfūrīya*) and sprinkle it with a small amount of ground cassia.[24]

(5) *Qaṭā'if* (Crepes) for Hārūn al-Rashīd
Choose ripe fresh walnuts (*jawz akhḍar*) whose shells can be rubbed off, and peel off their thin skins. Chop the walnuts with a knife, the way you chop date seeds (*abzār ruṭb*). Take a similar amount of rock sugar (*ṭabarzad*), pound it, and mix it with the walnuts. Sprinkle the mix with rose water of Jūr (*mā' ward Jūrī*),[25] and mix and bind the mixture with almond oil.

Use this walnut mix to fill *qaṭā'if* crepes. Let each piece be as small as a morsel (*luqma*). Arrange them in a silver or glass cup (*jām*) in attractively organized layers and pour freshly extracted almond oil on them. Sprinkle pounded white sugar (*sukkar abyaḍ madqūq*) over and between the layers. Put the cup in a big wide bowl (*ṭayfūrīya*) filled with ice, and present it, God willing.[26]

Recipes (1), (3), and (5) were created for ʿAbbasid caliphs Hārūn al-Rashīd, al-Ma'mūn, and al-Muʿtamid. Recipe (4) is a porridge (*harīsa*) with tripe created by Ibrāhīm, son of Caliph al-Mahdī. Recipes (2), (3), and (5) are cooked with sugar, white sugar, or rock sugar. Since other recipes also include sugars, we can presume that a considerable number of recipes, among the more than 200 recipes presented by Ibn Sayyār, made use of sugar. The several examples above plainly show that various innovative new dishes using sugar, which was still an expensive commodity, were created in the ʿAbbasid court in the latter half of the tenth century. According to Arabic tradition, the *tharīd* (chickpea broth) from recipe (1) was a favorite dish of the Prophet Muḥammad.[27] But, the dish

24 Ibn Sayyār, *Kitāb al-Ṭabīkh*, 139; Nasrallah tr., *Annals of the Caliphs' Kitchens*, p. 257.

25 Ibn Ḥawqal states that rose water (*mā' al-ward*) produced in the district of Jūr was exported to all parts of the world, including Maghrib, al-Rūm, al-Andalus, Firanja (Europe), Miṣr (Egypt), al-Yaman, al-Hind, and al-Ṣīn (*Kitāb Ṣūrat al-Arḍ*, 298). See also Le Strange, *The Lands of the Eastern Caliphate*, p. 293. Nasrallah notes that Jūr was a city in the region of Fāris (Fārs), famous for its export of excellent rose water (*Annals of the Caliphs' Kitchens*, p. 423).

26 Ibn Sayyār, *Kitāb al-Ṭabīkh*, 274; Nasrallah tr., *Annals of the Caliphs' Kitchens*, pp. 422–423.

27 Zaouali, *Medieval Cuisine*, p. 68. Al-Bukhārī states that the Prophet said, "As *tharīd* is better than any other dish, Fāṭima is superior to all other women." (*Ṣaḥīḥ al-Bukhārī*, 8 vols.,

he enjoyed might actually have been a simpler *tharīd* than that of the ʿAbbasid court.

Al-Baghdādī's Kitāb al-Ṭabīkh

The career of Muḥammad b. al-Ḥasan al-Kātib al-Baghdādī is mostly unknown, with the exception of his *Kitāb al-Ṭabīkh*, which he completed in 623/1226.[28] Judging from his name, we can presume that he was born in Baghdad or lived there for quite a while, serving either the ʿAbbasid caliphs or other influentials as a scribe (*kātib*). He completed his book only thirty-two years before the Mongol army under Hülegü ransacked Baghdad and murdered al-Mustaʿṣim (reigned 640–656/1242–58), the last ʿAbbasid Caliph. Compared to the era of Ibn Sayyār, Baghdad in the first half of the thirteenth century had declined and fallen considerably under the social disorder and economic stagnation of the eleventh and twelfth centuries. Let us see what kind of cookbook Muḥammad al-Baghdādī came up with under these historically harsh circumstances.

Al-Baghdādī states the following at the beginning of *Kitāb al-Ṭabīkh*. Here also, in interpreting the Arabic text, I quote Perry's new English translation, entitled *A Baghdad Cookery Book*, adding some Arabic terms and my own revisions.

> I have come across of a number of books composed on the preparation of dishes (*ṭabīkh*), which mention strange and unfamiliar things and include disapproved ingredients. When they are brought together, the soul is not reassured by them. Men disagree in their choice among the pleasures we have mentioned, some of them preferring food over the rest and some preferring other things, such as clothing (*malbas*), drink (*mashrūb*), sex (*nikāḥ*), and listening to music (*samāʿ*). I am one who prefers the pleasure of food (*faḍl ladhdha al-maʾākil*) over all the other pleasures, so I composed this book for myself, and for whoever may want to use it in the preparation of dishes. In it, I describe my personal preferences, perhaps leaving out some obvious and well-known dishes in the interests of brevity. Following those, I describe relishes (*ṣibāgh*), condiments (*ṭayyibāt*), pickles (*mukhallal*), fish (*samak*), puddings (*jūdhāb*), and sweets (*ḥalāwa*) that are also my preferences. I have aimed at brevity and succinctness

---

Beirut, n. d., VI, 207).

28 M. Rodinson, A.J. Arberry, and Ch. Perry ed., *Medieval Arab Cookery*, Trowbridge, 2006, p. 35; Zaouali, *Medieval Cuisine*, pp. 10–11; Brockelmann, *Geschichte der Arabischen Litteratur*, S. I, p. 904.

> rather than prolixity and longwindedness, and I pray God to give me aid and grant me success.[29]

While Ibn al-Sayyār wrote his book at the ʿAbbasid caliph's request, al-Baghdādī states unequivocally that he composed the book for himself, and that its contents reflect his personal preferences. The book is composed of ten chapters: Chapter One: Sour Dishes (*ḥāmiḍ*), Chapter Two: Simple Dishes (*sadhāja*), Chapter Three: Fried and Sauceless Dishes (*qalāyā wa-nāshif*), Chapter Four: Porridges (*harīsa*) with Shredded Meat, Chapter Five: Fried Dishes (*muṭajjana*), Cold Dishes (*bārida*), Egg Dishes (*maqlūba*), and Samosa (*sanbūsaj*), Chapter Six: Fish (*samak*), Chapter Seven: Pickles (*mukhallal*), Relishes (*ṣibāgh*), and Condiments (*muṭayyiba*), Chapter Eight: Puddings Served with Roast Meat (*jūdhāba*), Pudding Thickened with Flour or Crumbs (*khabīṣ*), and Their Varieties, Chapter Nine: Sweets (*ḥalāwa*) and Their Varieties, Chapter Ten: Crepes (*qaṭā'if*), Round Cookies (*khushkanānij*), and Other Items.

Al-Baghdādī presents 160 recipes, but does not include *tharīd* (chickpea broth), a favorite dish of the Prophet Muḥammad. We will choose several recipes from his book to compare with the above recipes from the work of Ibn Sayyār.

> (1) *Sikbāj* (Sour Lamb Stew)
> The way to make it is to cut up fat meat (*laḥm thamīn*) medium and put it in the pot with water to cover it, [a bunch of] green coriander leaves (*kusfara khaḍrā*), a stick of cinnamon and the necessary amount of salt. Then, when it boils, remove its scum and froth with a spoon and throw it away. Then white onions, Syrian leeks (*karrāth shāmī*) and carrots, if in season, or eggplant (if they are not), and skin them all. Quarter the eggplant lengthwise and half boil it in salt water in another pot, then dry it and leave them in the pot on top of the meat. When it is nearly done, take wine vinegar (*khall khamr*) and thick fruit-based syrup (*dibs*) – some people prefer to use honey (*ʿasal*), but thick fruit-based syrup is more appropriate – and mix them, balancing the sourness (*ḥamūḍa*) and sweetness (*ḥalāwa*). Then pour them into the pot and boil it for a while. When the fire needs to be cut, take some of the broth and mix it with the necessary amount of saffron. Pour it into the pot. Then take peeled sweet almonds (*lawz muqashshar ḥalw*) that have been split in half and leave them on top of the pot, with a few jujubes (*ʿunnāb*), raisins (*zabīb*), and

29 Al-Baghdādī, *Kitāb al-Ṭabīkh*, Mosul, 1934, 6; English tr. by Ch. Perry, *A Baghdad Cookery Book*, Trowbridge, 2005, p. 26.

dry figs (*tīn yābis*). Cover it awhile to grow quiet on the heat of the fire. Wipe the sides of the pot with a clean cloth and sprinkle rose water (*mā' ward*) on top. When it grows quiet on the fire, take it up.[30]

(2) *Ibrāhīmīya* (Ibrāhīm's Sour Meat Dish)
The way to make it is to cut up meat medium and put it in the pot with water to cover and the necessary amount of salt. Boil it so that it stews. Put in it a piece of strong linen, tied with pounded coriander, ginger, pepper and finely pounded [galingale] inside it. Then put pieces of cinnamon (*dār ṣīnī*) and mastic (*maṣṭakā*)[31] on it, and chop up two or three small onions finely and throw them in it. When the ingredients are done, remove that cloth that the spices are in. You make a sauce with the juice of aged mild sour grapes (*ḥiṣrim 'adhb 'atīq*); if there is none, with the juice of fresh sour grapes (*ḥisrim ṭarī*) squeezed by hand, without boiling, then strained. Beat sweet almonds (*lawz ḥalw*), which have been finely pounded to a liquid consistency with water. Pour the sour grape juice on it and sweeten it with white sugar (*sukkar abyaḍ*); let it not be strongly sour. Leave it on the fire awhile to grow quiet, and wipe the sides with a clean cloth. Then sprinkle the top of it with a little rose water, and when it is quiet, take it up.[32]

(3) *Harīsat al-Aruzz* (Rice Porridge)
It is called *al-'ursīya* (the dish for a wedding ceremony). The way to make it is to cut fat meat (*laḥm thamīn*) in elongated pieces, and make it like wheat *harīsa* [that is, put meat in the pot with water to cover it, and set it over a fire. When it boils, take the meat out, remove the bones, shred it, and then return it to the pot], except that there will be coarsely pounded rice (*aruzz madqūq*) in place of wheat (*ḥinṭa*). When the meat is thrown in it, follow the procedure mentioned in wheat *harīsa* [that is, kindle the fire under it continuously from the beginning of night until the first quarter of the night has passed, stirring it the whole time. Then leave it on a good fire, and throw jointed hens and sticks of cinnamon on it, and leave it until the middle of the night. Then beat it well until it becomes smoothly thickened. Throw the necessary amount of salt on it. If it needs water, add hot water. Leave it until dawn, then beat it again, then take it up].

30 Al-Baghdādī, *Kitāb al-Ṭabīkh*, 9–10; Perry tr., *A Baghdad Cookery Book*, pp. 30–31.
31 An evergreen lacquer tree originating in the Mediterranean world.
32 Al-Baghdādī, *Kitāb al-Ṭabīkh*, 10; Perry tr., *A Baghdad Cookery Book*, p. 31.

When you ladle it out, put melted chicken fat (*dahn al-dajāj al-masbūk*) on its surface and sprinkle sugar (*sukkar*) on it.[33]

(4) *Jūdhāb al-Khubz* (Bread Pudding)
Take the crumb of leavened bread (*khubz mukhtamar*) and soak it in water or fresh milk (*laban ḥalīb*) until it sours. Put sugar (*sukkar*) and ground almonds (*lawz madqūq*) over it and under it, color it with saffron and leave it on the fire until it gives off the aroma of its doneness. Stir it, then take it up, and when it is ladled out, sprinkle it with finely ground spiced sugar (*sukkar muṭayyab masḥūq*).[34]

(5) *Qaṭā'if* (Sweet Crepe Cake)
There are several kinds. One of them is the stuffed (*maḥshūwa*), which is the kind that is baked in elongated shapes. Put finely pounded almonds and sugar (*lawz wal-sukkar al-madqūq*) in them, roll them up and arrange them (on a plate). Throw sesame oil (*sīraj*), syrup (*julāb*), rose water (*mā' al-ward*) and finely pounded pistachios (*fustuq madqūq*) on them.

Another is the fried (*maqlawa*), which is the kind that is baked in (round) cakes. Knead finely pounded almonds and sugar with rose water and put it in them. Then fold them (around the filling) and fry them in sesame oil. Take them out, dip them in syrup and take them up.

And then there is the plain (*sādhija*), which is the kind that is put in a dish and sesame oil is poured on them, and then syrup, rose water, and finely pounded pistachios.[35]

In regards to the *sikbāj* in recipe (1), al-Baghdādī notes, "Some people prefer to use honey (*'asal*), but thick fruit-based syrup (*dibs*) is more appropriate," while Ibn Sayyār says, "Now add to the pot honey (*'asal al-naḥl*) or sugar syrup (*'asal al-sukkar*)." This difference may reflect the fact that Ibn Sayyār wrote his book exclusively for kings (*malik*), caliphs (*khalīfa*), lords (*sayyid*), and dignitaries (*ra'īs*), as opposed to al-Baghdādī, who wrote for himself and for anyone wanting to use his recipes to prepare food. The *Ibrāhīmīya* of recipe (2) is believed to be a dish invented by Ibrāhīm, son of Caliph al-Mahdī, several kinds of which are also found in the book by Ibn Sayyār: for example, porridge with

33 Al-Baghdādī, *Kitāb al-Ṭabīkh*, 52–53; Perry tr., *A Baghdad Cookery Book*, pp. 72–73.
34 Al-Baghdādī, *Kitāb al-Ṭabīkh*, 70; Perry tr., *A Baghdad Cookery Book*, pp. 92.
35 Al-Baghdādī, *Kitāb al-Ṭabīkh*, 80; Perry tr., *A Baghdad Cookery Book*, pp. 103.

tripe (*harīsa min kurūsh*),[36] a turnip dish (*shaljamīya*),[37] and bird stew (*zirbāja*).[38] Regarding the *harīsat al-aruzz* (rice porridge) of recipe (3), Ibn Sayyār describes the recipe with tripe (*kirsh*), while al-Baghdādī makes it with fat meat. Both, however, seem to be simple salted dishes using neither the traditional fruit-based syrup (*dibs*) nor the recently introduced sugar. Ibn Sayyār and al-Baghdādī do not vary in their descriptions of the procedures for *jūdhāb* and *jūdhāba* in recipe (4), but Ibn Sayyār is unique in putting a plump chicken (*dajāja samīna*) over the saturated and puffed bread in the pan, and letting it roast until done. The *qaṭāʾif* of recipe (5) is a sweet cake made with various nuts, like walnuts and almonds, with sugar or rose water added to, or sprinkled over, each dish.

In comparing the work of Ibn Sayyār (in the latter half of the tenth century) with that of al-Baghdādī (in the early thirteenth century), we find no major differences in the recipes, and in particular find the common use of white sugar or rock sugar in a large number of recipes given by both authors. Also, in addition to sugar-based sweeteners, we find liberal use of various spices and flavors, like pepper, cumin, coriander, clove, cinnamon, ginger, saffron, rose water, and sesame oil. This fact clearly shows that the upper classes in Muslim societies, along with wealthy people in European countries, were the main consumers of sugar and spices in the medieval ages. We will later discuss the issue of how and when white sugar and raw sugar consumption spread among the common people of the Islamic world.

Sugar in *The Thousand and One Nights*

Alf Layla wa-Layla, or *The Thousand and One Nights*, is a world-renowned collection of Middle Eastern folktales. In Japan also, it has been translated from European languages into Japanese by various translators since the beginning of the Meiji era. Shinji Maejima recently made the first translation into Japanese from the original Arabic, based on the Calcutta 2nd edition and the Bulaq edition.[39] When revisiting it, we are deeply impressed with the unexpected twists in the stories and the humanism articulated by them, the range of set-

36 Ibn Sayyār, *Kitāb al-Ṭabīkh*, 139; Nasrallah tr., *Annals of the Caliphs' Kitchens*, p. 257.

37 Ibn Sayyār, *Kitāb al-Ṭabīkh*, 147–148; Nasrallah tr., *Annals of the Caliphs' Kitchens*, pp. 267–269.

38 Ibn Sayyār, *Kitāb al-Ṭabīkh*, 152–154; Nasrallah tr., *Annals of the Caliphs' Kitchens*, pp. 274–277.

39 Translated by Sh. Maejima and O. Ikeda, *Arabian Naito*, 18 vols., Tokyo, 1966–92.

tings from the Indian Ocean to the Mediterranean Sea, and the colorful characters, from caliphs and wazirs to merchants, female slaves, porters, and thieves. We also find numerous references to sugar and sweets, examples of which are presented in the "*Foods Palatable and Nutritious*" section below.

The World of The Thousand and One Nights

First, let us examine the Arabic texts and their translations through history. *Alf Layla wa-Layla* originated in *The Thousand Tales* or *Hazār Afsāna* in Pahlavi Persian, which was translated into Arabic in the latter half of the eighth century under the title *Alf Khurāfa* (*One Thousand Fairy Tales*). The stories then gradually took on features particular to Islam, and the name was changed to *Alf Layla wa-Layla* around the twelfth century. After that, many new stories were added in Cairo throughout the Mamluk period, and the whole work was completed in its current form between the fifteenth and sixteenth centuries.[40]

The French Orientalist Antoine Galland (1646–1715) received an Arabic manuscript from Syria in 1701, and began to translate it into French. The published translation, *Les mille et une nuits*, first appeared in Europe in 1704 (vols. 1–6), 1706 (vol. 7), 1709 (vol. 8), 1712 (vols. 9–10), and 1715 (vols. 11–12).[41] The Galland translation prompted lively discussions about the origins of *The Thousand and One Nights*, and the publication of translations in other European languages. Translators such as Edward William Lane (1801–1876), John Payne (1842–1917), Richard Burton (1821–1890), and Joseph Charles Mardrus (1868–1949) attempted to distinguish themselves with their own translations based on the Bulaq edition, the Calcutta 2nd edition, or other newly attained manuscripts.[42] However, as Muhsin Mahdi shows based on the original Syrian manuscript, these editions and manuscripts contained more than a few stories reworked or invented after Galland had published his translation. In 1984, Mahdi edited the Syrian manuscript entitled *Kitāb Alf Layla wa-Layla*, composed of two hundred and eighty-two nights.[43]

---

40 *EI*[2], s.v. Alf Layla wa-Layla (E. Littmann).

41 Translated by Antoine Galland, *Les mille et une nuits contes traduits en français*, 12 vols., Paris, 1704–17.

42 Lane's translation is based on the Bulaq edition, *The Thousand and One Nights*, also known as *The Arabian Nights' Entertainments*, 3 vols., London, 1938–41; Payne's translation is based on the Calcutta 2nd edition, *The Book of the Thousand and One Nights*, 9 vols., London, 1882–84; Burton's translation is mainly based on the Calcutta 2nd edition, *A Plain and Literal Translation of the Arabian Nights' Entertainment*, 10 vols., Benares, 1885–86; Mardrus's translation is based on the Bulaq edition, *Le livre des mille nuits et une nuits*, 16 vols., Paris, 1900–04.

43 *Kitāb Alf Layla wa-Layla*, ed. M. Mahdi, Leiden, 1984.

Mahdi's main manuscript is the Galland manuscript, which Mahdi dates to the beginning of the fourteenth century. He believes that this core of the *Arabian Nights*, that is, the fourteenth-century Mamluk version, is most likely the only authentic part of the collection that has survived.[44] Based on this conclusion, it seems quite difficult to regard some tales in the *Arabian Nights* as reflecting the realities of tenth-century Baghdad or fourteenth-century Cairo. E. Littmann summarizes the literary stages of the *Arabian Nights* as follows:

(i) An eighth-century translation of the *Hazār Afsāna* into Arabic, entitled *Alf Khurāfa*
(ii) An eighth-century Islamized version of the *Hazār Afsāna* entitled *Alf Layla*
(iii) A ninth-century composite of *Alf Layla* containing both Persian and Arabic materials
(iv) *The Arabian Nights* of the late Fatimid period
(v) A twelfth-century collection augmented mostly by Egyptian tales
(vi) The final stages of the growing collection during the Mamluk period extending to the early sixteenth century[45]

According to this summary, the stories contained in the Mahdi edition roughly cover stages (i) to (v).

Foods Palatable and Nutritious

Now let us look at several mentionings of sweet dishes, pastries, sweets, and sherbets from Haddawy's English translation,[46] with some revisions via the Mahdi edition in consideration of their unclear historical authenticity.

(1) The Story of the Porter and the Three Ladies

(The Twenty-Eighth Night)
The Porter (*ḥammāl*) carried the basket and followed her until she came to the confectioner's (*ḥalwānī*), where she bought a whole tray full of every kind of pastry and sweet in the shop, such as Cairo rolls (*Qāhirīya*), open-worked Balkan rolls (*mushabbak baylqānīya*), stuffed and musk-scented crepes (*qaṭā'if bil-musk maḥshīya*), Umm Ṣāliḥ's tokens (*dalālat*

44 Marzolph and Van Leeuwen, *The Arabian Nights Encyclopedia*, s.v. Mahdi, Muhsin, II, pp. 632–633; M. Mahdi, *The Thousand and One Nights*, Leiden, 1995, pp. 141, 164.
45 *EI*[2], s.v. Alf Layla wa-Layla (E. Littmann).
46 Translated by H. Haddawy, *The Arabian Nights*, New York and London, 1990.

Umm Ṣāliḥ), ʿUthmānī rolls (*sakab ʿuthmānīya*),[47] and date rolls (*miqraḍa*), as well as soap cakes (*ṣābūnīya*), buns (*aqrāṣ*), rice pudding (*Maʾmūnīya*), amber combs (*amshāṭ al-ʿanbar*), ladyfingers (*aṣābiʿ bānīd*), widow's bread (*khubz al-arāmil*), Kadi's tidbits (*laqīmāt al-qāḍī*), eat-and-thanks (*kul wa-ushkur*), and dried dough (*kishk al-hawā*). When she placed all the sweets (*ḥalāwa*) in the basket, the porter said to her, "Mistress, if you had let me know, I would have brought with me a nag or a camel to carry all these purchases." She smiled and walked ahead until she came to the druggist's (*ʿaṭṭār*), where she bought ten bottles of scented waters, lily water, rose water scented with musk, and the like, as well as ambergris, musk, aloewood, and rosemary. She also bought two loaves of sugar (*ublūj sukkar*) and candles and torches.[48]

(2) The Story of the Two Viziers

(The Ninety-Fourth Night)
They (Vizier Shams al-Dīn and his daughter) spent the time at the Umayyad Mosque till close to the time of the afternoon prayer; then they walked through the Grand Market (*al-Sūq al-Kabīr*) and continued walking until they came to the shop of Badr al-Dīn Ḥasan (Shams al-Dīn's nephew) and found him standing there. He had prepared a pomegranate-seed dish (*ḥabb rummān*), preserved in almond and sweet julep (*julāb maḥallā*) and flavored with cardamom and rose water (*māʾ ward*), and the food was ready to serve.[49]
(The Ninety-Seventh Night)
Badr al-Dīn's mother said, "None has cooked this (pomegranate-seed) dish but my son Badr al-Dīn, for none knows how to cook it as well as he."[50]

---

47 The text has "*sakab ʿutmānīya*" (Mahdi ed., *Kitāb Alf Layla wa-Layla*, 127).

48 Mahdi ed., *Kitāb Alf Layla wa-Layla*, 127–128; Haddawy tr., *The Arabian Nights*, pp. 67–68. Regarding the various kinds of sweets in this paragraph, see Ch. Perry, "A Thousand and One 'Fritters': The Food of The Arabian Nights," M. Rodinson, A.J. Arberry, and Ch. Perry, *Medieval Arab Cookery*, Trowbridge, 2006, pp. 487–496.

49 Mahdi ed., *Kitāb Alf Layla wa-Layla*, 267–268; Haddawy tr., *The Arabian Nights*, p. 195.

50 Mahdi ed., *Kitāb Alf Layla wa-Layla*, 272; Haddawy tr., *The Arabian Nights*, p. 199. For the pomegranate-seed dish, see Perry, "A Thousand and One 'Fritters'," p. 494.

(3) The Christian Broker's Tale

(The One Hundred and Seventeenth Night)
I (the Christian broker *al-simsār al-Naṣrānī*) entered the hall, and hardly had I sat down, when the lady came up to me, bedecked in fine clothes and ornaments, with a diadem on her head. Her face was made up, and her eyes were penciled. When she saw me, she smiled at me, pressed me hard to her bosom and, setting her mouth to mine, sucked my tongue, and I did likewise. Then she said, "Can it be true, my little lord, that you have indeed come to me?" I replied, "Yes, I am with you and I am your slave." She said, "By God, since I first saw you, I have enjoyed neither food nor sleep." I said, "I have felt the same." Then we sat down to converse, while I kept my head bowed. Soon she set before me a tray with the most sumptuous dishes, such as sour meat stew (*sikbāj*), fricassee (*ṭabāhaja*), fritters (*qarmūsh maqlī*) soaked in honey, and chickens stuffed with sugar and pistachio nuts (*dajāj maḥshī sukkar wa-fustuq*), and we ate until we were satisfied.[51]

(4) The Steward's Tale: The Young Man from Baghdad and Lady Zubayda's Maid

(The One Hundred and Twenty-Eighth Night)
Then the Lady Zubayda (the wife of Caliph Hārūn al-Rashīd) consulted the caliph about the marriage of her waiting-woman, and he gave permission and assigned ten thousand dirhams for that purpose. Then the Lady Zubayda sent for the judge and witnesses, and they drew up the marriage contract, performed the ceremony, and for ten days thereafter celebrated our wedding with sumptuous meals and sweets. At the end of the ten days, the young lady entered the bath. In the meantime they set before me the supper tray, and as there was among the dishes a great platter of meat ragout (*zīrbāja*)[52] cooked with pistachio nuts, refined white sugar (*sukkar mukarrar*), rose water, and cumin, I did not hesitate but, by God, fell upon the ragout and ate until I was satisfied. Then I wiped my hands, for God had willed that I should forget to wash them.[53]

---

51 Mahdi ed., *Kitāb Alf Layla wa-Layla*, 298; Haddawy tr., *The Arabian Nights*, pp. 222–223.

52 For the *zīrbāj* or *zīrbāja*, see the following works. Zaouali, *Medieval Cuisine*, pp. 80–81, 200; Perry, "A Thousand and One 'Fritters'," pp. 494–495; Nasrallah tr., *Annals of the Caliphs' Kitchens*, p. 620.

53 Mahdi ed., *Kitāb Alf Layla wa-Layla*, 312; Haddawy tr., *The Arabian Nights*, p. 235.

(5) The Story of Nur al-Din Ali ibn Bakkar and the Slave Girl

> (The One Hundred and Seventy-Second Night)
> When the maid came, she said, "My lord Abū al-Ḥasan, my mistress Shams al-Nahar, the favorite of the Commander of the Faithful, Hārūn al-Rashīd, bids you and my lord Nūr al-Dīn 'Alī, in the name of God, to come to her." Abū al-Ḥasan rose, saying to Nūr al-Dīn 'Alī, "Very well, my lord, let us go." They disguised themselves and followed the girl at a distance until she entered the caliph's palace and brought them to the lodging of Shams al-Nahar, where the young man (*ghulām*) found himself in a room that looked like a chamber in Paradise, furnished with couches, cushions, and pillows, the like of which he had never seen before. After he and Abū al-Ḥasan were seated and settled in their places, the black maid set a table before them and waited on them. The young man ate and marveled at the fine food: suckling lambs (*kharūf rāḍiʿ*), fatted chickens (*dajāj musamman*), and other birds, such as grouse (*qaṭan*), quail (*summān*), and pigeons (*ḥamām*), all the sugar candies (*muʿallaqāt al-sukkar*), and the jar (*sukkardān*) full of assorted pickles (*mukhallala*).[54]

These accounts describe various pastries and sweets, lamb and chicken dishes, often flavored with rose water, lily water, cumin, ambergris, musk, aloewood, and rosemary. Excerpt (1), in particular, provides us with a long list of various pastry and sweets, such as Cairo rolls, Balkan rolls, stuffed and musk-scented crepes, Umm Ṣāliḥ's tokens, 'Uthmānī rolls, date rolls, soap cakes, buns, rice pudding, amber combs, ladyfingers, widow's bread, Kadi's tidbits, eat-and-thanks, and dried dough. Along with these, we find sweet julep (*julāb maḥallā*), sugar (*sukkar*), refined white sugar (*sukkar mukarrar*), sugar loaves (*ublūj sukkar*), honey (*ʿasal*), sherbets (*sharābāt*), and fruits (*fākiha*) throughout the stories of the *Arabian Nights*. It is also quite interesting that the dishes, like the pomegranate-seed in excerpt (2), the sour meat stew and chickens stuffed with pistachio nuts in excerpt (3), and the ragout in excerpt (4), are cooked with sugar, or preserved in sweet julep. The story in excerpt (4) explains that meat ragout (*zīrbāja*) is cooked with pistachio nuts, refined white sugar, rose water, and cumin. Let us compare that with the following recipe for *zīrbāj* taken from al-Baghdādī's *Cookery Book*.

> *Zīrbāj*. The way to make it is to cut up fat meat (*laḥm thamīn*) small and put it in the pot, with enough water on it to cover it and pieces of

54 Mahdi ed., *Kitāb Alf Layla wa-Layla*, 381–382; Haddawy tr., *The Arabian Nights*, p. 297.

> cinnamon, peeled chickpeas and a little salt. When it boils, take away its scum. Then throw on a *raṭl* (300 grams) of wine vinegar, a quarter of a *raṭl* of sugar (*sukkar*) and a *ūqīya* (37.4 grams) of peeled sweet almonds (*lawz ḥulw muqashshar*), pounded fine. Mix with rose water and vinegar, then throw them on the meat. Throw on a dirham (each) of ground coriander, pepper and sieved mastic, then color it with saffron. Put a handful of split [peeled] almond on top of the pot. Sprinkle a little rose water on it, wipe its sides with a clean cloth, leave it on the fire to grow quiet, and take it up. If you like to put chicken (*dajāj*) in it, take a plucked hen and wash it and joint it. When the pot comes to the boil, throw it on the meat to become done.[55]

Al-Baghdādī presents the recipe for *zīrbāj* as cooking meat not with pistachio nuts and cumin, but with chickpeas, wine vinegar, sweet almonds, coriander, pepper, and sieved mastic. However, both recipes are similar in boiling meat with salt, sugar, and spices, and then sprinkling rose water on it before serving it. It is worth noting that the recipe in the *Arabian Nights* is nearly identical to the recipe in the actual Baghdad cookbook from the ʿAbbasid period. We can therefore presume that the descriptions of dishes and sweets in Mahdi's *Arabian Nights* reasonably represent the dietary habits common to caliphs, sultans, and wealthy people in Muslim societies from the ʿAbbasid to the Mamluk periods.[56]

Sugar in Arabic Pharmacology

We know that within Arabic pharmacology, nutrition (*ghidhāʾ*) was studied for health maintenance and disease prevention. From the tenth century, physicians of the medieval Islamic world wrote many books on nutrition (*kitāb al-ghidhāʾ*) and pharmacology (*kitāb al-dawāʾ*). Here, we will look at three Arabic language books on health and disease: *Tacuini Sanitatis* (*Taqwīm al-Ṣiḥḥa*) by Ibn Buṭlān (d. 458/1066), a Christian physician and theologian in Baghdad; *The Prevention of Bodily Ills* (*Kitāb Dafʿ Maḍār al-Abdān*) by Ibn Riḍwān al-Miṣrī

---

55 Al-Baghdādī, *Kitāb al-Ṭabīkh*, 13–14; Perry tr., *A Baghdad Cookery Book*, p. 33.

56 Muhsin Mahdi notes, "They (the audience of the *Nights*) were only too willing to transform the fictional version back into history. The same would prove to be true of audiences in later times and other countries or cultures. But it seems to have been especially true of learned Orientalists who have used the *Nights* as a source for the study of the manners and customs of Oriental societies." (*The Thousand and One Nights*, p. 180).

(388–460/998–1068), an Egyptian rival of Ibn Buṭlān; and *The Purpose of Health Maintenance and Disease Prevention* (*Jāmiʿ al-Gharaḍ fī Ḥifẓ al-Ṣiḥḥa wa-Dafʿ al-Maraḍ*) by Ibn al-Quff al-Karakī (630–685/1233–86), a Syrian physician of the Ayyubid and Mamluk periods.

Taqwīm al-Ṣiḥḥa *by Ibn Buṭlān*

Ibn Buṭlān, also known as Abū al-Ḥasan al-Mukhtār and Yuwānis b. al-Ḥasan, was a Nestorian physician and theologian born in Baghdad in the middle ʿAbbasid period. In 440/1049, after he had given lectures on physics and theology in Baghdad, Ibn Buṭlān left his native home and arrived in Cairo under the Fatimids, by way of Aleppo, Antioch, and Yaffa. He found there a strong academic rival in Ibn Riḍwān. For more than three years, the two constantly challenged each other's knowledge of Greek medicine and theology. After his stay in Cairo, Ibn Buṭlān moved to Constantinople in 446/1054, where he was involved in further disputes between the Greek and the Latin Churches. Then, he left Constantinople, secluded himself in a monastery in Antioch, and devoted himself to writing books and leading a pious life. He died in 458/1066. His major work was *Taqwīm al-Ṣiḥḥa*, although he also published a noteworthy booklet entitled *Kitāb fī Shirāʾ al-Raqīq* (*Book for Purchasing Slaves*).[57]

At the beginning of *Taqwīm al-Ṣiḥḥa*, Ibn Buṭlān explains the six principles of health maintenance.

> *Taqwīm al-Ṣiḥḥa* contains six principles for maintenance of good health, and anyone who follows them properly will be in good health for many years. The first principle is to purify the air (*hawāʾ*) arriving in the lungs. The second is to balance food (*maʾkal*) with drink (*mashrab*). The third is to regulate exercise (*ḥaraka*) and rest (*sukūn*). The fourth is to refrain from excessive sleep (*nawm*) or waking (*yaqẓa*). The fifth is to control the quantity of excreta (*faḍla*). And the sixth is to willingly accept joy (*faraḥ*), anger (*ghaḍab*), fear (*fazaʿ*), and grief (*ghamm*).[58]

In the remainder of *Taqwīm al-Ṣiḥḥa*, Ibn Buṭlān outlines the health aspects of various items based on the above principles. He addresses 280 items, including edibles such as figs (*tīn*), grapes (*ʿinab*), pomegranates (*rummān*), quince

---

57 For the career of Ibn Buṭlān, see Ibn Abī Uṣaybiʿa, *ʿUyūn al-Anbāʾ*, II, 238–242; *EI*², s.v. Ibn Buṭlān (J. Schacht); Elkhadem tr., *Le Taqwīm al-Ṣiḥḥa*, pp. 9–13. *Kitāb fī Shirāʾ al-Raqīq* is fully examined in T. Sato, *Mamlūks: Muslim Rulers from the Non-Islamic World* (*Mamuruku: Ikyo no sekai kara kita Isuramu no shihaishatachi*, in Japanese), Tokyo, 1991, pp. 24–31.

58 Ibn Buṭlān, *Taqwīm al-Ṣiḥḥa*, 71; Elkhadem tr., *Le Taqwīm al-Ṣiḥḥa*, p. 146.

(*safarjal*), bananas (*mawz*), dates (*ruṭab*), walnuts (*jawz*), wheat (*ḥinṭa*), barley (*sha'īr*), rice (*aruzz*), broad-beans (*bāqillā*), lentils (*'adas*), bread (*khubz*), lettuce (*khass*), eggplant (*bādhinjān*), onions (*baṣal*), milk (*laban*), olives (*zaytūn*), eggs (*bayḍ*), lamb (*laḥm al-ḍa'n*), beef (*laḥm al-baqar*), chicken (*dajāj*), fish (*samak*) and salt (*milḥ*); dishes such as *sikbāj*, *harīsa*, *jīrbāja*, *tannūrīya*, and *kabāb*, as well as sugar (*sukkar*), honey (*'asal*), roses (*ward*), wine (*khamr*); moods like joy (*faraḥ*), and anger (*ghaḍab*); activities such as sleep (*nawm*), exercise (*ḥaraka*), rest (*sukūn*), and bathing (*ḥammām*); fragrances like musk (*misk*), amber (*'anbar*), rose water (*mā' al-ward*); the north and south winds (*rīḥ*); and the four seasons: spring (*rabī'*), summer (*ṣayf*), autumn (*kharīf*), and winter (*shitā'*).[59]

He lists each item's qualities (under Humorism theory: hot or cold, dry or moist), characteristics, medicinal efficacy, toxicity, alleviation of its toxicity, effects, effectiveness according to the physical constitution and age of the recipient, location where it is used, and the excerpts from the results of previous research. Item number 169 is sugar.

1. Number: 169
2. Name: sugar (*sukkar*)
3. Qualities: Oribasius (ca.325-ca.400): hot and dry
4. 'Īsā al-Baṣrī (3/9 c.): Old sugar is hot and dry.
5. Yūḥannā, Yaḥyā al-Naḥawī (1/7 c.): hot and moist
6. Degrees: hot and moist
7. Characteristics: fine, white
8. Medicinal effects: It relieves internal organ pain, particularly effective in relieving pain of the kidney (*ḥashā*) and bladder (*mathāna*).
9. Toxicity: It causes thirst (*'aṭash*) and increases yellow gall (*ṣafrā'*).
10. Alleviation of its toxicity: with sourish pomegranate (*rummān muzz*)
11. Effects: It cleanses the blood.
12. Physical constitution: It is effective on people of any physical constitution.
13. Age: It is effective on people of any age.
14. Season: It is effective in any season.
15. Location: It is used exclusively in urban areas (*al-ma'mūra*).
16. Ibn al-'Abbās al-Majūsī (d. 384/994) relates: The best quality of sugar is rock sugar (*ṭabarzad*), and the best quality and taste of *ṭabarzad* is that produced in the district of al-Masruqān.[60] It is a well-balanced

59 Ibn Buṭlān, *Taqwīm al-Ṣiḥḥa*, 75–113; Elkhadem tr., *Le Taqwīm al-Ṣiḥḥa*, pp. 150–229.

60 Masruqān was located on the east bank of the Dujayl River, north of Ahwāz in the province of Khūzistān, which was famous for sugar production in districts like Ahwāz, 'Askar

> food, with a quality inclined toward hot. It is quite similar to honey (*ʿasal*), but different in that it doesn't cause thirst and supplies more nutrition. After the scum is skimmed off the boiled juice, it reduces thirst and cough (*suʿāl*), and relieves pain of the stomach, kidney, and bladder.[61]

This account indicates that sugar in the tenth century was consumed in urban, rather than rural, areas, and was a luxury good and a high-priced medicine. Ibn al-ʿAbbās al-Majūsī was either a Manichean or the descendant of one, serving ʿAḍud al-Dawla (reigned 367–372/978–983), a Buwayhid ruler in Iraq and Fārs, as a physician. Ibn al-ʿAbbās wrote two books, *Perfect Medical Technology* (*Kāmil al-Ṣināʿat al-Ṭibbīya*) and *ʿAḍud Principles for Medicine* (*al-Qānūn al-ʿAḍudī fī al-Ṭibb*).[62] The account cited above, however, is not confirmed as coming from either book. As mentioned in Chapter One, the Māsakān area of southern Iran was well known in the tenth century Islamic world for its production of high quality white sugar. But here, it says that Masruqān in the province of Khūzistān was the first district to produce high quality rock sugar (*ṭabarzad*).[63]

Ibn al-ʿAbbās explains that sugar has hot and moist qualities, reduces thirst and cough, and relieves pain of the stomach, kidney, and bladder. This is similar to explanations given by Ibn al-Bayṭār and Ibn al-Nafīs. Also, he notes that if one consumes too much sugar, it causes thirst and increases yellow gall, again not diverging from Ibn al-Bayṭār's description. We can say that Ibn Buṭlān, while referencing medical authorities like Ibn al-ʿAbbās, is unique in compiling a straight-forward manual for health maintenance, with its 280 concise entries for edible items, foods, drinks, spices, activities, living environments, and more.

Kitāb Dafʿ Maḍār al-Abdān *by Ibn Riḍwān*

Next, Ibn Riḍwān ʿAlī al-Miṣrī, who was a worthy opponent of Ibn Buṭlān. According to Ibn Abī Uṣaybiʿa, Ibn Riḍwān was born to a poor baker in al-Jīza on the west bank of the Nile. Since he could not afford to pay for a formal education, Ibn Riḍwān taught himself, and mastered medicine by reading books. His

---

Mukram, and Māsakān. See Ibn Ḥawqal, *Kitāb Ṣūrat al-Arḍ*, 254; Yāqūt, *Muʿjam al-Buldān*, v, 125; Le Strange, *The Lands of the Eastern Caliphate*, pp. 236–237.

61 Ibn Buṭlān, *Taqwīm al-Ṣiḥḥa*, 98–99; Elkhadem tr., *Le Taqwīm al-Ṣiḥḥa*, pp. 198–199.

62 *EI*², s.v. ʿAlī b. al-ʿAbbās al-Madjūsī (C. Elgood); Pormann and Savage-Smith, *Medieval Islamic Medicine*, pp. 55–56; Chipman, *The World of Pharmacy and Pharmacists in Mamlūk Cairo*, pp. 25–31.

63 According to Yāqūt, Masruqān was the name of a river which flowed in Khūzistān, where many towns (*balad*) and villages (*qarya*) were found (*Muʿjam al-Buldān*, v, 125).

opponents later on criticized him for not having studied medicine under a recognized authority. Nevertheless, Fatimid Caliph al-Mustanṣir recognized his ability and appointed him as "the head of physicians in Cairo (*ra'īs aṭibbā' Miṣr*)." Thus, his life seemed satisfactory. But one day, an orphan girl (*yatīma*) he had been raising since a great famine[64] stole and ran away with property of his, including 20,000 dinars. This bitter experience brought out his fastidious side, and from then on, he was prone to argue with those around him. This includes the three years when he frequently sparred with Ibn Buṭlān. Ibn Riḍwān devoted himself to working both as a physician and a writer, never leaving Cairo and al-Fusṭāṭ in his lifetime. Let us look at his work *The Prevention of Bodily Ills* (*Kitāb Dafʿ Maḍār al-Abdān*).

Kitāb Dafʿ consists of fifteen chapters dealing with various aspects of physical health in Egypt. Chapter 1: A Description of Egyptian Land and its Temperament, Chapter 2: A Description of the Various Kinds of Air (*hawā'*) in Egypt, Chapter 3: Six Causes of Health (*ṣiḥḥa*) and Illness (*maraḍ*) in Egypt, Chapter 4: The Seasons of the Year (*fuṣūl al-sana*) in Egypt, Chapter 5: The Incorrectness of Most of Ibn al-Jazzār's [65] Reasons for the Unhealthy Air in Egypt, Chapter 6: The Peculiarities of the Capital City (*al-madīnat al-kubrā*) of Egypt, Chapter 7: A Description of the Causes of Pestilence (*wabā'*) and Epidemic Diseases, Chapter 8: A Summary of What Has Been Said and a Commentary on the Six Causes of Health and Sickness, Chapter 9: A General Strategy for Preserving Health and Treating Illnesses, Chapter 10: The Actions Required of Egyptian Physicians (*ṭabīb*) for the Body in Egypt, Chapter 11: Prescriptions to Regulate the Body (*tadbīr al-abdān*) in Egypt, Chapter 12: How to Improve Air, Water, and Food (*ghidhā'*) Quality in Egypt, Chapter 13: How to Avoid Epidemic Diseases (*al-amrāḍ al-wāfida*) in Egypt, Chapter 14: Prescriptions (*nusakh adwiya*) to Prevent Injury and Preserve Bodily Health, and Chapter 15: The Advantages of Living in Egypt.[66]

We will examine sections from the chapters that discuss sugar.

(1) From Chapter 3: Six Causes of Health and Illness in Egypt
The Egyptians have various kinds of nutrition (*ghidhā'*). The people in Upper Egypt get nutrition from dates (*tamr*) and sweets (*ḥalāwa*) produced from sugarcane. They bring them to al-Fusṭāṭ and other districts,

64 Since Ibn Buṭlān went to Cairo and met Ibn Riḍwān in 440/1049, this was not during "the seven-year great famine (457–462/1065–70)" under the reign of al-Mustanṣir.

65 Ibn al-Jazzār Aḥmad b. Ibrāhīm was a Tunisian doctor who died in about 395/1004–5. He compiled *A Book of Medicine for the Poor* (*Kitāb Ṭibb al-Fuqarā'*) and *A Book on the Stomach* (*Kitāb al-Maʿida*). *EI*², s.v. Ibn al-Djazzār (H.R. Idris).

66 Ibn Riḍwān, *Kitāb Dafʿ*, 1; English tr. by Dols, p. 78.

> where they are sold and eaten. The people in Lower Egypt, on the other hand, get nutrition from taro (*quruqās*) and peas (*jurubbān*). They also bring them to al-Fusṭāṭ and other districts, where they are sold and eaten.[67]

This account shows that the Egyptian people in around the eleventh century made sweets from sugarcane and consumed them for nutrition. It is worth noting that Ibn Riḍwān uses the expression "the people in Upper Egypt," implying that the consumers of sweets were not limited to the caliphs and wealthy persons. We can therefore presume that the common people in Upper Egypt came to consume sweets produced from cheap raw sugar (*qand*) and molasses (*ʿasal*) during this period. Aside from the accounts of persons of power and wealth, the Arabic sources tell us relatively little about how sugar was consumed in the medieval Islamic world. In this context, an account that seems to imply the popularization of sugar consumption in Egypt is quite significant.

> (2) From Chapter 12: How to Improve Air, Water, and Food Quality in Egypt
> When the air is hot, one should consume sweets (*ḥalwā*) made of camphor (*kāfūr*), rose water (*māʾ al-ward*), sugar (*sukkar*), syrup (*julāb*), and starch (*nashāʾ*). On the contrary, when it is cold, one should consume various kinds of sweets, like figs (*tīn*), dried grapes (*zabīb*), honey (*ʿasal*), sugar (*sukkar*), walnuts (*jawz*), almonds (*lawz*), hazelnuts (*bunduq*), and pistachios (*fustuq*).[68]

The kinds of sweets prescribed vary by season, but, interestingly enough, sugar is included in both cases. Also, as the author cites walnuts, almonds, hazelnuts, and pistachios as "sweet" foods, they were likely sweetened with sugar when eaten.[69]

> (3) From Chapter 14: Prescriptions to Prevent Injury and Preserve Bodily Health
> *Sakanjabīn*, which I (Ibn Riḍwān) prescribe, is particularly effective against the retention of urine (*sadad al-būl*). Seven dirhams (about 23 grams) of chicory (*hindibāʾ*), white clover (*kushūt abyaḍ*), fennel (*rājiyānj*),

67 Ibn Riḍwān, *Kitāb Dafʿ*, 8; English tr. by Dols, p. 92.

68 Ibn Riḍwān, *Kitāb Dafʿ*, 27–28; English tr. by Dols, pp. 133–134.

69 Ibn Khalṣūn explains that walnuts (*lawz*) and hazelnuts (*bunduq*) are eaten with sugar (*Kitāb al-Aghdhiya*, 101–102).

> and celery seed (*karafs*) are required for one prescription. They are soaked together in four *raṭl*s (1.2 kilograms) of wine vinegar (*khall khamr*) for four days. Next, bitter quince (*safarjal ʿafin*) and sour grape (*ḥiṣrim*) juice are added, and boiled in a ten-*raṭl* (3 kilograms) mixture of water and sugar until they become sticky. Lastly, after adding a drop of vinegar, they should be mixed thoroughly.[70]

As mentioned above, both Ibn al-Bayṭār and Ibn al-Nafīs state that sugar is effective against the retention of urine. Ibn Riḍwān also prescribes *sakanjabīn*, incorporating a large amount of sugar, as a diuretic. He also prescribes a medicated bath made of figs (*sharāb al-tīn*) with *fānīdh* and *sulaymānī* white sugar to reduce cough and aid recovery from liver ailments.[71] These nutritional prescriptions making use of sugar were innovations of the Islamic age, and were never mentioned by Greek and Roman physicians and pharmacologists such as Dioscorides and Galen.[72]

Jāmiʿ al-Gharaḍ fī Ḥifẓ al-Ṣiḥḥa wa-Dafʿ al-Maraḍ *by Ibn al-Quff*

Ibn al-Quff Abū al-Faraj al-Karakī (630–685/1233–86) was born in the citadel city of al-Karak in the late Ayyubid period. His father, Yaʿqūb, worked in a governmental office in al-Karak, and was transferred to Ṣarkhad ten years after the birth of Ibn al-Quff. While living in Ṣarkhad, his father Yaʿqūb became acquainted with Ibn Abī Uṣaybiʿa, the compiler of the *Biographical Dictionary of Doctors* (*ʿUyūn al-Anbāʾ fī Ṭabaqāt al-Aṭibbāʾ*). Ibn Abī Uṣaybiʿa took on Ibn al-Quff as an apprentice. When Yaʿqūb was transferred again, this time to Damascus, Ibn al-Quff accompanied his father to the Syrian capital, and continued his studies there toward a mastery of medicine. During the reign of Sultan Baybars, Ibn al-Quff was sent to the citadel of ʿAjlūn,[73] north of ʿAmmān, as a physician. He wrote his first book on medical science there. Ibn al-Quff was thereafter ordered to serve in Damascus, where he continued writing until his death in 685/1286.[74] Here, we will examine his main work, *Jāmiʿ al-Gharaḍ fī*

---

70 Ibn Riḍwān, *Kitāb Dafʿ*, 32; English tr. by Dols, p. 144.

71 Ibn Riḍwān, *Kitāb Dafʿ*, 33; English tr. by Dols, p. 145.

72 We find that sugar is often used as an ingredient in the syrups described in *Minhāj al-Dukkān* by Kūhīn al-ʿAṭṭār (6/13 c.) (Chipman, *The World of Pharmacy and Pharmacists in Mamlūk Cairo*, pp. 185–270).

73 As mentioned in the Preface, I had a chance to see firsthand a set of *ublūj*, cone-shaped pieces of unglazed earthenware pottery, at a museum in the citadel of ʿAjlūn, where Ibn al-Quff first served as a physician.

74 Ibn Abī Uṣaybiʿa, *ʿUyūn al-Anbāʾ*, III, 444–445.

Ḥifẓ al-Ṣiḥḥa wa-Dafʿ al-Maraḍ, which explains in great detail about health maintenance and disease prevention.

After explanations of health maintenance for children, boys, adults, and the elderly, Ibn al-Quff goes into detail on the various aspects of meat, fish, eggs, milk, grains, sweets, fruits, and drinks. Chapter 39: On sweets, reads as follows.

> White rock sugar (*sukkar ṭabarzad abyaḍ*)
> *Ṭabarzad* is pure white in color. The best quality *ṭabarzad* is hard. It is both hot and moist to the first degrees. It provides more nutrition than honey, and removes harmful substances from bladder (*mathāna*) and kidney (*kulya*). It protects against diseases of the breast, provides nutrition to the body, and opens clogging of the liver (*kibda*) and spleen (*ṭiḥāl*).
>
> *Fānīd* [*fānīdh*] white sugar
> It is made with one loaf of sugar (*sukkar*), and dissolves easily in the mouth. It has a hotter quality than *ṭabarzad.* It is effective against chest pain (*suʿāl*) and calms one's nerves by reducing cold substances in the chest.
>
> White sugar (*sukkar abyaḍ*)
> It is made of sugar (*sukkar*) before refining or consolidation. It is boiled until it congeals and turns red. White sugar [produced by separating molasses with an *ublūj*] calms one's nerves and cleanses the digestive organs (*maʿida wa-miʿāʾ*) by expelling solids. It is therefore also used for enemas (*ḥuqna*).[75]

Ibn al-Quff, at the beginning of the rock sugar (*ṭabarzad*) entry, denounces the views of Dioscorides and Galen.

> Neither Dioscorides nor Galen understood the nature of sugar. They said, "Sugar (*sukkar*) is a kind of honey (*ʿasal*), but solid. In fertile lands like al-Hind and al-ʿArab, it congeals on [sugar] cane."[76] But these are the words of men who did not truly know sugar.[77]

---

75 Ibn al-Quff, *Jāmiʿ al-Gharaḍ*, 313–315.

76 It is doubtful that the account given by Dioscorides refers to sugar made from sugarcane. Mintz also contests R.J. Forbes's view that the account provided by Dioscorides shows that sugar was produced during the first century (*Sweetness and Power*, p. 20).

77 Ibn al-Quff, *Jāmiʿ al-Gharaḍ*, 314.

That is, Ibn al-Quff indicates that the *sakcharon* (sugar) Dioscorides and Galen spoke of was not the extracted and refined crystal sugar resulting from the sugar production process, but merely a naturally occurring product, that which congeals on sugarcane. As mentioned in Chapter One, I concur, neither Dioscorides nor Galen provides a description that would lead us to believe a method for producing sugar crystals existed in the early first century.

Next, we will look at some of the foods and drinks recommended by Ibn al-Quff for the maintenance of good health.

(1) Rice Cooked with Milk (*aruzz bil-laban*)
For the best quality, use sheep's (*ḍa'n*) milk, sweetened with white sugar. This is an optimal dish, full of nutritional value. It is effective for those suffering from pain or fatigue, and is also suitable for those with discerning palates (*murtafih*). It provides nutrition to the body and revitalizes the brain (*dimāgh*). It also reduces pains in the lungs (*ri'a*) and chest area.[78]

(2) *Kabrītīya*
For the best quality, cook with eggplant (*bādhinjān*). Cut eggplant into long pieces, soak the pieces in salted water, and then put them on lamb cut into long thin pieces [and boil them]. Then sprinkle wine vinegar (*khamra*) on them, and stir them slowly after adding sugar (*sukkar*). This dish calms the nerves and strengthens the internal organs. It may, however, cause bad dreams. Also, as it is hard to digest, this dish may be inappropriate for the elderly. It should be eaten with bitter spices.[79]

(3) Lemon and Quince Sherbet (*sharāb laymūn safarjalī*)
It warms a cold stomach (*maʿida bārida*), clears the throat of phlegm (*balgham*), and is also effective against other diseases. Mix the juice of washed, good quality quince (*safarjal*) with the juice of unsalted, good quality lemons (*laymūn*). To three *ūqīya*s (112 grams) of the mixture, add syrup (*julāb*) made from one *raṭl* (300 grams) of clean sugar, and boil. Add more small pieces of quince, and remove it from the fire when it comes to a boil.[80]

---

78 Ibn al-Quff, *Jāmiʿ al-Gharaḍ*, 282. Ibn Khalṣūn also states that rice (*aruzz;* known as *rūz* by the common people) has ample nutrition when cooked with milk (*laban*), sugar (*sukkar*), and almond oil (*dahn al-lawz*) (*Kitāb al-Aghdhiya*, 83).

79 Ibn al-Quff, *Jāmiʿ al-Gharaḍ*, 286.

80 Ibn al-Quff, *Jāmiʿ al-Gharaḍ*, 396.

As shown in the accounts above, the book discusses various nutritious foods and drinks that include sugar, and describes their prescriptions and medicinal effects in detail. Since Ibn al-Quff served the lords in ʿAjlūn and Damascus in the early Mamluk period as a physician, we can assume that his primary responsibility was studying and explaining the health and diseases of the influential and wealthy people of that time. Yet, in the above accounts, we find he also gives consideration to commoners, including children and the elderly. To further our discussion of the spread of sugar consumption among commoners, we will compare the above account by Ibn Riḍwān with the following account by al-Maqrīzī.

Hanging Candies for Children

Hanging Candies in the Month of Rajab

Al-Maqrīzī, an Egyptian historian in the seventh–eighth/fouteenth–fifteenth centuries, gives a very interesting account of a "Sweets Merchants' Market (*Sūq al-Ḥalawīyīn*)" in Cairo.

> This market was set up to sell sweets (*ḥalawīyāt*) made from sugar. Now it is called the "Various Sweets Market (*Sūq Ḥalāwa Munawwaʿa*)". This was the most excellent market in Cairo, where the streets were lined on both sides with shops (*ḥānūt*) selling heavy copper trays (*ālāt al-naḥḥās*) of superb craftsmanship, and multi-colored sweets called "mosaics (*mujammaʿa*)". Here, one *qinṭār* (96.7 kilograms) of sugar (*sukkar*) cost 170 dirhams.[81] When Egypt suffered hardship (*miḥna*) [in 817/1414] that damaged waterwheels (*dūlāb*) in Upper Egypt and sugar refineries (*maṭbakh al-sukkar*) in al-Fusṭāṭ, the price of sugar increased and the production of sweets declined.[82] Also, many sweets makers (*ṣāniʿ*) died in the disaster. Previously, I had seen carried on the trays red jars containing milk and various kinds of cheese, and sugar candies shaped like cucumbers (*khi-*

81 According to al-ʿUmarī, in early fourteenth century Egypt, 1 *qinṭār* of regular sugar (*sukkar*) sold for 150 *dirhams*, and repeatedly refined sugar (*mukarrar*) for 250 *dirhams* (*Masālik al-Abṣār fī Mamālik al-Amṣār: Dawlat al-Mamālīk al-Ūlā*, 84).

82 During the Mamluk period, sugarcane cultivation in Egypt was centered in the provinces of Upper Egypt. Raw sugar (*qand*) produced in Upper Egypt was transported to sugar refineries (*maṭbakh al-sukkar*) in al-Fusṭāṭ, where it was refined into various kinds of high quality sugar, like white sugar, repeatedly refined white sugar, and rock sugar. See Chapter Six.

yār), bananas (*mawz*), and other things. And, there were other such outstanding goods on display that amazed all who saw them.

In the month of Rajab, a beautiful sight appeared in this market: hanging sugar candies (*ʿilāqa*) shaped like horses (*khayl*), lions (*sabʿ*), cats (*quṭṭa*), and more, were hung from threads in front of the shops.[83] They all sold out, as gifts for children, every size of candy, from 1/4 *raṭl* (113 grams) to 10 *raṭls* (4.5 kilograms) in weight. Both upper class (*jalīl*) and lower class (*ḥaqīr*) customers wanted them for their families and children (*ahlih wa-awlādih*). Other markets in Cairo and al-Fusṭāṭ, and even in the suburbs (*al-aryāf*), were full of similar sugar candies. These same candies were also produced in the month of Shaʿbān, a custom that continued until quite recently. For those who visited the markets during the festival of breaking the fast (*ʿīd al-fiṭr*), when they saw sweet cakes like *khushkanānij*, *basandūd*, and *mushāsh*, their hearts leapt for joy. When sweets production began each Ramaḍān, the markets of al-Fusṭāṭ, Cairo, and the suburbs were full of these kinds of sweets. But in 817/1414, such a joyous scene could no longer be found [because of the hardship faced by Cairo.][84] Praise the Lord who changes the situation as He wishes. There is no god except Him.[85]

This account describes an annual custom in the month of Rajab in Cairo, al-Fusṭāṭ, and the suburbs of making sugar candies for children in shapes like horses, lions, and cats, and displaying them in front of shops. Ouerfelli presents this same account in his work *Le sucre*, but only as an example of sugar consumption during the festival seasons.[86] Nonetheless, the sale of sugar candies for children began in the sacred month of Rajab, and continued through the months of Shaʿbān and Ramaḍān until the festival of breaking the fast (*ʿīd al-fiṭr*). It was an annual polychromatic celebration of sugar candies that

---

83 This account describes the candies sold in the Sweets Market as being shaped like horses, lions, and cats, as well as cucumbers, bananas, and other items. We find similar items in contemporary Egypt in the *Mawlids* of the Prophet Muḥammad and sufi saints.

84 Al-Maqrīzī states in his *Kitāb al-Sulūk* that in Muḥarram 817/March 1414 strong winds and heavy rains pummeled al-Fusṭāṭ (IV, 280), and in Muḥarram 818/March 1415 plague (*ṭāʿūn*) began to spread in Cairo (IV, 301). He says crop prices then rose sharply in Egypt and Syria (IV, 330–331), and many people died due to a shortage of bread in the markets (IV, 335). According to Ibn Taghrībirdī, in 818/1415 plague appeared in Cairo, and spread further the following year (*al-Nujūm al-Zāhira*, XIV, 26, 41).

85 Al-Maqrīzī, *al-Khiṭaṭ*, II, 99–100.

86 Oeurfelli, *Le sucre*, p. 571. Regarding sweets in the month of Rajab, we also find a brief account in Ashtor, "Levantine Sugar Industry in the Later Middle Ages," p. 95.

continued on and off for three months from the beginning of Rajab to the end of Ramaḍān.

The Generalities of Sugar Consumption

Al-Maqrīzī states in the above account, "Both upper class (*jalīl*) and lower class (*ḥaqīr*) customers wanted them (sugar candies) for their families and children." Reflecting on Islamic history, we do not see the terms *jalīl* and *ḥaqīr* indicating any actual social classes in Muslim societies. Generally speaking, the Muslim societies of medieval Islam were classified into the *khāṣṣa* and the *ʿāmma*: the *khāṣṣa* consisted of caliphs and their families, sultans and their families, amirs, *mamlūk*s, high officials, and major merchants (*tājir*), while the *ʿāmma* consisted of minor merchants (*sūqa*) and artisans (*ṣāniʿ*) in the markets, religious intellectuals (*ʿulamāʾ*), scribes (*kātib*), and notaries public (*shāhid*).[87] It is reasonable to presume that the above *jalīl* roughly implies the *khāṣṣa*, and the *ḥaqīr*, the *ʿāmma*. We note that in fourteenth-fifteenth century Cairo and al-Fusṭāṭ, not just the privileged classes of influential and wealthy people, but also common people without property wanted to buy sugar candies for their families and children.

Ibn Riḍwān, in eleventh century Cairo, states that the people of Upper Egypt get their nutrition from dates (*tamr*) and sweets (*ḥalāwa*) produced from sugarcane, which suggests that the common people had adopted a habit of eating cheap sweets made from raw sugar and molasses. Ibn al-Quff, in the thirteenth century, explains about various nutrients employing sugar, and medicinal prescriptions for the commoners. In considering these accounts along with al-Maqrīzī's above description of sugar candies, we can presume that the consumption of raw sugar and molasses, not refined sugar, had already begun to spread among the common people of Egypt around the eleventh century.

Up until now, researchers on sugar production, trade, and consumption in medieval Islamic history had presumed that sugar was a luxury good, something that was only consumed as sweets in the homes of the privileged classes, and given as gifts from the ruling authorities during festival seasons. Which is to say that the only time common people would encounter sugar was as a medicine when they were severely ill. Ashtor, for example, states, "Although a large quantity of sugar was consumed in the courts and by the privileged persons, Egypt and Syria during the thirteenth century could export the surplus sugar to

87 For the terms *khāṣṣa* and *ʿāmma* in Muslim societies, see the following works: R. Mottahedeh, *Loyalty and Leadership in an Early Islamic Society*, Princeton, 1980, pp. 154–155; Sato, *State and Kingship in Islam* (*Isurāmu no kokka to oken*, in Japanese), Tokyo, 2004, pp. 90–94; Durand-Guédy, *Iranian Elites and Turkish Rulers*, pp. 27–29, 254.

European countries."[88] According to Ashtor, and as was my understanding as well, since sugar was an important commercial product under the control of the government, the common people would only have had chances to taste sugar when they were ill, or during the festival seasons.[89] However, based on the research results discussed above, I now believe that the availability of inexpensive sweets gradually expanded from the *khāṣṣa* to the *ʿāmma* of Egypt in about the eleventh century. As sugar production increased, changes in diet first appeared in the *khāṣṣa*, and later extended to the *ʿāmma*.

88 Ashtor, "Levantine Sugar Industry in the Later Middle Ages," pp. 95–96; id., *A Social and Economic History*, p. 306.

89 Sato, *State and Rural Society*, p. 215.

Epilogue

The Revival of Sugar Production in Egypt

Sugar production in Egypt and Syria declined rapidly as the Mamluk economy stagnated in the fifteenth century. As we saw in Chapter Five, al-Maqrīzī cites three main causes for the famine and price increases: political corruption, the land tax increases, and the circulation of copper coins. In contrast to al-Maqrīzī's explanation, A. Udovitch speculates that the repeated outbreaks of plague from the mid-fourteenth century would have reduced the rural and urban populations of Egypt. Since agricultural products were generally less expensive than artisanal products, the *muqṭa*ʿs that relied on land tax in kind would have suffered a great loss of tax revenue. So, they had to resort to increasing taxes to recover their *iqṭā*ʿ revenues. This, according to Udovitch, indicates that the "political corruption" suggested by al-Maqrīzī may actually have been a *result* of economic decline, rather than the *cause* of it.[1]

Nevertheless, Egyptian peasants were annually given land to farm according to a *qabāla* contract with their *muqṭa*ʿs, and most peasants were provided with seeds (*taqāwī*) for farming (*ʿimāra*). Also, the *muqṭa*ʿs were obliged to provide maintenance for the irrigation systems, which meant employing peasants in corvée (*sukhra*) labor every winter.[2] These facts indicate that Egyptian agriculture was closely tied to administrative affairs (*tadbīr*). We can also see that there was a close relationship between a just or unjust government and agricultural success or failure in the Islamic Middle East.[3] Thus, we cannot simply

1 A. Udovitch, "England to Egypt, 1350–1500: Long-term Trends and Long-distance Trade, IV. Egypt," M.A. Cook ed., *Studies in the Economic History of the Middle East*, London, 1970, pp. 115–128. E. Ashtor also discusses the technological decline of the sugar industry in the Levant in the later middle ages, indicating some relationship between technological decline and demographic decline. See "Levantine Sugar Industry in the Late Middle Ages," pp. 117–120.

2 Sato, *State and Rural Society*, pp. 177–233.

3 Ann K.S. Lambton stresses that the absence of effective government often led to a decline in agricultural prosperity in medieval Iran ("Reflections on the Role of Agriculture in Medieval Persia," A.L. Udovitch ed., *The Islamic Middle East, 700–1900*, 1981, pp. 283–312). Stuart J. Borsch also indicates that al-Maqrīzī's observations should be given due credit, stressing his account that *Kitāb al-Sulūk* describes the decay of the irrigation system and links it to corruption (*fasād*) in the administration (*The Black Death in Egypt and England: A Comparative Study*, Cairo, 2005, p. 43). See also the revisionary view in Udovitch's new article, A.L. Udovitch, "Technology, Land Tenure, and Rural Society: Aspects of Continuity in the Agricultural History

 | DOI 10.1163/9789004281561_010

dismiss al-Maqrīzī's view on the grounds that he mistook the results for the cause.

To produce sugar in Egypt, a government also needed a firm grasp on power in order to build and maintain the irrigation systems and guard against pillaging by the Bedouins (*ʿUrbān*). But, as explained in Chapter Three, by the fifteenth century the Mamluk government had lost the ability to maintain the social order needed for stable economic activities. So, for a fuller understanding of the socio-economic decline of the late Mamluk period, we also need to think about the problems associated with keeping social order, not just the plague-related population declines.

Historical research to date has shown that the economic decline of Ottoman Egypt continued from the early sixteenth century to the dissolution of the Mamluk regime following Napoléon's invasion of Egypt in 1798. The production of sugar from sugarcane followed a similar downward trajectory, steadily declining until the beginning of the "modern era" at the end of the eighteenth century. Nelly Hanna, on the other hand, disputes this commonly held view. In her recent work entitled *Making Big Money in 1600*, she argues that Egyptian sugar production largely recovered during the sixteenth and seventeenth centuries. Allow me to summarize her findings, which are based on Arabic court records housed at Dār al-Wathāʾiq in Cairo.

The revival and growth of the sugar industry is particularly significant because it was linked to demand and financed by the merchants who eventually exported sugar to other parts of the Ottoman Empire. It was probably their financial support that helped the industry come out of the deep crisis it had experienced in the fifteenth century. The revival of the economy at the end of the sixteenth and beginning of the seventeenth century is a clear indication that the three centuries from that time to the dissolution of the Ottoman Empire should not be viewed as one long line of unrelenting decline. Such an approach can only blur the complex realities of the period. The Egyptian merchants in this period replaced the *Kārimī* merchants of the Mamluk period as the bringers of both raw materials like rice and grain, and finished products like sugar and linen, to Anatolia, the Holy Cities of Mecca and Medina, and the European markets.[4]

Among these commodities, traditional sugar from Egypt and the newly appearing coffee from Yemen were particularly important to the growth of the Egyptian economy. Ismāʿīl Abū Ṭāqīya (d. 1034/1624) and his family played a

of the Pre-Modern Middle East," id. ed., *The Islamic Middle East, 700–1900: Studies in Economic and Social History*, Princeton, 1981.

4 Hanna, *Making Big Money*, pp. 6, 12–14.

major role in the commercial revival of sixteenth to seventeenth century Egypt. Abu Ṭāqīya, who was active for about forty years in the 1580–1620's, invested capital in sugarcane plantations and the sugar industry in the provinces of al-Manūfīya and al-Gharbīya in Lower Egypt. He profited greatly from the export of refined sugar to Istanbul, Damascus, Jedda, al-Bilād al-Rūmīya, and Venice. In 1613, Abū Ṭāqīya was appointed as "head of the merchants' guild (*shāhbandar al-tujjār*)" apparently due to his successful sugar business.[5]

However, the situation changed drastically during the eighteenth century, when the refineries of Marseille, Trieste, and Fiume started exporting their own sugar to a number of centers in the Ottoman Empire, thus depriving the Egyptian sugar industry of some of its major outlets. After the middle of the nineteenth century, Egypt was forced to produce raw materials and import finished products from the European countries, with the development of a dependent economy.[6]

The above summarizes Hanna's findings on the revival of the Egyptian economy, specifically the sugar industry, in the sixteenth and seventeenth centuries. Halil Inalcik, the author of *The Ottoman Empire*, also states, "After the conquest of Egypt in 1516–17, Egypt and Syria were vital to the economy of Istanbul and the empire. Provisions for the sultan's Palace, such as rice, wheat, barley, spices, or sugar, came by galleon from Egypt, and in the sixteenth century Syria annually sent 50,000 kg. of soap to the Palace."[7] Hanna further notes that the sugar produced in rural areas was known as dark sugar (*sukkar khām*), which was both consumed locally and exported. Whereas the imperial palace in Istanbul would presumably have used the most luxurious kind of sugar, the white refined sugar (*sukkar mukarrar*) that was primarily produced in Cairo.[8] This is significant because it leads us to conclude, as discussed in the previous chapter, that the consumption of raw sugar (*qand*) and molasses (*ʿasal*) gradually began to expand to the common people (*ʿāmma*) in Egypt from around the eleventh century. Also, it is believed that the edge-type mill for pressing sugarcane was replaced by the roller-type mill as a part of the process of revitalizing the sugar industry. However, this technological innovation is not fully explained in this work. It remains an important subject for future research using the Arabic and Ottoman Turkish source materials.

5 Hanna, *Making Big Money*, pp. 36, 79, 90–91.

6 Hanna, *Making Big Money*, pp. 6, 170–171.

7 H. Inalcik, *The Ottoman Empire: The Classical Age 1300–1600*, English tr. by N. Itzkowitz and C. Imber, London, 1973, p. 128.

8 Hanna, *Making Big Money*, p. 88.

The Expansion of Sugar Production to the Caribbean Islands and South America

The sugar industry that had developed in the Eastern Islamic world expanded through North Africa and the Mediterranean Islands to al-Maghrib and al-Andalus, where in the fifteenth century the Portuguese and the Spanish adopted the technologies used to produce sugar. As A.W. Mintz tells us in *Sweetness and Power*, "In the fifteenth century both powers (Portugal and Spain) looked for favorable locales for sugar production: while Portugal seized São Tomé and other islands, Spain captured the Canaries. After about 1450, Madeira was the leading supplier, followed by São Tomé; by the 1500's, the Canary Islands had also become important. And both powers experienced a growing demand for sugar."[9] That is, Portugal and Spain fought and captured new territories where they steadily farmed and produced sugar through the fifteenth century.

Mintz goes on to explain, "The sugar industries in the Spanish and Portuguese Atlantic islands were characterized by slave labor, a tradition supposedly transferred from the Mediterranean sugar plantations of the Arabs and Crusaders."[10] However, as discussed in Chapter Two, we lack conclusive evidence that slaves were employed at the sugarcane farms and sugar refineries of the medieval Islamic world. Regarding the Madeira archipelago under Portuguese rule, Norio Kinshichi says, "From the middle of the fifteenth century, the arable lands used for sugarcane increased at the expense of reduced wheat farming. Henry the Navigator (1394–1460) helped settlers get quality sugarcane plants from Sicily, and installed water wheels for sugar production in 1452. This resulted in sugar becoming the leading industry on the main island of Madeira."[11] Henry, a well-known prince of Portugal, led expeditions to West Africa and into the Atlantic Ocean, emboldening Portuguese advances overseas.

By the 1530's, sugar production had shifted to the Caribbean Islands, and began to decline on the Madeira Islands. Sugarcane was first brought to the New World by Christopher Columbus (ca. 1451–1506) on his second voyage in 1493. He transported sugarcane from the Canary Islands to Spanish Santo Domingo, where it would first be grown in the New World, and from whence [raw] sugar was first shipped back to Europe, beginning in around 1516.[12] According to N. Deerr, monarchs Ferdinand and Isabella, who had captured Granada in

9 Mintz, *Sweetness and Power*, pp. 31–32.

10 Mintz, *Sweetness and Power*, p. 32.

11 N. Kinshichi, *Henry the Navigator* (*Enrike kokai oji*, in Japanese), Tokyo, 2004, p. 86.

12 Mintz, *Sweetness and Power*, p. 32.

1492, issued orders the following year that Columbus "should take with him twenty field experts in cultivation and a supply of all sorts of seeds and plants [including sugarcane]." "In Isabella (a settlement founded by Columbus) were sown the first seeds brought by Columbus, and such was the fertility of the soil that the planters saw in a few days potent proof of the unbelievable rapidity with which grew the vines, the wheat, and the sugarcanes."[13] It is said that Venetian merchants provided ample funds for Spain's new venture, sending Columbus to "the Fertile Asia."

Columbus remained firmly under the misconception that the Caribbean Islands he visited were a part of India. His misunderstanding nevertheless resulted in a revolutionary enterprise. The Caribbean Islands rapidly developed large-scale sugarcane plantations, typically utilizing African slave labor. By the 1520's, Brazil was shipping raw sugar to Lisbon, and soon the sixteenth century became the century of Brazilian sugar.[14] England took possession of Barbados and Jamaica for sugarcane farms, expelling the Portuguese from the area. Most of the raw sugar produced there was shipped to Liverpool, Bristol, London, Amsterdam, Nantes, and Marseille, where it was refined and then distributed to the European markets. But even into the seventeenth century, a mass demand for sugar in Europe failed to materialize. Citing Mintz again, "Until the eighteenth century, sugar was really the monopoly of a privileged minority, and its uses were still primarily as a medicine, as a spice, or as a decorative (display) substance."[15]

Sugar Meets Coffee and Tea

As coffee houses began appearing in London and Paris in the mid-seventeenth century, and then as the custom of drinking tea spread through Europe, the use of sugar rapidly became commonplace. There have been numerous studies on the advent of coffee and tea in Europe. Let us look at sugar as the sweetener in the coffee and tea of those studies. One of the first points worth noting is that in seventeenth and eighteenth century Europe, sugar from the New World, produced with techniques from the Islamic world, was used in coffee from the Arabian Peninsula and green tea (later red tea) from Asia.

As R.S. Hattox discusses in great detail in his *Coffee and Coffeehouses*, coffee (*qahwa*) was first consumed by the sufis of the Arabian Peninsula in

13 Deerr, *The History of Sugar*, vol. 1, pp. 116–117.

14 Mintz, *Sweetness and Power*, p. 33.

15 Mintz, *Sweetness and Power*, p. 45.

the mid-fifteenth century when the Ethiopian coffee plant was brought to the Mocha (al-Mukhā) region of western Yemen. They roasted the beans of the plant (*bunn*), ground them, and drank the boiled grounds as coffee. This may very well have originated with the Shādhilīya sufi order, who believed that anything that could help them stay awake and alert could be seen as an aid to nightly devotional activities.[16] However, as coffee was said to be in the same category as wine (*khamr*), some ʿulama repeatedly forbade its consumption in accordance with the Islamic law prohibition of alcohol. Nevertheless, the custom of drinking coffee soon spread to Mecca, the central city of Islam. Thereafter, coffeehouses (*maqhā*) first appeared in Cairo in the early sixteenth century,[17] and similar coffeehouses (*kahvekhane*) in Istanbul in 1554. From all historical accounts, in these early days of coffee, sugar was seldom if ever used, and milk was almost never added.[18]

The first coffeehouse in Europe appeared in Oxford. It was started in 1650 by a Jewish man named Jacob (Yacob). It was Turkish in style,[19] which indicates that the coffeehouses of Istanbul may have served as a model. Jacob soon relocated his new business to London, and other coffeehouses then opened in Oxford. Shortly thereafter, coffeehouses began appearing in Cambridge, too. All these coffeehouses were exclusively for men.[20] It is said that by the end of the eighteenth century, the English had begun to add milk and sugar to their coffee.

The first café in France opened in Marseille, the entrepôt of Levant trade, around the middle of the seventeenth century. Many cafés then opened in Paris in the 1680's, where members of the new bourgeoisie class passionately debated politics and the arts. According to J. Grehan, during Napoléon's occupation of Egypt (1798–1801), the Egyptians mocked the French soldiers for

16 R.S. Hattox, *Coffee and Coffeehouses: The Origins of a Social Beverage in the Medieval Near East*, Seattle and London, 1985, pp. 14, 23, 24–25.

17 Coffee is also said to have been first introduced in Egypt by sufis in the early 16th century, who used it to keep awake during their *dhikr*. See N. Hanna, "Coffee and Coffee Merchants in Cairo 1580–1630," M. Tuchscherer ed., *Le commerce du café avant l'ère des plantations coloniales*, Cairo, 2001, p. 94.

18 Hattox, *Coffee and Coffeehouses*, pp. 46–52, 77, 83.

19 A. Kobayashi, *Coffeehouses: Urban Life in Eighteenth Century London* (*Kofi hausu: Toshi no seikatsushi 18 seiki no London*, in Japanese), Tokyo, 1984, pp. 16–17. According to S.D. Smith, the first Oxford coffee house opened between 1649 and 1650 ("The Early Diffusion of Coffee Drinking in England," M. Tuchscherer ed., *Le commerce du café avant l'ère des plantations coloniales*, Cairo, 2001, p. 248).

20 Kobayashi, *Coffeehouses*, pp. 41–42.

sweetening their coffee with sugar.[21] This shows that the French had embraced the custom of drinking coffee with sugar by the end of the eighteenth century.

In 1610, a ship owned by the Dutch East India Company carried Japanese green tea from Hirado in Nagasaki to the Netherlands. The custom of drinking tea subsequently caught on in the Netherlands, later spreading to France and England. People purchased their tea from the above-mentioned coffeehouses. In particular, a coffeehouse in London named Garraway sold high quality teas that were believed effective in preventing and recovering from disease. In the eighteenth century, the custom of drinking green tea with sugar spread among the ladies of the upper classes of England. Then, in the nineteenth century, the practice of enjoying tea with added milk and sugar made its way into the working and lower middle classes. Sugar consumption rose sharply as black tea replaced green tea among the common people. S. Tsunoyama tells us in *A World History of Tea*, "In early eighteenth century England, people had already developed the custom of drinking tea with the inevitable milk and sugar. The sugar in those days was a cone-shaped hard loaf to be broken into pieces when used."[22] "A cone-shaped hard loaf of sugar" may well indicate sugar refined with the cone-shaped earthenware (*ublūj*) widely used in the Islamic world. This shows that the medieval Islamic technology for refining sugar was brought not only to the New World, but also to early modern England.

In November 1806, when Napoléon Bonaparte issued the Berlin Decree that mandated a continental blockade against England, European countries began using sugar beets instead of sugarcane to produce sugar. Faced with no more raw sugar coming from the West Indies, the European states acted quickly and decisively to develop an industrialized method of producing sugar from domestic beets. Since sugar beets grow well in cold climates, production today has spread to Western Europe, Eastern Europe, Russia, North America, Turkey, Northern China, and Japan (Hokkaido), while sugarcane is still primarily grown in the subtropical climates of Brazil, India, South China, Thailand, Mexico, and Egypt. In 2008, global sugar production amounted to about 162,500,000 tons, with sugarcane accounting for 129,650,000 of those tons (79.8%), and sugar beets accounting for the remaining 32,850,000 tons (20.2%).[23]

---

21 J. Grehan, *Everyday Life and Consumer Culture in 18th-Century Damascus*, Seattle and London, 2007, p. 137.

22 S. Tsunoyama, *A World History of Tea* (*Cha no sekaishi*, in Japanese), Tokyo, 1980, p. 93.

23 International Sugar Organization, *Sugar Year Book*, 2009.

Coffee, Tea, and Sugar in Contemporary Muslim Societies

As mentioned above, the custom of drinking coffee began in the Arabian coastal town of al-Mukhā at the beginning of the fifteenth century, and subsequently spread to Cairo and Istanbul by way of Mecca around the middle of that century. But then, what about Damascus and Aleppo, which lie between Cairo and Istanbul? According to Abdul-Karim Rafeq, coffee drinking became the norm in both Damascus and Aleppo under Ottoman rule in around the 1530's, a bit later than in Cairo. The chief Ottoman judges in both cities repeatedly banned coffee, not because they thought consuming coffee was wrong, but because coffee would have become unfairly associated with persons of ill repute.[24] Some coffeehouses, mostly frequented by soldiers, were located near the citadel in Damascus, and others were established in caravansaries serving merchants and travelers, or were built close to mosques and sufi shrines.[25] Rafeq goes on to say that from the 1730's, the traditional Yemeni coffee imported into Syria began to encounter competition from the new colonial coffee. And more than a century later in the 1870's, we find that a cup of coffee *without* sugar at any of the coffeehouses in Damascus cost five *paras*, which implies that coffee *with* sugar was also common in that era.[26]

Next, let us look the debut of tea in the Islamic world. By the middle of the eighth century, some Muslim merchants were traveling as far as the southeast China coastal cities. These merchants brought their knowledge of Chinese tea and its consumption back to the Muslim peoples of the Middle East. For example, an anonymous compilation from 237/851, titled *Akhbār al-Ṣīn wal-Hind*, tells us that the king of China secured income (*ma'din*) for the state with monopolistic policies on salt (*milḥ*) and herbs (*ḥashīsh*). The herbs, called tea (*sākh*), were drunk with hot water and sold at high prices in every town.[27] However, other Arabic geographical works written in around the tenth century make no mention of importing tea from China or a custom of drinking tea in the Islamic world. Neither Ibn Buṭlān nor Ibn Riḍwān makes any reference to drinking tea to prevent disease or as a medical treatment. Berthold Laufer, the author of *Sino-Iranica*, speculates, not based on any particular reliable sources, that the custom of drinking tea seems to have spread to western Asia no earlier

---

24 A. Rafeq, "The Socioeconomic and Political Implications of the Introduction of Coffee into Syria. 16th-18th Centuries," M. Tuchscherer ed., *Le commerce du café avant l'ère des plantations coloniales*, Cairo, 2001, p. 129.

25 Rafeq, "The Socio-economic and Political Implications," p. 131.

26 Rafeq, "The Socio-economic and Political Implications," pp. 131, 139.

27 Anon., *Akhbār al-Ṣīn wal-Hind*, ed. and French tr. by J. Sauvaget, Paris, 1948, 18.

than the thirteenth century, and that it was perhaps the Mongols who assumed the role of propagators.[28]

Laufer, meanwhile, cites the travel accounts of J.A. de Mandelslo, published in 1662, as stating that the Persians drank *kahwa* (coffee) rather than *thè* (*tea*).[29] In Ottoman Egypt as well, we find coffee, sugar, and tobacco, rather than green tea or black tea, on an inventory of goods traded by Ismāʿīl Abū Ṭāqīya from the 1580's to the 1620's.[30] The people of Istanbul, who had exclusively drunk coffee in the *kahvekhane*s that appeared in the mid-sixteenth century, began drinking tea only when the price of coffee rose after the First World War. Nor does Edward W. Lane refer to tea drinking in his work *An Account of the Manners and Customs of the Modern Egyptians*, which describes in minute detail the social life of Egypt in the early nineteenth century.[31] Based on these instances, we can presume that the custom of drinking tea with sugar took root in the Islamic world only after the eighteenth or nineteenth centuries.

In contemporary Cairo, each year as the Birthday of the Prophet (*Mawlid al-Nabī*, 12 Rabīʿ I) draws near, bridal figurines made from colorful sugar candies, and boxes filled with sweets shaped like radishes, carrots, eggplants, strawberries, and other things are displayed in the fronts of shops. We can presume that this tradition comes from "the hanging sugar candies for children" described by al-Maqrīzī in *al-Khiṭaṭ*. Also, Ṭanṭā in Lower Egypt has the well-known mausoleum of Aḥmad al-Badawī (d. 675/1276), a popular sufi saint of the Muslims of medieval Egypt. On his three birthday celebrations (17 or 18 January, the Vernal Equinox, and about one month after the summer solstice),[32] his devotees visit the mausoleum, buying sweets made from chickpeas as they exit. When they return home, they divide them up as gifts for their families and neighbors, believing the sweets to be filled with the blessings (*baraka*) of the sufi saint.

Nowadays, sugar is omnipresent in Egypt. When the sugar production season arrives each winter, small pieces of the cone-shaped raw sugar (*jallāb*) are sold in the shops along the streets. Boiled sugar juice is poured into the bowl of a hookah (*arghīla*, *narjīla*) until it solidifies into *jallāb*. It is quite interesting to see that popular sweets are made using parts from the hookahs that are ubiquitous in the day-to-day life of the common people.

---

28 Laufer, *Sino-Iranica*, p. 553.

29 Laufer, *Sino-Iranica*, p. 554.

30 Hanna, *Making Big Money*, pp. 78–79.

31 Lane, *An Account of the Manners and Customs of the Modern Egyptians*.

32 These three great festivals are held annually in Ṭanṭā as the result of the indigenization of Muslim veneration in Egypt. See *EI*^{2}, s.v. Aḥmad al-Badawī (K. Vollers and E. Littmann).

Glossary

The asterisk mark (*) indicates a term that is explained under its own, separate heading.

amīr, pl. umarāʾ	A military officer who was obliged to retain a fixed number of soldiers based on his *iqṭā** revenue. In the Mamluk era, the ranks of the amirs were systematized into amirs of ten (*amīr ʿashara*), forty (*amīr ṭablkhāna*), one hundred (*amīr miʾa*), etc.
amīr al-ḥājj	The amirs who oversaw the Meccan pilgrimages from Iraq, Syria, and Egypt, and provided protection for the pilgrims. Annually appointed by the sultan.
ʿāmma	The common people, as opposed to the *khāṣṣa**, including the merchants and artisans of the markets, *imāms* and *khaṭībs* of the mosques, scholars, notary publics, scribes, etc.
ardabb, irdabb	A unit of volume. One *ardabb* is equal to six *waybas*, or about 90 liters.
aruzz, ruzz	Rice cultivated mainly in the coastal areas south of the Caspian Sea, Southern Iraq, al-Fayyūm in Upper Egypt, and later, the provinces of Lower Egypt.
ʿasal	The molasses separated out from the *qand** after the first boiling of pressed sugarcane juice. The refined molasses obtained after the second boiling was called *quṭāra*. Honey was also called *ʿasal*.
ʿashshāb	A herbalist or pharmacologist.
ʿaṭṭār	A druggist or perfumer in the markets who sold spices, perfumes, and various kinds of sugar as medicine. It is said that an *ʿaṭṭār* would have been knowledgeable about drugs (*ʿaqqār*), medicines (*dawā**), drinks (*sharāb**), and flavors (*ṭīb*).
ʿazq	The act of loosening soil to remove weeds from fields, specifically for sugarcane cultivation.
bāʾiʿ, pl. bāʿa	A small scale bazaar merchant dealing in small capital transactions, also known as a *sūqa**. See also *tājir*.
baqar, pl. abqār	Oxen used to plough or drive waterwheels (*dūlāb**, or *sāqiya**) for irrigation and pressing sugarcane.
bayt al-dafn	The "burial house" for *ublūjs**, where *ublūjs* containing boiled sugarcane juice were covered with soil and then sprayed with water to separate out the molasses.

bayt al-nuwab	The house where the cleaned sugarcane was cut into small pieces in preparation for pressing with edge mills (*ḥajar**).
Dār al-qand	A storehouse for raw sugar (*qand**), first constructed in al-Fusṭāṭ in the Fatimid period. The raw sugar produced at high officials' estates or amirs' *iqṭā*ʿs was transported to the *Dār al-qand*, where various taxes were levied. This storehouse was under the control of the Fatimid, Ayyubid, and Mamluk governments.
dār ṣīnī	Cinnamon. The Arabic name originating from "a fragrant wood grown in China."
dawāʾ, pl. adwiya	A drug. Classified into two types: simple drugs (*adwiya mufrada*) and compound drugs (*adwiya murakkaba*).
dhirāʿ, pl. adhruʿ	A unit of length. In medieval Egypt, one *dhirāʿ* was equal to 24 *iṣba*ʿs, or about 58 centimeters.
dibs	A traditional thick syrup or molasses made from boiled grapes, figs, apricots, dates, etc. It was the most common sweetening additive before sugar from sugarcane.
dīnār, pl. danānīr	A denomination of gold coin currency. One dinar was equal to 14 silver dirhams* during the Buwayhid period, around 38 dirhams during the Ayyubid period, and 20 dirhams in the first half of the Mamluk period.
dirham, pl. darāhim	A denomination of silver coin currency. For exchange rates in gold coins, see *dīnār*.
dīwān, pl. dawāwīn	An administrative office. During the Ayyubid and Mamluk periods, various governmental offices, such as *dīwān al-kharāj*, *dīwān al-rasāʾil*, and *dīwān al-barīd*, played important roles in central administration. The amirs of the Mamluk period also had *dīwān al-amīr*s that managed their *iqṭā*ʿs.
ḍiyāfa	Items like grain, fowl, goats, clover, dough, and cakes, that were given by peasants to their *muqṭaʿ* as a tribute. In Syria, this was called the "tax on festivals and Thursday" (*rasm al-aʿyād wal-khamīs*).
dūlāb, pl. dawālīb	A waterwheel on the banks of the Nile used to irrigate cultivated fields or press harvested sugarcane to produce raw sugar (*qand**).
faddān, pl. fadādīn	This term originally meant a pair of cows for plowing. In Egypt, it meant a unit of cultivated land equal to 6,006 m^2 during the Ayyubid period, and 6,368 m^2 during the Mamluk period.
fallāḥ, pl. fallāḥūn	A peasant; specifically an independent farmer or tenant farmer who farmed land under a *qabāla* contract by means of family

	labor, essentially synonymous with *muzāriʿ**, legally different from a slave.
fānīdh	White sugar, sometimes spelled *fānīd. Fānīdh māsakānī* from Māsakān was particularly well-known in the medieval Islamic world.
fasād	Social disorder or disasters caused by *ʿUrbān* or peasant uprisings in rural areas, and civil discord (*fitna*) in urban areas. See *ʿimāra*.
funduq	The Arabic term for a hotel, from which the Italian term "*fóndaco*" originated.
Geniza	A Hebrew term meaning a storage space for documents. A massive collection of Arabic documents written in Hebrew script, found at a synagogue in al-Fusṭāṭ in 1889, are commonly referred to as "the Cairo Geniza Documents."
ghidhā, pl. aghdhiya	Various kinds of nourishment, both for maintaining health and preventing disease.
ghulām, pl. ghilmān	Originally it meant a youth, servant, or page, but after the ʿAbbasid period, it was also used to mean a young slave soldier, synonymous with a *mamlūk*. The non-slave youths or servants who worked in the sugar factories of Egypt were also called *ghilmān* in Arabic papyri.
ḥajar	A stone mill for pressing small pieces of sugarcane. The edge type mill was widely used in the medieval Islamic world, rather than the roller type mill.
ḥalāwa, ḥalwā	Various kinds of sweets.
ḥalwānī	A merchant who traded various kinds of sweets (*ḥalwā**).
harīsa	Gruel with meat.
ḥawḍ, pl. aḥwāḍ	The annually occurring basin of irrigation water that formed after the flooding of the Nile. After the mud had settled, the water would be released back to the Nile with the breaking of the dikes (*jisr**).
ḥawṭa	The attachment of a property by the government, usually followed by its confiscation (*muṣādara**).
ḥiml	The load a camel carries, approximately 250 kilograms.
ḥisba	The function of a person who is effectively entrusted with supervising the moral behavior and markets of a town. A person entrusted with *ḥisba* was called a *muḥtasib**.
Ibrāhīmīya	A dish bearing the name of Ibrāhīm Ibn al-Mahdī, an ʿAbbasid prince said to have created it.

ʿīd al-aḍḥā	The Feast of Immolation, or Greater Bairam, after the completion of the *ḥajj* pilgrimage to Mecca.
ʿīd al-fiṭr	The Feast of the End of the Ramaḍān Fast, or Lesser Bairam.
ifṭār	The daily after-sunset breaking of the Ramaḍān fast. Also, the breaking of the Ramaḍān fast on the first sighting of the new moon in Shawwāl. A large amount of sugar and sweets are consumed for the *ifṭār.*
ʿilāqa	The hanging sugar candies shaped like horses (*khayl*), lions (*sabʿ*), cats (*quṭṭa*), and other things, hung by strings in the fronts of shops in the markets of Cairo and al-Fusṭāṭ in the month of Rajab.
ʿimāra	Generally this term means "building" or "prosperous conditions." The *muqṭa*'s were required to practice *ʿimāra*; that is, to construct hospitals, mosques, and schools, and to manage the irrigation systems used for farming. See also *fasād.*
iqṭāʿ, pl. iqṭāʿāt	The land or, rarely, taxes allocated by a great amir or sultan to soldiers in return for military service (*khidma**). *Khubz** (bread) was synonymous with this term. The holder of the *iqṭāʿ* was called a *muqṭaʿ* in Arabic and an *iqṭāʿdār* in Persian.
iqṭāʿ darbastā	The term *darbastā* is derived from the Persian *dar-basta* (complete). The *iqṭāʿ darbastā* was a privileged *iqṭāʿ* holding; that is, its holder had the right to receive all associated revenues, including poll taxes and the property of heirless persons in addition to the land tax (*kharāj**).
jarīb, pl. ajriba	A unit of area used in Iraq and Iran. During the Buwayhid period, one *jarīb* was equal to 10 *qafīz*s (about 1,592 m^2).
jisr, pl. jusūr	An irrigation dike designed to contain water and form a temporary basin (*ḥawḍ**) after the annual flooding of the Nile. They were classified as either *al-jusūr al-sulṭānīya*, under government control, or *al-jusūr al-baladīya*, under the control of *muqṭa*'s and peasants.
jūdhāba	A pudding made with a flat loaf of bread, honey, rock sugar, and saffron.
julāb	Fruit juice.
kabrītīya	Stewed lamb with added wine, vinegar, and sugar.
kaʿk	A round or ring-shaped biscuit made of flour or starch, sweetened with sugar, and flavored with musk or rose water.
kammūn	Cumin. There are many different species of cumin plant, named for their region of origin: *kammūn fārisī, kammūn shāmī, kammūn ḥabashī*, etc.

Kārimī — The Muslim merchants who traded spices, perfumes, sugar, pottery, textiles, and other goods between the Indian Ocean and the Mediterranean Sea during the Ayyubid and Mamluk periods.

kātib, pl. kuttāb — A scribe. Some *kuttāb* worked at *dīwān*s* as administrators, while others served amirs as managers of *iqṭā*ʿs*. In medieval Egypt, the requisite knowledge and techniques of the secretariat (*kitāba*) were passed down through distinguished Coptic families.

kattān — Flax or linen. Linen textiles remained popular among the Egyptians even in the Ayyubid and Mamluk periods. Flax and linen were also the main raw materials for the paper (*kāghad*) produced in the Islamic world.

khābiya — A large boiler for boiling the juice from pressed sugarcane. One *khābiya* held 3,000 *raṭl*s, which is about 2,880 kilograms.

khalīj, pl. khuljān — A canal, larger than *turʿa** canal. For example, in al-Fayyūm province in the thirteenth century, 58 *khalīj*s branched off from the Yūsuf canal. These canals allowed water to flow into the fields through smaller channels (*turʿa*).

kharāj — The land tax levied on peasants; the most important tax collected by a government or *muqṭaʿ*. During the Mamluk period the *kharāj* in Lower Egypt was partly levied in cash. See also *ʿushr*.

khāṣṣa — A privileged class composed of a caliph or sultan, their families, amirs, high officials, and wealthy merchants. See also *ʿāmma*.

khawājā — An Arabic adaptation of *hoca*, the Turkish term for "teacher." During the Mamluk period, this title was given to influential merchants who came from outside the territory.

khawlī, pl. khawala — An overseer of agricultural production in Egypt who was knowledgeable about crops and farming. This person was responsible for providing support to farms and, along with the village *shaykh*s, for breaking open irrigation dikes.

khidma, pl. khidam — Services rendered to the sultan in return for *iqṭāʿ* holdings. In addition to military service, *khidma* also implied obligations to construct citadels, assist in irrigation work, and attend the sultan's banquets (*simāṭ**).

khilfa — Sugarcane from the second of two consecutive growing seasons. The second-year sugarcane yielded a smaller harvest than *raʾs**, but made better quality sugar.

khubz, pl. akhbāz	Literally "bread," the staple food made from wheat (*qamḥ*) in the Middle East. In Egypt and Syria after the Ayyubid period, it was often used to denote *iqṭāʿ**, in the sense of *iqṭāʿ* being the foundation of a soldier's day-to-day life.
khushkanānij	A round cake or cookie with almonds and pistachios.
kiswa	The black silk drape used to cover the Kaʿba, embroidered with verses from the Qur'an. The Egyptian sultans of the Mamluk period had the privilege of presenting a new *kiswa* each year during the *ḥajj* pilgrimage season.
kuḥl	Antimony sulfide or lead sulfide, used to color the eyelids. It was traditionally sold together with sugar, which was believed to prevent irritation of the eyes.
kunāfa	A cake covered with vermicelli, baked in sugar, butter, and honey. One of the sweets typically eaten at night during Ramaḍān.
kuzbara	Coriander, also known as *kusbara*.
laban	Milk. When the juice from pressed sugarcane was boiled, *laban ḥalīb* (cow's milk) was added to absorb impurities.
layālī al-waqūd al-arbaʿ	The four bonfire nights from the beginning of Shaʿbān to the end of Ramaḍān. Starting in the Fatimid period, on these four nights, authorities donated various sweets to historically important mosques in Cairo and al-Fusṭāṭ.
māʾ al-rāḥa	The "water of repose". A rural Egyptian term for the water periodically irrigated for sugarcane.
māʾ al-ward	Rose water. Classified into two kinds; one for scents, and the other for cooking.
maḥāla, pl. maḥal	An Egyptian word for a wooden waterwheel used to elevate irrigation water, also called a *sāqiya**.
maḥmil	A palanquin used in caravans travelling to Mecca for the *ḥajj* pilgrimage, symbolizing the protective role of the Mamluk and Ottoman sultans, also commonly known as a *maḥmal*.
maks, pl. mukūs	Miscellaneous taxes, also called *rasm* (pl. *rusūm*), such as the port tariffs on grains (*maks sāḥil al-ghalla*), the tax on the Storehouse for Raw Sugar (*rusūm dār al-qand*), the governor's tax (*rusūm al-wilāya*), the tax on sugarcane (*sajn al-aqṣāb*), and so on.
maqhā	A coffee house, first appearing in Cairo and Istanbul in the first half of the sixteenth century, and later appearing in European cities like Oxford, London, and Paris from the mid-seventeenth century. In Istanbul, they were known as *kahvekhane*.

maʿṣara li-qaṣab al-sukkar A sugarcane pressing factory, usually located adjacent to cultivated fields. After the roots and leaves were cut off the cane, it was pressed in a stone mill (*ḥajar*) worked by oxen. The resulting juice was boiled to produce raw sugar (*qand*) and molasses (*ʿasal*). See also *maṭbakh al-sukkar* and *ublūj.*

maṣlaḥa, pl. maṣāliḥ Social welfare; as opposed to social disorder (*fasād**) or calamity (*miḥna**). This meant administrative measures to promote prosperity and welfare through the practice of *ʿimāra**; that is, the management and control of irrigation systems and the construction of mosques, hospitals, and markets.

maṭbakh al-sukkar A sugar factory producing raw sugar (*qand**). Also used to indicate a sugar refinery where raw sugar was repeatedly boiled to produce a range of types of sugar, from brown to white varieties. Al-Fusṭāṭ had many refineries owned by sultans, amirs, the *Kārimī*s, and Jewish merchants. See also *maʿṣara li-qaṣab al-sukkar.*

miḥna, pl. miḥan Calamity or hardship brought about by widespread crop failures, wind storms, locusts, inflation, plagues, etc. Contrast with *ʿimāra** and *maṣlaḥa**.

miḥrāth, pl. maḥārīth A plough pulled by oxen or camels. A typical peasant (*fallāḥ**) would have a plough and a pair of oxen. See also *muqalqila.*

mubāshir The officials working at the central and provincial *dīwāns**. The *iqṭāʿ* officials employed in *dīwān al-amīr* were also called *mubāshir*s. Many of them were chosen from among the Copts in medieval Egypt.

muḥtasib A person responsible for maintaining social order, specifically to ensure fair commercial transactions in the markets. His office was called *ḥisba**.

muqalqila, pl. muqalqilāt A large plough; originally denoting "something that shakes or disturbs." As sugarcane plantations spread into Egypt, the *muqalqila* was invented for deeper cultivation. See also *miḥrāth.*

muqṭaʿ An *iqṭā** holder; *iqṭāʿdār* in Persian sources, a person obliged to perform military service (*khidma**) for the sultan in return for an *iqṭāʿ* holding.

murābiʿ, pl. murābiʿūn A tenant farmer who had the right to keep one fourth of his crop yield. In Egypt during the Ayyubid and Mamluk periods, most of them grew sugarcane. They were subordinate to the *muzāriʿūn** who formed the majority of Egyptian rural society.

muṣādara To confiscate property. The Muslim governments from the ninth century regarded *muṣādara* as a means of supplementing fiscal

	deficits. During the ʿAbbasid period, a special office (*dīwān al-muṣādara*) was instituted to manage and control confiscation by officials.
Muslimānī al-Qibṭ	Coptic converts to Islam. During the Ayyubid and Mamluk periods, a significant number of the *Qibṭ* converted to Islam to get preferential treatment from the bureaucratic governments.
mustawfī al-dawla	The state treasurer. This person served in the central offices (*dīwān**) managing fiscal affairs. Typically chosen from among the Copts, who handed down the knowledge and techniques required for regional governance in Egypt.
muzāriʿ, pl. muzāriʿūn	A farmer. In the early Islamic period, it meant a tenant farmer who had made a *muzāriʿ* contract with the government or a landlord. Under the *iqṭāʿ* system, this term was synonymous with a *fallāḥ** (farmer or tenant), legally different from a slave. See also *murābiʿ*.
qabāla	An annual farming contract made between the proprietors (the government or a *muqṭaʿ*) and peasants after the annual flooding of the Nile.
qamḥ	Wheat; also called *ḥinṭa*; planted in October and harvested in April and May. The main ingredient in the chief staple food, bread (*khubz**).
qand	The raw sugar produced from the first boiling of pressed sugarcane juice, often called red sugar (*sukkar aḥmar*). The *qand* produced in rural areas was transported to al-Fusṭāṭ where it was refined into white sugar. European candy derives from *qand*. See also *ʿasal* and *sukkar*.
qaṣab al-sukkar	Sugarcane; sometimes called "Persian cane" (*qaṣab fārisī*) or *qaṣab* for short in Arabic; *nāy-shakar* in Persian; grown mainly in southwestern Iran, southern Iraq, Syrian coastal districts, and Egypt. The sugarcane harvested in the first year was called *raʾs**, and the harvest in the second year *khilfa**.
qaṭāʾif	Sweet crepes, with added walnuts, rock sugar, white sugar, rose water, and almonds. One of the sweets typically eaten at night during Ramaḍān.
qinṭār	A unit of weight. one *qinṭār* was equal to 45 kilograms in medieval Egypt. Sugar was customarily weighed in *qinṭār*s *jarwī* (about 96.7 kilograms).
quṭāra	A fine molasses obtained through repeated boilings and refinings with an *ublūj**.
raʾīs al-ʿashshābīyīn	Chief Pharmacologist. An honorary post given by the Ayyubid and Mamluk sultans to eminent pharmacologists.

ra'īs al-aṭibbā'	Chief Physician. An honorary post given by the Ayyubid and Mamluk sultans to superb physicians.
ra'īs al-tujjār	Chief Merchant. An honorary post given by the Mamluk sultans to influential merchants. In Ottoman Egypt, this post was called *shāhbandar*.
ra's	Sugarcane harvested in the first of consecutive growing seasons. It yielded more than *khilfa**, but produced lesser quality sugar. See also *qaṣab al-sukkar*.
rasm al-aʿyād wal-khamīs	Literally the "tax on festivals and Thursday"; goods given by Syrian peasants as tribute to their *muqṭaʿ* or to government officials. In Egypt, these were known as *ḍiyāfa**.
raṭl	1/100 *qinṭār**; about 300 grams during the ʿAbbasid period, and 450 grams during the Ayyubid and Mamluk periods. Sugar in Egypt was customarily weighed in *raṭl jarwī* (967 grams).
rawk	A cadastral survey; originating from the Coptic *rosh* meaning "land survey." In addition to land surveys (*misāḥa*), it was also used to denote an assessment of annual revenue (*ʿibra*), and reallocation of *iqṭā*'s to amirs and *mamlūk* cavalrymen. In Egypt and Syria under the *iqṭāʿ* system, three main *rawk*s were carried out: *al-Rawk al-Ṣalāḥī* (567–577/1171–2–1181–2), *al-Rawk al-Ḥusāmī* (697/1298), and *al-Rawk al-Nāṣirī* (713–725/1313–1325).
rishwa, pl. rishan	Bribery; also known as *badhl* or *barṭala*. During the latter half of the Mamluk period, men often used bribery to obtain positions such as judge (*qāḍī*), professor (*mudarris*), or governor (*wālī*, *nā'ib*).
safarjal	Quince. Sherbet mixed with boiled quince juice and sugar was used as a health drink, as was rose water (*mā' al-ward**).
sakanjabīn	A sweet vinegar; effective against urinary retention.
sāqiya	A waterwheel operated with oxen, donkeys, or camels. Buckets for drawing up water by hand were called *shādūf*s.
shādd	An *iqṭāʿ* official; also called a *mubāshir**. His duties were overseeing cultivation, collecting unpaid taxes, and punishing criminals.
sharāb, pl. sharābāt	Sweet drinks with the juice of pressed lemons, figs, oranges, apples, etc., with added sugar and water. The English term "sherbet" originated from *sharābāt*.
sharāb al-tīn	Fig drinks to strengthen liver function and reduce coughing.
sikbāj	A lamb and eggplant dish cooked with salt, coriander, cinnamon, wine vinegar, and *dibs** or sugar. Sour meat stew.
simāṭ	A tablecloth; also used at banquets (*walīma*) held by sultans and amirs to present a wide variety of sugar and sweets. Attendance

	at such banquets was considered a *muqṭaʿ*'s service (*khidma**) to the sultan.
simsār, pl. samāsīr	A broker; especially one who dealt in crops.
ṣīnīya	A large, round, brass or copper tray, as made in medieval Egypt.
sukhra	The corvée labor required of peasants to dig and repair canals (*khalīj**) and construct irrigation dikes (*jisr**) each winter. See the term *ʿimāra*.
sukkar	The Arabic word for sugar; adapted from *shakar* in Persian, which came from *sarkarā* in Sanskrit. English *sugar*, French *sucre*, and German *Zucker* all originated from *sukkar* in Arabic.
sukkar abyaḍ	The white sugar obtained from repeated refinings; synonymous with *sukkar mukarrar**.
sukkar aḥmar	The red sugar synonymous with *qand**. In Ottoman Egypt, it was also called *sukkar khām* (raw sugar).
sukkar fānīdh	*Fānīdh** white sugar, also known as *sukkar fānīd*.
sukkar māsakānī	The white sugar produced in Māsakān in southern Iran.
sukkar mukarrar	The white sugar obtained through repeated refinings.
sukkar al-nabāt	Rock sugar. Twigs from a date plant were added to a pot of the high-grade molasses (*quṭāra*) obtained from repeated boilings of pressed sugarcane juice. The pure sugar stuck to the twigs, forming small angular crystals (*ḥajar ṣaghīr*). Rock sugar thereby came to be called *sukkar al-nabāt*, or plant sugar.
sukkar qifṭī	High quality white sugar produced in the province of Qifṭ in Upper Egypt.
sukkar sulaymānī	White sugar made in the province of Sulaymān in Southwestern Iran.
sukkar ṭabarzad	Solid white sugar. It is also called *sukkar ublūj**. The Arabic word *ṭabar* is borrowed from the Persian word for a hatchet or an axe used to break a solid, cone-shaped loaf of sugar into small pieces.
sukkar ublūj	The cone-shaped loaf of white sugar produced through refinings with an *ublūj**, also called *sukkar ṭabarzad**.
sukkardān, pl. sukkardānāt	A container for keeping sugar. The *dān* part of the word is from a Persian affix denoting a container.
sukkarī	A Muslim or Jewish merchant specializing in sugar.
sūqa	A small-scale bazaar merchant, also known as a *bāʾiʿ**. See also *tājir*.
taḥkīr	The monopolistic policy used by Mamluk sultans to control the sales of pepper and sugar. This policy dealt a severe blow to the *Kārimī** merchants who had enjoyed privileged commerce be-

	tween the Indian Ocean and the Mediterranean Sea during the Ayyubid and Mamluk periods.
ṭāḥūn, pl. ṭawāḥīn	A mill operated with oxen, donkeys, or water.
tājir, pl. tujjār	A major merchant with ample capital who dealt in various commodities. See also *bāʾiʿ* and *sūqa*.
taqāwī, sing. taqwīya	The seeds or cash given or rented to peasants before crop planting in autumn.
ṭarḥ	The government control of merchant transactions.
ṭāʿūn	The plague; during the Ayyubid and Mamluk periods, Egypt and Syria were repeatedly hit by *ṭāʿūn* and *wabā** (epidemics).
turʿa, pl. turaʿ	A small canal or watercourse carrying water from a larger *khalīj** canal to the cultivated fields after the annual flooding of the Nile.
ublūj, pl. abālīj	A cone-shaped piece of earthenware pottery used to separate sugar from molasses (*ʿasal**). A loaf of sugar produced with this device was also called an *ublūj* in Arabic and an *āblūj* in Persian. One *ublūj* was a ninth of a *qinṭār** *jarwī* (about 10 kilograms) in Egypt during the Mamluk period. The *ublūj* of Mamluk Egypt was adopted by China during the Yüan dynasty, where it was called a *wa liu* (瓦溜) meaning "an earthenware pot."
ūqīya	A unit of weight for drugs and rock sugar; about 37.4 grams.
ʿUrbān	Arab cattlebreeders or sometimes farmers. They kept order in the regional provinces, providing horses, camels, and information on the borders to the government, but also tended to rob travellers on the pilgrimage to Mecca and comercial caravans. They lead peasant revolts against heavy taxation.
ʿushr, pl. aʿshār or ʿushūr	The tithe of ten percent according to Islamic law. The early *fiqh* works define *ʿushr* as a tax on the land owned by Muslims, or as a tax on commercial goods to be paid by both Muslims and non-Muslim merchants.
wabāʾ	The various epidemics, including the plagues (*ṭāʿūn**) that intermittently ravaged Egypt and Syria from the early Islamic period.
Zanj	Black slaves brought in from the coastal regions of East Africa during the ʿAbbasid period. They were employed solely to revitalize the salt-damaged soil (*sibākh*) of southern Iraq, but not forced to work on sugarcane farms.
zīrbāj	A sweet and sour dish of meat or chicken prepared with fruit or nuts.

Bibliography

Arabic Manuscripts

Anon., *Kitāb al-Ḥāwī lil-Aʿmāl al-Sulṭānīya*, Paris, Bibliothèque Nationale, MS. Arabe 2462.

Al-ʿAynī, Badr al-Dīn Abū Muḥammad Maḥmūd b. Aḥmad (762–855/1361–1451), *ʿIqd al-Jumān fī Taʾrīkh Ahl al-Zamān*, Istanbul, Süleymaniye Kütüphanesi, MS. Haci Beşir Ağa 457.

Al-Bakrī, Abū ʿUbayd ʿAbd Allāh b. ʿAbd al-ʿAzīz (d. 487/1094), *Kitāb al-Masālik wal-Mamālik*, Wien, Österreichische Nationalbibliothek, MS. Cod Mixt 779.

Baybars al-Manṣūrī, Rukn al-Dīn al-Dawādārī (d. 725/1325), *al-Tuḥfat al-Mulūkīya fī al-Dawlat al-Turkīya*, Cairo, Maʿhad al-Makhṭūṭāt al-ʿArabīya, MS. Taʾrīkh 614.

———, *Zubdat al-Fikra fī Taʾrīkh al-Hijra*, London, British Library, MS. Add. 2332511.

Ḥasan al-Ḥanafī, Ḥasan b. Ḥusayn (9/15 c.), *al-Nuzhat al-Sanīya fī Akhbār al-Khulafāʾ wal-Mulūk al-Miṣrīya*, Istanbul, MS. Konstantiniye 1302.

Al-Ḥusaynī, Shams al-Dīn Muḥammad (d. 676/1277), *Majmaʿ al-Akhbār fī Manāqib al-Akhyār*, Cairo, Dār al-Kutub al-Miṣrīya, MS. Taʾrīkh 1245.

Ibn Abī al-Damm (d. 642/1244), *al-Shamārīkh min al-Taʾrīkh*, Oxford, Bodleian Library, MS. Marsh 60.

Ibn Abī al-Hayjāʾ (d. 589/1193), *Taʾrīkh Ibn Abī al-Hayjāʾ*, Cairo, Maʿhad al-Makhṭūṭāt al-ʿArabīya, MS. Taʾrīkh 945.

Ibn al-ʿAwwām, Abū Zakariyā Yaḥyā b. Muḥammad (6–7/12–13c.), *Kitāb al-Filāḥat al-Musulimīn al-Andalusīyīn*, Paris, Bibliothèque Nationale, MS. Arabe 2804.

Ibn Aybak al-Dawādārī, Abū Bakr b. ʿAbd Allāh (d. 8/14 c.), *Durar al-Tījān wa-Ghurar Tawārīkh al-Azmān*, Istanbul, Süleymaniye Kütüphanesi, MS. Damad Ibrahim Paşa 911–912.

Ibn Dāwūd al-Ayyūbī, al-Ḥasan b. Dāwūd (d. 656/1258), *al-Fawāʾid al-Jallīya fī al-Farāʾid al-Nāṣirīya*, Cairo, Dār al-Kutub al-Miṣrīya, MS. Adab 2293.

Ibn Dāwūd al-Miṣrī, Nūr al-Dīn (d. 779/1377), *Kitāb al-Luʾluʾ al-Manḍūd fī Mā bi-Miṣr*, Istanbul, Süleymaniye Kütüphanesi, MS. Süleymaniye 838.

Ibn Ḥabīb al-Ḥalabī, Badr al-Dīn Abū Muḥammad al-Ḥasan (d. 779/1377), *Kitāb Durrat al-Aslāk fī Dawlat al-Atrāk*, Istanbul, Süleymaniye Kütüphanesi, MS. Damad Ibrahim Paşa 911–912.

Ibn Ḥajar al-ʿAsqalānī, Shihāb al-Dīn Aḥmad (773–852/1372–1449), *Badhl al-Māʿūn fī Fawāʾid al-Ṭāʿūn*, University of London, School of Oriental and African Studies, Arabic Manuscripts, No. 13998.

Ibn Iyās, Zayn al-Dīn Muḥammad al-Jarkasī (852–ca.930/1448–ca.1524), *Kitāb Nuzhat al-Umam fī ʿAjāʾib wal-Ḥikam*, Istanbul, Süleymaniye Kütüphanesi, MS. Ayasofya 3500.

———, *Nashq al-Azhār fī ʿAjāʾib al-Aqṭār*, Istanbul, Süleymaniye Kütüphanesi, MS. Haci Beşir Ağa 497–498.

———, *ʿUqūd al-Jumān fī Waqāʾiʿ al-Azmān*, Istanbul, Süleymaniye Kütüphanesi, MS. Ayasofya 3311.

Ibn Mammātī, *Kitāb Qawānīn al-Dawāwīn*, Damascus, Maktabat al-Asad, MS. Microfilm No. 672

Ibn Minkalī, Muḥammad (d. 784/1382), *al-Aḥkām al-Mulūkīya fī al-Ḍawābiṭ al-Nāmūsīya*, Cairo, Dār al-Kutub al-Miṣrīya, MS. Furūsīya Taymūr 23.

Ibn Mubārak, Aḥmad b. Mubārak (d. 867/1458), *Muntakhabāt fī ʿIlm al-Filāḥa*, Istanbul, Süleymaniye Kütüphanesi, MS. Şehezade Mehmet 81.

Ibn Taghrībirdī, Jamāl al-Dīn Abū Maḥāsin Yūsuf (ca.812–874/ca.1409–1470), *Kitāb Mawrid al-Laṭāfa fī Man Waliya al-Salṭana wal-Khilāfa*, Damascus, Maktabat al-Asad (Dār al-Kutub al-Ẓāhirīya), MS. ʿĀmma 3395.

Ibn Waḥshīya, Abū Bakr Aḥmad b. ʿAlī al-Kasdānī (3/10 c.), *Kitāb al-Filāḥat al-Nabaṭīya*, Oxford, Bodleian Library, MS. Hunt 340.

Ibn Waṣīf Shāh (d. 599/1202–3), *Taʾrīkh Akhbār al-Diyār al-Miṣrīya*, Cairo, Dār al-Kutub al-Miṣrīya, MS. Taʾrīkh Dhakīya 57.

Ibn Wāṣil, Jamāl al-Dīn Muḥammad b. Sālim (d. 697/1298), *Kitāb al-Taʾrīkh al-Ṣāliḥī*, Istanbul, Süleymaniye Kütüphanesi, MS. Fatih 4224.

———, *Mufarrij al-Kurūb fī Akhbār Banī Ayyūb*, Paris, Bibliothèque Nationale, MS. Arabe 1702.

ʿImād al-Dīn al-Iṣfahānī, Abū ʿAbd Allāh Muḥammad (d. 597/1201), *al-Barq al-Shāmī*, Oxford, Bodleian Library, MS. Bruce 11 (vol. 3), Marsh 425 (vol. 5).

Al-Jawharī, ʿAlī b. Dāwūd (d. 887/1482), *al-Durar al-Thamīn fī Mā Warada fī Miṣr*, Paris, Bibliothèque Nationale, MS. Arabe 1813.

Al-Khazrajī, Aḥmad b. Muḥammad (d. 875/1471), *Kitāb Nayl al-Rāʾid fī al-Nīl al-Zāʾid*, Istanbul, Süleymaniye Kütüphanesi, MS. Ayasofya 3528.

Al-Khazrajī, Muḥammad b. Ibrāhīm (d. 656/1258), *Taʾrīkh Dawlat al-Akrād wal-Atrāk*, Istanbul, Süleymaniye Kütüphanesi, MS. Hekimoğlu Ali Paşa 695.

Al-Makhzūmī, Abū al-Ḥasan ʿAlī b. ʿUthmān (d. 585/1189), *Minhāj fī ʿIlm Kharāj Miṣr*, London, British Library, MS. Add. 23483.

Al-Nuwayrī, Shihāb al-Dīn Aḥmad b. ʿAbd al-Wahhāb (677–733/1279–1333), *Nihāyat al-Arab fī Funūn al-Adab*, Cairo, Dār al-Kutub al-Miṣrīya, MS. Maʿrifa ʿĀmma 549.

Al-Qāḍī al-Fāḍil, ʿAbd al-Raḥīm al-Baysānī (d. 596/1200), *al-Fāḍil min Kalām al-Qāḍī al-Fāḍil*, London, British Library, MS. Add. 7307.

Al-Ṣafadī, Ṣalāḥ al-Dīn Khalīl Ibn Aybak (d. 764/1363), *Nuzhat al-Mālik wal-Mamlūk*, London, British Library, MS. Or. 6267.

Al-ʿUmarī, Shihāb al-Dīn Aḥmad Ibn Faḍl Allāh (700–749/1301–1349), *Masālik al-Abṣār fī Mamālik al-Amṣār*, Istanbul, Topı Kapı Saray Müzesi, Yeni Kütüphanesi, MS. Ahmed III 2797-a3; Facsimile edition by Fuat Sezgin, 27 vols., Frankfurt am Main, 1988–89.

Printed Primary Sources

Anon., *Akhbār al-Dawlat al-ʿAbbāsīya*, ed. ʿAbd al-ʿAzīz al-Dūrī and ʿAbd al-Jabbār al-Muṭṭalabī, Beirut, 1971.

Anon., *Akhbār al-Ṣīn wal-Hind*, ed. and French tr. by J. Sauvaget, Paris, 1948; Japanese tr. by Hikoichi Yajima (*Chugoku to Indo no Shojoho*), Tokyo, 2007.

Anon., *Alf Layla wa-Layla*, 2 vols., Bulaq, 1252H.; repr. Baghdad, n. d.; *Kitāb Alf Layla wa-Layla*, ed. Muhsin Mahdi, Leiden, 1984; English tr. by Husain Haddawy, *The Arabian Nights*, New York and London, 1990; Japanese tr. based on the Culcatta 2nd ed. by Shinji Maejima and Osamu Ikeda, *Arabian Naito*, 18 vols., Tokyo, 1966–92.

Anon., Une chronique Syrienne du VIe/XIIe siècle: *Le "Bustān al-Jāmiʿ,"* ed. Cl. Cahen, *BEO*, 7–8 (1937–38), 113–158. See ʿImād al-Dīn al-Iṣfahānī, *al-Bustān al-Jāmiʿ*.

Anon., *Ḥudūd al-ʿĀlam*, Tehran, 1962; English tr. and Commentary by V. Minorsky, *Ḥudūd al-ʿĀlam: The Regions of the World*, Gibb Memorial Series XI, London, 1970.

Anon., *Ḥujjat Tamlīk wa-Waqf*, ed. Ḥasanayn Muḥammad Rabīʿ, *Majallat al-Jamʿīyat al-Miṣrīya lil-Dirāsāt al-Taʾrīkhīya*, 12 (1964–65), 191–202.

Anon., *Kitāb al-Anwāʾ*, originally published by R. Dozy; new ed. by Ch. Pella, *Le calendrier de Cordoue*, Leiden, 1961.

Anon., *Kitāb al-Istibṣār fī ʿAjāʾib al-Amṣār*, ed. S.Z. ʿAbd al-Ḥamīd, Alexandria, 1958.

Anon., *Miftāḥ al-Rāḥa li-Ahl al-Filāḥa*, ed. M.I. Ṣāliḥīya and I.S. al-ʿAmad, Kuwait, 1984.

Anon., *al-Nujūm al-Zāhira fī Ḥulā Ḥaḍrat al-Qāhira*, ed. Ḥusayn Naṣṣār, Cairo, 1970.

Anon., *Nūr al-Maʿārif fī Nuẓum wa-Qawānīn wa-Aʿrāf al-Yaman fī al-ʿAhd al-Muẓaffarī al-Wārif*, 2 vols., Sanaa, 2003–05.

Anon., *Taʾrīkh al-Malik al-Ashraf Qāytbāy*, ed. ʿUmar ʿAbd al-Salām Tadmurī, Beirut, 2003.

ʿAbd al-Laṭīf al-Baghdādī, Muwaffaq al-Dīn Abū Muḥammad (557–629/1162–3–1231), *Kitāb al-Ifāda wal-Iʿtibār*, Arabic text and English tr. by K.H. Zand and I.E. Videan, *The Eastern Key*, London, 1965.

Al-Abshīhī, Shihāb al-Dīn Muḥammad (d. 850/1446), *Mustaṭraf fī Kull Fann Mustaẓraf*, ed. M.M. Qumayḥa, 2 vols., Beirut, 1986.

Abū al-Faḍāʾil, Muḥammad al-Ḥamawī (d. 7/13), *al-Taʾrīkh al-Manṣūrī*, Facsimile ed., Moscow, 1963; ed. A. Dūdū, Damascus, 1982.

Abū al-Fidāʾ, ʿImād al-Dīn Ismāʿīl b. ʿAlī (d. 732/1331), *al-Mukhtaṣar fī Akhbār al-Bashar*, 4 vols., Cairo, 1325H.

———, *Taqwīm al-Buldān*, ed. M. Reinaud and M. de Slane, Paris, 1840.

Abū Ḥāmid al-Qudsī, Muḥibb al-Dīn Muḥammad b. Khalīl al-Shāfiʿī (d. 888/1483), *Kitāb Duwal al-Islām al-Sharīfat al-Bahīya*, ed. Ulrich Haarmann, Beirut, 1997.

Abū Sahl, ʿĪsā b. Yaḥyā al-Masīḥī (d. ca. 401/1010), *Kitāb al-Miʾa fī al-Ṭibb*, ed. Floréal Sanagustin, 2 vols., Damascus, 2000.

Abū Shāma, Shihāb al-Dīn 'Abd al-Raḥmān al-Dimashqī (d. 665/1268), *al-Dhayl 'alā al-Rawḍatayn*, ed. Muḥammad Zāhid al-Bakūtharī, Beirut, 1947.

———, *Kitāb al-Rawḍatayn fī Akhbār al-Dawlatayn al-Nūrīya wal-Ṣalāḥīya*, ed. Muḥammad Ḥilmī Muḥammad Aḥmad, vol. I-1/2, Cairo, 1956–62.

Abū Ṣāliḥ al-Armanī (7/13 c.), *The Churches and Monasteries of Egypt*, English tr. by B. Evetts, Oxford, 1969.

Abū Yūsuf, Ya'qūb b. Ibrāhīm (d. 182/798), *Kitāb al-Kharāj*, 3rd ed., Cairo, 1382H.; English tr. by A. Ben Shemesh, *Taxation in Islam*, vol. 3, Leiden, 1969.

Aḥmad b. Ibrāhīm al-Hanbalī (d. 876/1471), *Shifā' al-Qulūb fī Manāqib Banī Ayyūb*, ed. N. Rashīd, Baghdad, 1978.

Al-'Aynī, Badr al-Dīn Abū Muḥammad Maḥmūd b. Aḥmad (762–855/1361–1451), *Awḍaḥ al-Ishārāt fī Man Tawallā Miṣr al-Qāhira min al-Wuzarā' wal-Bāshāt, al-Mulaqqab bil-Ta'rīkh al-'Aynī*, ed. 'Abd al-Raḥīm 'Abd al-Raḥmān 'Abd al-Raḥīm, Cairo, 1978.

———, *'Iqd al-Jumān fī Ta'rīkh Ahl al-Zamān: 'Aṣr Salāṭīn al-Mamālīk*, ed. Muḥammad Muḥammad Amīn, 4 vols., Cairo, 1987–1992; *'Iqd al-Jumān fī Ta'rīkh Ahl al-Zamān*, ed. 'Abd al-Rāziq al-Ṭanṭāwī al-Qarmūṭ, 2 vols., Cairo, 1985–89; *'Iqd al-Jumān fī Ta'rīkh Ahl al-Zamān: al-'Aṣr al-Ayyūbī*, ed. Maḥmūd R. Maḥmūd, 2 vols., Cairo, 2003–04; *al-Sulṭān Barqūq: Mu'assis Dawlat al-Mamālīk al-Jarākisa 784–801/1382–98, min Khilāl Makhṭūṭ 'Iqd al-Jumān fī Ta'rīkh Ahl al-Zamān*, ed. Īmān 'Umar Shukrī, Cairo, 2003.

———, *al-Sayf al-Muhannad fī Sīrat al-Malik al-Mu'ayyad "Shaykh al-Maḥmūdī,"* ed. Fahīm Muḥammad Shaltūt, Cairo, 1967.

Al-'Aẓīmī, Muḥammad b. 'Alī al-Ḥalabī (482–556/1090–1161), *Ta'rīkh Ḥalab*, ed. Ibrāhīm Za'rūr, Damascus, 1984.

Al-Badrī, Abū al-Baqā' 'Abd Allāh (d. 909/1503), *Nuzhat al-Anām fī Maḥāsin al-Shām*, Beirut, 1980.

Al-Baghdādī, Muḥammad b. al-Ḥasan al-Kātib (7/13 c.), *Kitāb al-Ṭabīkh*, Mosul, 1934; English tr. by A.J. Arberry, *A Baghdad Cookery Book*, 1939; repr. in *Medieval Arab Cookery*, Trowbridge, 2001; repr. 2006; New English tr. by Ch. Perry, *A Baghdad Cookery Book*, Trowbridge, 2005.

Baḥshal, Aslam b. Sahl al-Wāsiṭī (d. 292/905), *Ta'rīkh Wāsiṭ*, ed. Kūrkīs 'Awwād, Baghdad, 1967.

Al-Bakrī, Abū 'Ubayd 'Abd Allāh b. 'Abd al-'Azīz (d. 487/1094), *Kitāb al-Masālik wal-Mamālik*, ed. A. P. van Leeuwen and A. Ferre, 2 vols., Tunis, 1992; *Jughrāfiyat Miṣr min Kitāb al-Mamālik wal-Masālik*, ed. 'Abd Allāh Y. al-Ghānim, Kuwait, 1980.

———, *Kitāb Mu'jam Mā Ista'jama*, ed. F. Wüstenferd, 2 vols., Göttingen, 1876- 77; repr. Osnabrük, 1976.

Al-Balādhurī, Abū al-'Abbās Aḥmad (d. 279/892), *Futūḥ al-Buldān*, ed. 'Abd Allāh A. al-Ṭabbā' and 'Umar A. al-Ṭabbā', Beirut, 1957; English tr. by P.K. Hitti, *The Origins of the Islamic State*, New York, 1916; repr., Beirut, 1966.

Banyāmīn al-Tuṭīlī (Benjamin of Tudela) (6/12 c.), *Riḥlat Banyāmīn (1165–1173)*, Arabic tr. by ʿIzrā Ḥaddād, Baghdad, 1945.

Bar Hebraeus, Abū al-Faraj (d. 685/1286), *The Chronography of Gregory Abū'l Faraj commonly known as Bar Hebraeus*, Syriac text ed. and English tr. by E.A. Wallis Budge, 2 vols., London, 1932; repr. Piscataway, 2003.

Baybars al-Manṣūrī, Rukn al-Dīn al-Dawādārī (d. 725/1325), *al-Tuḥfat al-Mulūkīya fī al-Dawlat al-Turkīya*, ed. ʿAbd al-Ḥamīd Ṣ. Ḥamdān, Cairo, 1987.

———, *Zubdat al-Fikra fī Taʾrīkh al-Hijra*, ed. D.S. Richards, Beirut, 1998; ed. Zubayda Muḥammad ʿAṭā, Cairo, n. d.

Al-Bayhaqī, Abū al-Faḍl Muḥammad b. Ḥusayn (d. 470/1077), *Taʾrīkh-i Bayhaqī*, ed. Ghanī and Fayāḍ, Tehran, 1324Kh.

Al-Bīrūnī, Abū al-Rayḥān Muḥammad b. Aḥmad al-Khwārizmī (d. 440/1048), *al-Āthār al-Bāqiya ʿan al-Qurūn al-Khāliya*, ed. C.E. Sachau, Leipzig, 1923.

Al-Bukhārī, Muḥammad b. Ismāʿīl (194–256/810–870), *Ṣaḥīḥ al-Bukhārī*, 8 vols., Beirut, n. d.

Al-Bundārī, Qiwām al-Dīn al-Fatḥ b. ʿAlī (7/13 c.), *Sanā al-Barq al-Shāmī*, ed. Fatḥīya al-Nabrāwī, Cairo, 1979; ed. Ramazan Şeşen, Istanbul, 2004.

Al-Būzjānī, Abū al-Wafāʾ Muḥammad (d. 388/998), *Kitāb al-Manāzil al-Sabʿ*, ed. A. Saʿīdīn, Amman, 1971.

Al-Damīrī, Kamāl al-Dīn Muḥammad (d. 808/1405), *Ḥayāt al-Ḥayawān al-Kubrā*, 2 vols., Cairo, 1969–70.

Al-Dhahabī, Shams al-Dīn Abū ʿAbd Allāh Muḥammad (d 748/1348), *al-ʿIbar fī Khabar Man Ghabara*, ed. Ṣalāḥ al-Dīn al-Munajjid, 5 vols., Kuwait, 1960–66.

———, *Kitāb Tadhkirat al-Ḥuffāẓ*, 4 vols. and Supplement, Beirut, 1374H.

———, *Siyar Aʿlām al-Nubalāʾ*, ed. Shuʿayb al-Arnūt, Ḥusayn al-Asad, etc. 25 vols., 3 rd ed., Beirut, 1985–92.

———, *Taʾrīkh al-Islām wa-Wafayāt al-Mashāhīr wal-Aʿlām*, ed. ʿUmar ʿAbd al-Salām Tadmurī, 35 vols., Beirut, 1987–94.

Al-Dimashqī, Abū al-Faḍl Jaʿfar (5/11c.), *Kitāb al-Ishāra ilā Maḥāsin al-Tijāra*, Cairo, 1900.

Al-Dimashqī, Shams al-Dīn Muḥammad (d. 727/1327), *Nukhbat al-Dahr fī ʿAjāʾib al-Barr wal-Baḥr*, Petersburg, 1866; repr. Osnabrück, 1982.

Al-Dimashqī, Taqī al-Dīn ʿAbd Allāh b. Muḥammad (d. 909/1503), *Nuzhat al-Anām fī Maḥāsin al-Shām*, Cairo, 1341H.

Al-Dīnawarī, Abū Ḥanīfa Aḥmad b. Dāwūd (d. 282/895), *Kitāb al-Nabāt*, II, ed. Muḥammad Ḥamīdullāh, Cairo, 1973; *Kitāb al-Nabāt*, III, V-1, ed. B. Lewin, Wiesbaden, 1974; V, ed. B. Lewin, Uppsala, 1953.

Dioscorides (1c.), *Materia Medica*, English tr. by R.T. Gunther, *The Greek Herbal of Dioscorides*, Oxford, 1933; repr. London and New York, 1968.

Al-Fāriqī, Ibn al-Azraq Aḥmad b. Yūsuf (d. after 572/1176), *Ta'rīkh al-Fāriqī*, ed. Badawī 'Abd al-Laṭīf 'Awaḍ, Cairo, 1959; Partial Arabic text and English tr. by C. Hillenbrand, *A Muslim Principality in Crusader Times: The Early Artuqid State*, Leiden, 1990.

Grohmann, A. ed., *Arabic Papyri in the Egyptian Library*, 6 vols., Cairo, 1934–62; Arabic Text and Arabic tr., *Awrāq al-Bardī al-'Arabīya bi-Dār al-Kutub al-Miṣrīya*, 6 vols., Cairo, 1994.

Al-Hamdānī, Badr al-Dīn Muḥammad (7–8/13–14 c.), *Kitāb al-Simṭ al-Ghālī al-Thaman*, ed. G.R. Smith, Gibb Memorial Series, New Series XXXVI, 2 vols., London, 1974.

Al-Hamadānī, Muḥammad b. 'Abd al-Malik (d. 521/1127), *Takmilat Ta'rīkh al-Ṭabarī*, ed. A.Y. Kan'ān, Beirut, 1958; in *Dhuyūl Ta'rīkh al-Ṭabarī*, ed. Muḥammad Abū al-Faḍl Ibrāhīm, Cairo, n. d.

Ḥamza b. al-Ḥasan al-Iṣfahānī (4/10 c.), *Ta'rīkh Sinī Mulūk al-Arḍ wal-Anbiyā'*, Beirut, 1961.

Hilāl al-Ṣābī, Abū al-Ḥusayn Hilāl b. al-Muḥassin al-Ḥarrānī (359–448/970–1056), *Rusūm Dār al-Khilāfa*, ed. Mīkhā'īl 'Awwād, Baghdad, 1964; English tr. by Elie A. Salem, *The Rules and Regulations of the 'Abbasid Court*, Beirut, 1977; Japanese tr. by Junichi Taniguchi and Kazuhiro Shimizu, *Karifu kyutei no shikitari*, Kyoto, 2003.

———, *Tuḥfat al-Umarā' fī Ta'rīkh al-Wuzarā'*, ed. 'Abd al-Sattār A. Farāj, Cairo, 1958.

Ibn 'Abbād, Abū al-Qāsim Ismā'īl (326–385/938–995), *Rasā'il al-Ṣāḥib b. 'Abbād*, ed. 'Abd al-Wahhāb 'Azzām and Shawqī Ḍayf, Cairo, 1947.

Ibn 'Abd al-Ẓāhir, Muḥī al-Dīn Abū al-Faḍl 'Abd Allāh al-Miṣrī (620– 692/1223–93), *al-Rawḍ al-Zāhir fī Sīrat al-Malik al-Ẓāhir*, Arabic text and English tr. by S.F. Sadeque, *Baybars The First of Egypt*, Dacca, 1956; *al-Rawḍ al-Zāhir fī Sīrat al-Malik al-Ẓāhir*, ed. 'Abd al-'Azīz al-Khuwaytir, Riyad, 1976.

———, *al-Rawḍat al-Bahīyat al-Zāhira fī Khiṭaṭ al-Mu'izzīyat al-Qāhira*, ed. Ayman Fu'ād Sayyid, Cairo, 1996.

———, *Tashrīf al-Ayyām wal-'Uṣūr fī Sīrat al-Malik al-Manṣūr*, ed. Murād Kāmil, Cairo, 1961.

Ibn Abī al-Faḍā'il, Mufaḍḍal (8/14 c.), *Kitāb al-Nahj al-Sadīd wal-Durr al-Farīd*, Arabic text and French tr. by E. Blochet, *Patrologia Orientalis*, 12, 14, 20 (1919–28), 345–550, 375–672, 3–267.

Ibn Abī Jarrāda, Kamāl al-Dīn 'Umar b. Aḥmad (588–660/1192–1262), *Zubdat al-Ḥalab min Ta'rīkh Ḥalab*, ed. Suhayl Zakkār, 2 vols., Damascus, 1997.

Ibn Abī Uṣaybi'a, Abū al-'Abbās Aḥmad al-Khazrajī (d. 668/1270), *'Uyūn al-Anbā' fī Ṭabaqāt al-Aṭibbā'*, 3 vols., Beirut, 1956–57.

Ibn al-'Adīm, Kamāl al-Dīn Abū al-Qāsim 'Umar (588–660/1192–1262), *Bughyat al-Ṭalab fī Ta'rīkh Ḥalab*, ed. Suhayl Zakkār, 11 vols., Damascus, 1988; ed. Ali Sevim, Ankara, 1976.

———, *al-Wuṣla ilā al-Ḥabīb fī Waṣf al-Ṭayyibāt wal-Ṭayyib*, ed. Sulaymī Maḥbūb and Darīya al-Khaṭīb, 2 vols., Aleppo, 1986–88.

Ibn al-ʿAmīd, al-Makīn (d. 672/1273), *Akhbār al-Ayyūbīyīn*, ed. Cl. Cahen, *BEO*, 15 (1958), 127–184.

Ibn ʿAsākir, Abū al-Qāsim ʿAlī al-Shāfiʿī (d. 571/1176), *Taʾrīkh Madīnat Dimashq*, ed. Ṣalāḥ al-Dīn al-Munajjid etc., vols. 1–15, Damascus, 1963–91; Partial tr. by N. Elisséeff, *La description de Damas d'Ibn ʿAsākir*, Damascus, 1959.

Ibn al-Athīr, Ḍiyāʾ al-Dīn al-Jazarī (d. 637/1239), *Rasāʾil Ibn al-Athīr*, ed. A. al-Maqdisī, Beirut, 1959.

Ibn al-Athīr, ʿIzz al-Dīn Abū al-Ḥasan ʿAlī (535–630/1160–1233), *al-Kāmil fī al-Taʾrīkh*, ed. C.J. Tornberg, 12 vols., Leiden, 1853; repr. Beirut, 1965–66; *al-Fahāris*, Beirut, 1967; Partial English tr. by D.S. Richards, *The Chronicle of Ibn al-Athīr for the Crusading Period from al-Kāmil fiʾl-Taʾrīkh*, 3 vols., Aldershot, 2006–08.

———, *al-Taʾrīkh al-Bāhir fī al-Dawlat al-Atābakīya*, ed. ʿAbd al-Qādir Aḥmad Ṭulaymāt, Cairo, 1963.

Ibn Aybak al-Dawādārī, Abū Bakr b. ʿAbd Allāh (d. 8/14 c.), *Kanz al-Durar wa-Jāmiʿ al-Ghurar:* VI. *al-Durrat al-Maḍīya fī Akhbār al-Dawlat al-Fāṭimīya*, ed. Ṣalāḥ al-Dīn al-Munajjid, Cairo, 1961; VII. *al-Durr al-Maṭlūb fī Akhbār Mulūk Banī Ayyūb*, ed. Saʿīd A. ʿĀshūr, Cairo, 1972; VIII. *al-Durrat al-Zakīya fī Akhbār al-Dawlat al-Turkīya*, ed. U. Haarman, Cairo, 1971; IX. *al-Durr al-Fākhir fī Sīrat al-Malik al-Nāṣir*, ed. H.R. Roemer, Cairo, 1960.

Ibn al-Balkhī (5–6/11–12 c.), *Kitāb Fārs Nāma*, Gibb Memorial Series, New Series I, ed. G. Le Strange and R.A. Nicholson, London, 1921; repr. London, 1968.

Ibn Bassām, Shams al-Dīn Muḥammad al-Tinnīsī (6–7/12–13 c.), *Anīs al-Jalīs fī Akhbār Tinnīs*, ed. Jamāl al-Dīn al-Shayyāl, *Majjallat al-Majmaʿ al-ʿIlmī al-ʿIrāqī*, 14 (1967), 151–189.

Ibn Baṭṭūṭa, Abū ʿAbd Allāh Muḥammad al-Lawātī al-Ṭanjī (703–770 or 779/1304–1368–9 or 1377), *Tuḥfat al-Nuẓẓār fī Gharāʾib al-Amṣār*, Arabic text and French tr. by C. Défremery and B.R. Sanguinetti, *Voyages d'Ibn Battûta*, 4 vols., Paris, 1854; repr. Paris, 1969; English tr. by H.A.R. Gibb, *The Travels of Ibn Baṭṭūṭa*, 3 vols., Cambridge, 1956–71; Japanese tr. by Hikoichi Yajima, *Dairyokoki*, 8 vols., Tokyo, 1996–2002.

Ibn al-Bayṭār, Ḍiyāʾ al-Dīn ʿAbd Allāh al-Andalusī (d. 646/1248), *al-Jāmiʿ li-Mufradāt al-Adwiya wal-Aghdhiya*, 4 vols., Bulaq, 1874; repr. Baghdad, n. d.

Ibn Buṭlān, al-Mukhtār (or Yuwānis) b. al-Ḥasan (d. 458/1066), *Taqwīm al-Ṣiḥḥa*, Arabic Text and French tr. by H. Elkhadem, *Le Taqwīm al-Ṣiḥḥa (Tacuini Sanitatis) d'Ibn Buṭlān*, Leuven, 1990.

Ibn Diḥya, Abū al-Khaṭṭāb ʿUmar b. al-Ḥasan al-Kalbī (d. 633/1235), *Kitāb al-Nibrās fī Taʾrīkh Khulafāʾ Banī al-ʿAbbās*, ed. ʿAlī al-ʿAzzāwī, Baghdad, 1946.

Ibn al-Dubaythī, Abū ʿAbd Allāh Muḥammad b. Saʿīd (558–637/1163–1239), *Dhayl Taʾrīkh Madīnat Baghdād*, ed. Bashshār A. Maʿrūf, 2 vols., Baghdad, 1974–79.

Ibn Duqmāq, Ṣārim al-Dīn Ibrāhīm b. Muḥammad al-ʿAlāʾī al-Miṣrī (d. 809/1406), *al-Jawhar al-Thamīn fī Siyar al-Mulūk wal-Salāṭīn*, ed. Muḥammad Kamāl al-Dīn ʿIzz al-Dīn ʿAlī, 2 vols., Beirut, 1985.

———, *Kitāb al-Intiṣār li-Wāsiṭat ʿIqd al-Amṣār*, ed. K. Vollers, 2 vols., Cairo, 1893.

———, *Nuzhat al-Anām fī Taʾrīkh al-Islām*, ed. Samīr Ṭabbāra, Beirut, 1999.

Ibn al-Faqīh, Abū Bakr Aḥmad b. Muḥammad al-Hamadhānī (3/9 c.), *Baghdād Madīnat al-Salām*, Baghdad, n. d.

———, *Mukhtaṣar Kitāb al-Buldān*, BGA. V, ed. M.J. de Goeje, 2nd ed., Leiden, 1967.

Ibn al-Furāt, Nāṣir al-Dīn Muḥammad (d. 807/1405), *Taʾrīkh Ibn al-Furāt*, ed. Ḥasan Muḥammad al-Shammāʿ, vols. 4–5/i, Basra, 1967–70; ed. Qusṭanṭīn Zarīq, vols. 7–9, Beirut, 1936–42; Arabic text and English tr. by U. Lyons, M.C. Lyons, and J. Riley-Smith, *Ayyubids, Mamluks and Crusaders*, 2 vols., Cambridge, 1971.

Ibn al-Fuwaṭī, Kamāl al-Dīn Abū al-Faḍl ʿAbd al-Razzāq (d. 723/1323), *al-Ḥawādith al-Jāmiʿa wal-Tajārib al-Nāfiʿa fī al-Miʾat al-Sābiʿa*, ed. Mahdī al-Najm, Beirut, 2003.

Ibn Ḥabīb, al-Ḥasan b. ʿUmar al-Dimashqī (d. 779/1377), *Tadhkirat al-Nabīh fī Ayyām al-Manṣūr wa-Banīh*, ed. Muḥammad Muḥammad Amīn, 3 vols., Cairo, 1976–86.

Ibn Ḥajar al-ʿAsqalānī, Shihāb al-Dīn Aḥmad (773–852/1372–1449), *Dhayl al-Durar al-Kāmina*, ed. A. Darwīsh, Cairo, 1992.

———, *al-Durar al-Kāmina fī Aʿyān al-Miʾat al-Thāmina*, ed. M.S. Jād al-Ḥaqq, 5 vols., Cairo, 1966–67.

———, *Inbāʾ al-Ghumr bi-Anbāʾ al-ʿUmr*, ed. Ḥasan Ḥabashī, 4 vols., Cairo, 1969–98.

———, *Kitāb Nuzhat al-Albāb fī al-Alqāb*, ed. M.M. ʿAzab, Beirut, 1991.

———, *Rafʿ al-Iṣr ʿan Quḍāt Miṣr*, 2 vols., Cairo, 1957.

Ibn al-Ḥājj, Abū ʿAbd Allāh Muḥammad al-Fāsī (d. 737/1336), *al-Madkhal ilā Tanmiyat al-Aʿmāl bi-Taḥsīn al-Nīyāt*, 4 vols., Beirut, 1981.

Ibn Ḥajjī, Shihāb al-Dīn Abū al-ʿAbbās Aḥmad al-Dimashqī (751–816/1350–1413), *Taʾrīkh Ibn Ḥajjī*, ed. Abū Yaḥyā ʿAbd Allāh al-Kundurī, 2 vols., Beirut, 2003.

Ibn Ḥawqal, Abū al-Qāsim al-Naṣībī (4/10c.), *Kitāb Ṣūrat al-Arḍ*, BGA. II, ed. J.H. Krammers, 3rd ed., Leiden, 1967; French tr. by J.H. Krammers and G. Wiet, *Configuration de la terre*, 2 vols., Paris, 1964.

Ibn ʿImād al-Ḥanbalī, Abū al-Falāḥ ʿAbd al-Ḥayy al-ʿAkarī (d. 1089/1678), *Shadharāt al-Dhahab fī Akhbār Man Dhahaba*, 8 vols., Beirut, n. d.

Ibn al-ʿImrānī, Muḥammad b. ʿAlī (d. 580/1184), *al-Inbāʾ fī Taʾrīkh al-Khulafāʾ*, ed. Q. al-Sāmarrāʾī, Leiden, 1973.

Ibn Iyās, Zayn al-Dīn Muḥammad al-Jarkasī (852–ca.930/1448–ca.1524), *Badāʾiʿ al-Zuhūr fī Waqāʾiʿ al-Duhūr*, 3 vols., Bulaq, 1893; ed. M. Muṣṭafā, 5 vols., Wiesbaden, 1960–75; *al-Fahāris* by M. Muṣṭafā, 3 vols., Cairo, 1984.

———, *Nuzhat al-Umam fī al-ʿAjāʾib wal-Ḥikam*, ed. Muḥammad Zaynahum M. ʿAzab, Cairo, 1995.

Ibn al-Jawzī, Jamāl al-Dīn Abū al-Faraj ʿAbd al-Raḥmān b. ʿAlī (510–597/1126–1200), *Kitāb al-Quṣṣāṣ wal-Mudhakkirīn*, ed. and English tr. by M.S. Swartz, Beirut, 1986.

———, *al-Miṣbāḥ al-Muḍī fī Khilāfat al-Mustaḍī*, ed. Nājiya A. Ibrāhīm, Baghdad, 1976.

———, *al-Muntaẓam fī Taʾrīkh al-Mulūk wal-Umam*, vols. 5–10, Hyderabad, 1357–58H.

———, *Talbīs Iblīs*, Cairo, n. d.

———, *ʿUyūn al-Ḥikāyāt*, ed. ʿAbd al-ʿAzīz S.H. al-Ghazūlī, Beirut, 2003.

Ibn al-Jazarī, Shams al-Dīn Abū ʿAbd Allāh Muḥammad (d. 738/1338), *Taʾrīkh Ḥawādith al-Zamān wa-Anbāʾih*, ed. ʿUmar A. Tadmurī, 3 vols., Beirut, 1998.

Ibn al-Jazzār, Abū Jaʿfar Aḥmad b. Ibrāhīm al-Qayrawānī (d. 395/1004–5), *Kitāb fī al-Maʿida wa-Amrāḍihā wa-Muwādātihā*, ed. Salmān Qaṭāba, Baghdad, 1980.

Ibn al-Jīʿān, Sharaf al-Dīn Yaḥyā b. al-Maqarr (d. 885/1480), *Kitāb al-Tuḥfat al-Sanīya bi-Asmāʾ al-Bilād al-Miṣrīya*, Cairo, 1898.

Ibn Jubayr, Abū al-Ḥusayn Muḥammad b. Aḥmad al-Kinānī al-Andalusī (540–614/1145–1217), *Riḥlat Ibn Jubayr*, Beirut, 1964; English tr. by R. Broadhurst, *The Travels of Ibn Jubayr*, London, 1952.

Ibn Kathīr, ʿImād al-Dīn Abū al-Fidā Ismāʿīl al-Qurashī (ca.700–774/ca.1300–73), *al-Bidāya wal-Nihāya*, 14 vols., Beirut, 1966.

Ibn Khaldūn, Walī al-Dīn ʿAbd al-Raḥmān b. Muḥammad (732–808/1332–1406), *Kitāb al-ʿIbar*, 7 vols., Beirut, 1959–61; Japanese translation of *al-Muqaddima* by Kosei Morimoto, *Rekishi Josetsu*, 3 vols., Tokyo, 1979–87.

Ibn Khalīl al-Asadī, Muḥammad b. Muḥammad (9/15 c.), *al-Taysīr wal-Iʿtibār wal-Taḥrīr wal-Ikhtiyār fī Mā Yajibu min Ḥusn al-Tadbīr wal-Taṣarruf wal-Ikhtiyār*, ed. ʿAbd al-Qādir Aḥmad Ṭulaymāt, Cairo, 1968.

Ibn Khalīl al-Ḥalabī, Shams al-Dīn Muḥammad (d. 881/1476), *Taʾrīkh al-Amīr Yashbak al-Ẓāhirī*, ed. ʿAbd al-Qādir Aḥmad Ṭulaymāt, Cairo, 1973.

Ibn Khalṣūn, Muḥammad b. Yūsuf al-Andalusī (7/13 c.), *Kitāb al-Aghdhiya*, Arabic text and French tr. by Suzanne Gigandet, Damascus, 1996.

Ibn Mammātī, al-Aswad b. Muhadhdhab (d. 606/1209), *Kitāb Qawānīn al-Dawāwīn*, ed. A.S. Atiya, Cairo, 1943.

Ibn al-Maʾmūn, Jamāl al-Dīn Mūsā (d. 588/1192), *Nuṣūṣ min Akhbār Miṣr*, ed. Ayman Fuʾād Sayyid, Cairo, 1983.

Ibn Manẓūr, Jamāl al-Dīn Abū al-Faḍl Muḥammad al-Ifrīqī al-Miṣrī (d. 711/1312), *Lisān al-ʿArab*, 15 vols., Beirut, 1955–56.

Ibn al-Nadīm, Abū al-Faraj Muḥammad b. Isḥāq al-Warrāq al-Baghdādī (d. 385/995), *Kitāb al-Fihrist*, ed. G. Flügel, Leipzig, 1867; repr. Beirut, 1964; English tr. by B. Dodge, *The Fihrist of al-Nadīm*, 2 vols., New York, 1970.

Ibn al-Nafīs, ʿAlāʾ al-Dīn Ibn al-Nafīs al-Qurashī (d. 687/1288), *al-Shāmil fī al-Ṣināʿat al-Ṭibbīya*, 30 vols., Abu Dhabi, n.d.

Ibn Nāẓir al-Jaysh, Taqī al-Dīn ʿAbd al-Raḥmān (d. 786/1384), *Kitāb Tathqīf bil-Muṣṭalaḥ al-Sharīf*, ed. R. Vesely, Cairo, 1987.

Ibn Qāḍī Shuhba, Taqī al-Dīn Abū Bakr al-Dimashqī (779–851/1377–1448), *Ta'rīkh Ibn Qāḍī Shuhba*, ed. ʿAdnān Darwīsh, 4 vols., Damascus, 1977–97.

Ibn al-Qalānisī, Abū Yaʿlā Ḥamza (d. 555/1160), *Dhayl Ta'rīkh Dimashq*, Leiden, 1908; Partial English tr. by H.A.R. Gibb, *The Damascus Chronicle of the Crusades*, London, 1967.

Ibn Qayyim al-Jawzīya, Shams al-Dīn Abū ʿAbd Allāh Muḥammad (691–751/1292–1350), *al-Furūsīya*, Cairo, n. d.

———, *al-Ṭibb al-Nabawī*, English tr. by Penelope Johnstone, *Medicine of the Prophet*, Cambridge, 1998.

Ibn al-Quff, Amīn al-Dawla Abū al-Faraj al-Karakī (630–685/1233–86), *Jāmiʿ al-Gharaḍ fī Ḥifẓ al-Ṣiḥḥa wa-Dafʿ al-Maraḍ*, ed. Sāmī Kh. al-Ḥamārna, Amman, 1989.

Ibn al-Qunfudh, Abū al-ʿAbbās Aḥmad al-Qusanṭīnī (d. 810/1407–8), *Kitāb al-Wafayāt*, ed. A. Nuwayhiḍ, Beirut, 1971.

Ibn al-Rafʿa, al-ʿAbbās al-Anṣārī (d. 710/1310), *Kitāb al-Iḍāḥ wal-Tibyān fī Maʿrifat al-Mikyāl wal-Mīzān*, ed. Muḥammad al-Ḥalabī, Damascus, 1990.

Ibn Riḍwān, ʿAlī al-Ṭabīb al-Miṣrī (388–460/998–1068), *Kitāb Dafʿ Maḍār al-Abdān*, Arabic Text ed. by A.S. Gamal and English tr. by M.W. Dols, London, 1984.

Ibn Saʿīd al-Maghribī, Abū al-Ḥasan ʿAlī b. Mūsā (d. 673/1274 or 685/1286), *Kitāb al-Jughrāfiyā*, ed. Ismāʿīl al-ʿArabī, Beirut, 1970.

Ibn Sarābiyūn, Suhrāb (4/10 c.), *Kitāb ʿAjā'ib al-Aqālīm al-Sabʿa*, ed. H. von Mžik, Leipzig, 1929.

Ibn Ṣaṣrā, Muḥammad b. Muḥammad (8/14 c.), *al-Durrat al-Muḍī'a fī al-Dawlat al-Ẓāhirīya*, 2 vols.: vol.1 English tr. by William M. Brinner, *A Chronicle of Damascus 1389–1397*, vol. 2, Arabic text ed. By W. Brinner, Berkeley and Los Angeles, 1963.

Ibn al-Ṣayrafī, Amīn al-Dīn Abū al-Qāsim ʿAlī (d. 542/1147), *al-Ishāra ilā Man Nāla al-Wizāra*, ed. A. Mukhliṣ, Cairo, 1924.

Ibn al-Ṣayrafī, al-Khaṭīb al-Jawharī ʿAlī b. Dāwūd (d. 900/1495), *Nuzhat al-Nufūs wal-Abdān fī Tawārīkh al-Zamān*, ed. Ḥasan Ḥabashī, 4 vols., Cairo, 1970–94.

Ibn Sayyār al-Warrāq (4/10 c.), *Kitāb al-Ṭabīkh*, ed. K. Öhrnberg and S. Mroueh, Helsinki, 1987; English tr. with Introduction and Glossary by N. Nasrallah, *Annals of the Caliphs' Kitchens: Ibn Sayyār al-Warrāq's Tenth-Century Baghdadi Cookbook*, Leiden, 2007.

Ibn Shaddād, Bahā' al-Dīn Abū al-Maḥāsin Yūsuf (d. 632/1235), *al-Nawādir al-Sulṭānīya wal-Maḥāsin al-Yūsufīya*, ed. Jamāl al-Dīn al-Shayyāl, Cairo, 1964; English tr. by D.S. Richards, *The Rare and Excellent History of Saladin*, Aldershot, 2002.

Ibn Shaddād, ʿIzz al-Dīn Abū ʿAbd Allāh Muḥammad al-Ḥalabī (613– 684/1217–1285), *al-Aʿlāq al-Khaṭīra fī Dhikr Umarā' al-Shām wal-Jazīra: Dimashq*, ed. S. al-Dahhān, Damascus, 1956; *Ḥalab*, ed. D. Sourdel, Damascus, 1953; *Lubnān*, ed. Sāmī al-Dahhān, Damascus, 1963; *al-Jazīra*, ed. Z. ʿAbbāra, 2 vols., Damascus, 1978; *Shimāl Sūrīya*, ed. A.M. Eddé, *BEO*, 32–33 (1980–81), 268–402.

———, *Ta'rīkh al-Malik al-Ẓāhir*, ed. Aḥmad Ḥuṭayṭ, Wiesbaden, 1983.

Ibn Shāhanshā, Muḥammad al-Ayyūbī (d. 617/1221), *Miḍmār al-Ḥaqā'iq wa-Sirr al-Khalā'iq*, ed. Ḥasan Ḥabashī, Cairo, 1968.

Ibn Shāhīn, ʿAbd al-Bāsiṭ b. Khalīl al-Malaṭī (844–920/1440–1514), *Nuzhat al-Asāṭīn fī Man Waliya Miṣr min al-Salāṭīn*, ed. Muḥammad Kamāl al-Dīn ʿAlī, Cairo, 1987.

Ibn Shākir al-Kutubī, Ṣalāḥ al-Dīn Muḥammad (d. 764/1363), *Fawāt al-Wafayāt*, ed. Iḥsān ʿAbbās, 5 vols., Beirut, 1973–74.

———, *ʿUyūn al-Tawārīkh*, ed. Nabīla A. Dāwūd and Faysal al-Sāmir, vols. 12, 21, Baghdad, 1977–84.

Ibn al-Shiḥna, Muḥammad al-Ḥalabī (d. 890/1485), *al-Durr al-Muntakhab fī Ta'rīkh Mamlakat Ḥalab*, Beirut, 1909; repr. Damascus, 1984. *Ta'rīkh Ḥalab*, ed. K. Ohta, Tokyo, 1990.

Ibn al-Ṣuqāʿī, Faḍl Allāh b. Abī al-Fakhra (d. 725/1325), *Tālī Kitāb Wafayāt al-Aʿyān*, ed. J. Sublet, Damascus, 1974.

Ibn Taghrībirdī, Jamāl al-Dīn Abū al-Maḥāsin Yūsuf (ca.812–874/ca.1409–1470), *al-Dalīl al-Shāfī ʿalā al-Manhal al-Ṣāfī*, ed. Fahīm Muḥammad ʿAlawī Shaltūt, 2 vols., Cairo, 1998.

———, *Ḥawādith al-Duhūr fī Madā al-Ayyām wal-Shuhūr*, ed. W. Popper, 4vols., Berkeley, 1930–42.

———, *Kitāb Tahdhīb al-Tahdhīb*, 12 vols., Hyderabad, 1325–27H.

———, *al-Manhal al-Ṣāfī wal-Mustawfī baʿda al-Wāfī*, ed. Muḥammad Muḥammad Amīn etc., 12 vols., Cairo, 1956–2006.

———, *al-Nujūm al-Zāhira fī Mulūk Miṣr wal-Qāhira*, vols. 1–12, Cairo, 1963; vols. 13–16, ed. Fahīm M. Shaltūt etc., Cairo, 1970–72; English tr. by W. Popper, *History of Egypt 1382–1469 AD*, 10 vols., Berkeley, 1954–63.

Ibn Ṭawq, Shihāb al-Dīn Aḥmad (834–915/1430–1509), *al-Taʿlīq: Yawmīyāt Shihāb al-Dīn Aḥmad b. Ṭawq*, ed. Jaʿfar al-Muhājir, 3 vols., Damascus, 2000–04.

Ibn Taymīya, Taqī al-Dīn Aḥmad al-Dimashqī (d. 728/1328), *al-Ḥisba fī al-Islām*, Cairo, 1387H.

Ibn al-Ṭiqṭaqā, Muḥammad al-ʿAlawī (7/13c.), *al-Fakhrī fī al-Ādāb al-Sulṭānīya*, Beirut, 1966.

Ibn Ṭūlūn, Shams al-Dīn Muḥammad al-Ṣāliḥī (d. 953/1546), *Iʿlām al-Warā bi-Man Waliya Nā'iban min al-Atrāk*, ed. Muḥammad Aḥmad Dahmān, Damascus, 1964.

———, *al-Qalā'id al-Jawharīya fī Ta'rīkh al-Ṣāliḥīya*, ed. Muḥammad Aḥmad Dahmān, 2 vols., Damascus, 1980–81.

———, *Rasā'il Ta'rīkhīya*, 4 vols., Damascus, 1348H.

Ibn al-Ṭuwayr, Abū al-Murtaḍā ʿAbd al-Salām al-Qaysrānī (524–617/1130–1220), *Nuzhat al-Muqlatayn fī Akhbār al-Dawlatayn*, ed. Ayman Fu'ād Sayyid, Beirut, 1992.

Ibn al-Ukhuwwa, Muḥammad al-Qurashī (d. 729/1329), *Kitāb Maʿālim al-Qurba fī Aḥkām al-Ḥisba*, ed. Muḥammad M. Shaʿbān and Ṣadīq A. al-Muṭīʿī, Cairo, 1976.

Ibn Waḥshīya, Abū Bakr Aḥmad b. ʿAlī al-Kasdānī (4/10 c.), *al-Filāḥat al-Nabaṭīya*, ed. Tawfīq Fahd, 3 vols., Damascus, 1993–98.

Ibn al-Wardī, Zayn al-Dīn ʿUmar (d. 749/1348), *Taʾrīkh Ibn al-Wardī*, 2 vols., Najaf, 1969; *Tatimmat al-Mukhtaṣar fī Akhbār al-Bashar*, ed. A.R. al-Badrāwī, 2 vols., Beirut, 1970.

Ibn Wāṣil, Jamāl al-Dīn Muḥammad b. Sālim (d. 697/1298), *Mufarrij al-Kurūb fī Akhbār Banī Ayyūb*, Jamāl al-Dīn al-Shayyāl and Ḥasanayn M. Rabīʿ, vols. 1–5, Cairo, 1953–77; ed. ʿUmar ʿAbd al-Salām Tadmurī, vol. 6, Beirut, 2004.

Ibn Ẓāfir, Jamāl al-Dīn ʿAlī (d. 613/1216), *Akhbār al-Duwal al-Munqaṭiʿa*, ed. A. Ferré, Cairo, 1972.

Ibn Ẓahīra, Abū al-Ṭayyib Aḥmad, (d. 885/1480), *al-Faḍāʾil al-Bāhira fī Maḥāsin Miṣr wal-Qāhira*, ed. M. al-Saqā and K. al-Muhandis, Cairo, 1969.

Ibrāhīm al-Ṣābī, Abū Isḥāq Ibrāhīm b. Hilāl (d. 384/994), *al-Mukhtār min Rasāʾil Abī Isḥāq Ibrāhīm al-Ṣābī*, ed. A. Sh. Arslān, Beirut, n. d.

———, *Rasāʾil al-Ṣābī wal-Sharīf al-Raḍī*, ed. Muḥammad Yūsuf Najm, Kuwait, 1961.

Al-Idrīsī, Abū ʿAbd Allāh Muḥammad (493–560/1100–65), *Kitāb Nuzhat al-Mushtāq fī Ikhtirāq al-Āfāq*, 9 vols., Napoli-Roma, 1970–84.

ʿImād al-Dīn al-Iṣfahānī, Abū ʿAbd Allāh Muḥammad (d. 597/1201), *al-Bustān al-Jāmiʿ li-Jamīʿ Tawārīkh Ahl al-Zamān*, ed. ʿUmar ʿAbd al-Salām Tadmurī, Beirut, 2002.

———, *al-Fatḥ al-Qussī fī al-Fatḥ al-Qudsī*, ed. M.M. Ṣubḥ, Cairo, 1965; French tr. by H. Massé, *Conquête de la Syrie et de la Palestine par Saladin*, Paris, 1972.

———, *Kitāb al-Barq al-Shāmī*, ed. Ramazan Şeşen, vol. 5, Istanbul, 1979.

Al-Iṣṭakhrī, Abū Isḥāq Ibrāhīm (4/10c.), *Kitāb Masālik al-Mamālik*, ed. M.J. de Goeje, Leiden, 1967.

Al-Jāḥiẓ, Abū ʿUthmān ʿAmr al-Baṣrī (ca.160–255/ca.776–868–9), *al-Bukhalāʾ*, ed. Ṭāha al-Ḥājirī, Cairo, n. d.; English tr. by Fedwa Malti-Douglas, *Structures of Avarice: The Bukhalāʾ in Medieval Arabic Literature*, Leiden, 1985.

———, *Kitāb al-Tabaṣṣur bil-Tijāra*, ed. H.A. al-Tūnisī, Cairo, 1935.

———, *Manāqib al-Turk*, ed. ʿAbd al-Salām Muḥammad Hārūn, *Rasāʾil al-Jāḥiẓ*, 4 vols., Cairo, 1979, III, 161–220.

Al-Jahshiyārī, Abū ʿAbd Allāh Muḥammad (d. 331/942), *Kitāb al-Wuzarāʾ wal-Kuttāb*, ed. Muṣṭafā al-Saqā, Ibrāhīm al-Abyārī, and ʿAbd al-Ḥafīẓ Shalabī, Cairo, 1938.

Al-Jurjānī, ʿAlī b. Muḥammad (d. 816/1413), *Kitāb al-Taʿrīfāt*, ed. G. Flügel, Leipzig, 1845; repr. Beirut, 1969.

Al-Juwaynī, Muʾayyad al-Dawla Badīʿ Atābak (6/12 c.), *Kitāb ʿAtabat al-Kataba*, ed. Muḥammad Qazwīnī, Tehran, 1329Kh.

Al-Khaṭīb al-Baghdādī, Abū Bakr Aḥmad b. ʿAlī (d. 463/1071), *Taʾrīkh Baghdād*, 14 vols., Cairo, 1931; repr. Beirut, n. d.; *Fahāris*, Beirut, 1986.

Al-Khwārizmī, Abū ʿAbd Allāh Muḥammad (d. 387/997), *Kitāb Mafātīḥ al-ʿUlūm*, ed. G. van Vloten, Leiden, 1895.

Al-Khwārizmī, Abū Bakr Muḥammad (d. 383/993), *Rasā'il Abī Bakr al-Khwārizmī*, Beirut, 1970.

Al-Kindī, Abū ʿUmar Muḥammad b. Yūsuf (d. 350/961), *Kitāb al-Wulāt wa-Kitāb al-Quḍāt*, ed. R. Guest, Leiden and London, 1912.

Al-Makhzūmī, Abū al-Ḥasan ʿAlī b. ʿUthmān (d. 585/1189), *al-Muntaqā min Kitāb al-Minhāj fī ʿIlm Kharāj Miṣr*, ed. Cl. Cahen, Cairo, 1986.

Al-Maqrīzī, Taqī al-Dīn Abū al-ʿAbbās Aḥmad (ca.766–845/ca.1364–1442), *al-Bayān wal-Iʿrāb ʿammā bi-Arḍ Miṣr min al-Aʿrāb*, ed. ʿAbd al-Majīd ʿĀbidīn, Cairo, 1961.

———, *al-Dhahab al-Masbūk fī Dhikr Man Ḥajja min al-Khulafā' wal-Mulūk*, ed. Jamāl al-Dīn al-Shayyāl, Cairo, 1955.

———, *Durar al-ʿUqūd al-Farīda fī Tarājim al-Aʿyān al-Mufīda*, ed. Muḥammad Kamāl al-Dīn ʿAlī, 2 vols., Beirut, 1992.

———, *Ittiʿāẓ al-Ḥunafā' bi-Akhbār al-A'immat al-Fāṭimīyīn*, ed. Jamāl al-Dīn Shayyāl and Muḥammad Ḥilmī M. Aḥmad, 3 vols., Cairo, 1967–73.

———, *Kitāb Ighāthat al-Umma bi-Kashf al-Ghumma*, ed. Muḥammad M. Ziyāda and Jamāl al-Dīn M. al-Shayyāl, Cairo, 1940; French tr. by G. Wiet, *Le traité des famines de Maqrīzī*, *JESHO*, 5 (1962), pp. 1–90; English tr. by A. Allouche, *Mamluk Economics*, Salt Lake City, 1994.

———, *Kitāb al-Mawāʿiẓ wal-Iʿtibār bi-Dhikr al-Khiṭaṭ wal-Āthār*, 2 vols., Bulaq, 1270H.; repr. Baghdad, 1970; *al-Mawāʿiẓ wal-Iʿtibār bi-Dhikr al-Khiṭaṭ wal-Āthār*, ed. Ayman Fu'ād Sayyid, 6 vols., London, 2002–04.

———, *Kitāb al-Muqaffā al-Kabīr*, ed. Muḥammad al-Yaʿlānī, 8 vols., Beirut, 1991.

———, *Kitāb al-Sulūk li-Maʿrifat Duwal al-Mulūk*,ed. Muḥammad Muṣṭafā Ziyāda, vols. 1–2, Cairo, 1939–58; ed. Saʿīd ʿAbd al-Fattāḥ ʿĀshūr, vols. 3–4, Cairo, 1970–73.

———, *Niḥal ʿIbar al-Naḥl*, ed. Jamāl al-Dīn al-Shayyāl, Cairo, 1946.

———, *al-Nuqūd al-Islāmīya al-Musammā bi-Shudhūr al-ʿUqūd fī Dhikr al-Nuqūd*, ed. Muḥammad Baḥr al-ʿUlūm, Najaf, 1967.

———, *Rasā'il al-Maqrīzī*, ed. Ramaḍān al-Badrī and Aḥmad M. Qāsim, Cairo, 1998.

Marco Polo (1254–1324), *The Travels of Marco Polo*, English tr. from the text of L.F. Benedetto by Aldo Ricci, London, 1931; repr. London, 2005; English tr. and ed. by H. Yule and H. Cordier, *The Book of Ser Marco Polo*, 2 vols., 3rd ed., London, 1929; Japanese tr. by Matsuo Otagi, *Toho Kenbunroku*, 2 vols., Tokyo, 1970–71.

Al-Masʿūdī, Abū al-Ḥasan ʿAlī b. al-Ḥusayn (d. 346/956), *Akhbār al-Zamān*, 2nd ed., Beirut, 1966.

———, *Murūj al-Dhahab wa-Maʿādin al-Jawhar*, ed. Muḥammad M. ʿAbd al-Ḥamīd, 4 vols., Cairo, 1964–67; French tr. by Ch. Pellat, *Les prairies d'or*, 7 vols., Beirut, 1966–79.

———, *al-Tanbīh wal-Ashrāf*, ed. ʿAbd Allāh Ismāʿīl al-Ṣāwī, Cairo, 1938; repr. Baghdad, n. d.

Al-Māwardī, Abū al-Ḥasan ʿAlī b. Muḥammad al-Baṣrī al-Baghdādī (d. 450/1058), *al-Aḥkām al-Sulṭānīya wal-Wilāyāt al-Dīnīya*, 2nd ed., Cairo, 1966; English tr. by Wafaa H. Wahba, *The Ordinances of Government*, Reading, 1996; Japanese tr. by Takeshi Yukawa, *Tochi no shokisoku*, Tokyo, 2006.

Miskawayh, Abū ʿAlī Aḥmad b. Muḥammad al-Rāzī (d. 421/1030), *Kitāb Tajārib al-Umam*, Facsimile ed. by L. Caetani, 3 vols., Leiden, 1909–17; *Kitāb Tajārib al-Umam*, Arabic text and English tr. by H.F. Amedroz and D.S. Margoliouth, *The Eclipse of the ʿAbbasid Caliphate*, 7 vols., London, 1920–21; repr. Baghdad, n. d.; *Tajārib al-Umam*, ed. Abū al-Qāsim Imāmī, 8 vols., Tehran, Dār Surūsh, 2001–02.

Al-Mundhirī, Zakī al-Dīn Abū Muḥammad ʿAbd al-ʿAẓīm (d. 656/1258), *al-Takmila li-Wafayāt al-Naqala*, ed. Bashshār ʿAwwād Maʿrūf, vols. 1–4, Najaf, 1968–71; vols. 5–6, Cairo, 1975–76.

Al-Muqaddasī, Abū ʿAbd Allāh Muḥammad (4/10c.), *Aḥsan al-Taqāsīm fī Maʿrifat al-Aqālīm*, *BGA*. III, ed. M.J. de Goeje, Leiden, 1906; English tr. by Basil Collins, *The Best Divisions for Knowledge of the Regions*, Reading, 2001.

Al-Musabbiḥī, ʿIzz al-Malik Muḥammad (366–420/977–1029), *Akhbār Miṣr*, ed. Ayman Fu'ād Sayyid, T. Bianquis, and Ḥusayn Naṣṣār, 2 vols., Cairo, 1978–84.

Al-Mutanabbī, Abū al-Ṭayyib Aḥmad (303–354/915–965), *Dīwān Abī al-Ṭayyib al-Mutanabbī*, ed. ʿAbd al-Wahhāb ʿAzzām, Cairo, 1944.

Al-Nābulusī, Abū ʿAmr ʿUthmān b. Ibrāhīm al-Ṣafadī (d. 660/1261), *Kitāb Lumaʿ al-Qawānīn al-Muḍīya fī Dawāwīn al-Diyār al-Miṣrīya*, ed. C. Becker and Cl. Cahen, *BEO*, 16 (1958–60), 1–78.

———, *Ta'rīkh al-Fayyūm wa-Bilādih*, ed. B. Moritz, Cairo, 1898; repr. Beirut, 1974.

Nāṣir Khusraw, Abū Muʿīn Qubādhiyānī (394 – between 465 and 471/1004 – between 1072 and 78), *Safar Nāma*, Berlin, 1340H.; ed. Muḥammad Dabīr Siyāqī, Tehrān, 1387H.

Niẓām al-Mulk, Abū ʿAlī Ḥasan (d. 485/1092), *Siyāsat Nāma*, ed. J. Shiʿār, Tehran, 1348H.; English tr. by H. Darke, *The Book of Government or Rules for Kings*, London, 1960.

Al-Nuʿaymī, Muḥī al-Dīn Abū al-Mufākhir ʿAbd al-Qādir (d. 927/1521), *al-Dāris fī Ta'rīkh al-Madāris*, ed. J. al-Ḥusnī, 2 vols., Damascus, 1948–51.

Al-Nuwayrī, Shihāb al-Dīn Aḥmad b. ʿAbd al-Wahhāb (677–733/1279–1333), *Nihāyat al-Arab fī Funūn al-Adab*, vols. 1–18, Cairo, 1954; ed. Muḥammad Muḥammad Amīn etc., vols. 19–33, Cairo, 1975–97.

Al-Nuwayrī al-Iskandarānī, Muḥammad b. Qāsim (d. after 775/1372), *Kitāb al-Ilmām bil-Iʿlām*, ed. E.T. Combe, 7 vols., Hyderabad, 1968–76.

Piloti, Emmanuel (15 c.). *L'Égypte au commencement du quinzième siècle*, ed. and notes by P.H. Dopp, Cairo, 1950.

Al-Qalqashandī, Shihāb al-Dīn Abū al-ʿAbbās Aḥmad b. ʿAlī (756–821/1355–1418), *Nihāyat al-Arab fī Maʿrifat Ansāb al-ʿArab*, ed. ʿAlī al-Khāqānī, Baghdad, 1958.

———, *Qalā'id al-Jumān fī al-Taʿrīf bi-Qabā'il ʿArab al-Zamān*, ed. I. al-Abyarī, Cairo, 1964.

———, *Ṣubḥ al-Aʿshā fī Ṣināʿat al-Inshāʾ*, 14 vols., Cairo, 1963; *Fahāris Kitāb Ṣubḥ al-Aʿshā*, Cairo, 1972.

Al-Qazwīnī, Zakariyāʾ b. Muḥammad (ca.600–682/ca.1203–83), *Āthār al-Bilād wa-Akhbār al-ʿIbād*, Beirut, 1960.

Al-Qifṭī, Abū al-Ḥasan ʿAlī (d. 646/1248), *Taʾrīkh al-Ḥukamāʾ*, ed. J. Lippert, Leipzig, 1903.

Qummī, Ḥasan b. Muḥammad (4/10 c.), *Kitāb Taʾrīkh-i Qumm*, ed. Sayyid Jamāl al-Dīn Tehrānī, Tehran, 1353H.

Al-Qurṭubī, ʿArīb b. Saʿd (4/10 c.), *Ṣilat Taʾrīkh al-Ṭabarī*, ed. M.J. de Goeje, Leiden, 1897; in *Dhuyūl Taʾrīkh al-Ṭabarī*, ed. Muḥammad Abū al-Faḍl Ibrāhīm, Cairo, n. d.

Al-Rūdhrāwarī, Ẓahīr al-Dīn Abū Shujāʿ Muḥammad (d. 488/1095), *Dhayl Kitāb Tajārib al-Umam*, ed. H.F. Amedroz, Oxford, 1921.

Al-Ṣafadī, Ṣalāḥ al-Dīn Khalīl Ibn Aybak (696–764/1297–1363), *Kitāb al-Wāfī bil-Wafayāt*, ed. S. Dedering, Shukrī Fayṣal, B. Jokisch, etc., 31 vols., Wiesbaden, 1949–2010.

Al-Sakhāwī, Shams al-Dīn Abū al-Khayr Muḥammad (d. 902/1497), *al-Buldānīyāt*, ed. Ḥusām b. Muḥammad al-Qaṭṭān, Riyad, 2001.

———, *al-Ḍawʾ al-Lāmiʿ li-Ahl al-Qarn al-Tāsiʿ*, 12 vols., Beirut, 1934–36.

———, *al-Iʿlān bil-Tawbīkh li-Man Dhamma al-Taʾrīkh*, ed. F. Rosenthal, repr. Baghdad, 1963.

———, *Kitāb al-Tibr al-Masbūk fī Dhayl al-Sulūk*, Bulaq, 1896; repr., Cairo, 1974.

Ṣāliḥ b. Yaḥyā (9/15c.), *Taʾrīkh Bayrūt*, ed. K.S. al-Ṣalībī and F. Hours, Beirut, 1969.

Al-Sallāmī, Taqī al-Dīn Muḥammad Ibn Rāfiʿ (d. 774/1372), *al-Wafayāt*, ed. Ṣāliḥ Mahdī ʿAbbās, 2 vols., Beirut, 1982.

Shāfiʿ b. ʿAlī, Nāṣir al-Dīn al-Kātib al-Miṣrī (649–730/1252–1330), *al-Faḍl al-Maʾthūr min Sīrat al-Sulṭān al-Malik al-Manṣūr Qalāwūn*, ed. ʿUmar A. Tadmurī, Beirut, 1998; ed. P.B. Lewicka, *Šāfi Ibn ʿAlī's Bibliography of the Mamluk Sultan Qalāwūn*, Warsaw, 2000.

———, *Kitāb Ḥusn al-Manāqib al-Sirrīyat al-Muntazaʿa min al-Sīrat al-Ẓāhirīya*, ed. ʿAbd al-ʿAzīz al-Khuwayṭir, Riyad, 1976.

Al-Shāfiʿī, Abū ʿAbd Allāh Muḥammad b. Idrīs (150–204/767–820), *Kitāb al-Umm*, 8 vols., Beirut, n. d.

Al-Shayyāl, Jamāl al-Dīn ed. *Majmūʿat al-Wathāʾiq al-Fāṭimīya*, vol. 1, 2nd ed., Cairo, 1965.

Al-Shayzarī, Jalāl al-Dīn ʿAbd al-Raḥmān (d. 589/1193), *Nihāyat al-Rutba fī Ṭalab al-Ḥisba*, ed. al-Sayyid al-Bāz al-ʿArīnī, Beirut, 1969; English tr. by R.P. Buckley, *The Book of the Islamic Market Inspector*, Oxford, 1999.

Al-Shujāʿī, Shams al-Dīn al-Miṣrī (8/14 c.), *Taʾrīkh al-Malik al-Nāṣir Muḥammad b. Qalāwūn al-Ṣāliḥī*, Arabic text and German tr. by B. Schäfer, 2 vols., Wiesbaden, 1978–85.

Sibṭ Ibn al-Jawzī, Shams al-Dīn Abū al-Muẓaffar Yūsuf (d. 654/1256), *Mirʾāt al-Zamān fī Taʾrīkh al-Aʿyān*, vol. VIII-1/2, Hyderabad, 1951–52; *Mirʾāt al-Zamān fī Taʾrīkh al-Aʿyān (448–480 H.)*, ed. Ali Sevim, Ankara, 1968; *Mirʾāt al-Zamān fī Taʾrīkh al-Aʿyān (345–447 H.)*, ed. Janān J.M. al-Hamūndī, Baghdad, 1990; *Mirʾāt al-Zamān (395–411 H.)*, ed. Juliette Rassi, Damascus, 2005.

Song Yingxing (宋應星), *Tenko Kaibutsu* (*Tien-kung kai-wu*), Japanese tr. by Kiyoshi Yabuuchi, Tokyo, 1969.

Strabo (64 or 63 BC–ca.23 AD), *The Geography of Strabo*, ed. & tr. H.L. Jones, 8 vols., London and New York, 1917–32.

Al-Subkī, Tāj al-Dīn Abū Naṣr ʿAbd al-Wahhāb (d. 771/1370), *Kitāb Muʿīd al-Niʿam wa-Mubīd al-Niqam*, ed. David W. Myhrman, London, 1908; repr. New York, 1978.

———, *Ṭabaqāt al-Shāfiʿīyat al-Kubrā*, ed. Muḥammad M. al-Ṭanāḥī and ʿAbd al-Fattāḥ M. Ḥulw, 8 vols., Cairo, 1964.

Al-Ṣūlī, Abū Bakr Muḥammad b. Yaḥyā (d. 335/947), *Adab al-Kuttāb*, ed. Muḥammad b. al-Atharī, Cairo, 1341H.

———, *Akhbār al-Rāḍī wal-Muttaqī*, ed. J.H. Dunne, Cairo, 1935.

Al-Suyūṭī, Abū al-Faḍl Jalāl al-Dīn ʿAbd al-Raḥmān (849–911/1445–1505), *Ḥusn al-Muḥāḍara fī Taʾrīkh Miṣr wal-Qāhira*, ed. Muḥammad Abū al-Faḍl Ibrāhīm, 2 vols., Cairo, 1967–68.

———, *Kawkab al-Rawḍa fī Taʾrīkh al-Nīl wa-Jazīrat al-Rawḍa*, ed. Muḥammad al-Shashtāwī, Cairo, 2002.

———, *Naẓm al-ʿIqyān fī Aʿyān al-Aʿyān*, ed. Philip K. Hitti, New York, 1927.

———, *al-Raḥma fī al-Ṭibb wal-Ḥikma*, Beirut, 1983.

———, *Taʾrīkh al-Khulafāʾ*, ed. M.M. ʿAbd al-Ḥamīd, Cairo, 1964.

Al-Ṭabarī, Abū Jaʿfar Muḥammad b. Jarīr (d. 310/923), *Taʾrīkh al-Rusul wal-Mulūk*, ed. M.J. de Goeje, 15 vols., Leiden, 1879–1901; repr., Leiden, 1964.

Al-Tanūkhī, Abū ʿAlī al-Muḥassin b. ʿAlī (d. 384/994), *al-Faraj baʿda al-Shidda*, 2 vols., Cairo, 1955.

———, *Nishwār al-Muḥāḍara wa-Akhbār al-Mudhākara*, ed. A. al-Shāljī, 8 vols., Beirut, 1971–73.

Al-Ṭarsūsī, Marḍī b. ʿAlī (6/12 c.), *Tabṣirat Arbāb al-Albāb*, Arabic text and French tr. by Cl. Cahen, *BEO*, 12 (1948), 103–163.

Al-Ṭarsūsī, Najm al-Dīn (d. 758/1357), *Kitāb Tuḥfat al-Turk*, Arabic text and French tr. by Muḥammad Minaṣrī, Damascus, 1997.

Al-Tawḥīdī, Abū Ḥayyān ʿAlī b. Muḥammad (d. 414/1023), *al-Imtāʿ wal-Muʾānasa*, ed. Aḥmad Amīn and Aḥmad al-Zayn, 3 vols., Beirut, n. d.

———, *Mathālib al-Wazīrayn: Akhlāq al-Ṣāḥib b. ʿAbbād wa-Ibn al-ʿAmīd*, ed. Ibrāhīm al-Kaylānī, Damascus, 1961.

———, *Thalāth Rasāʾil li-Abī Ḥayyān al-Tawḥīdī*, ed. Ibrāhīm al-Kaylānī, Damascus, 1951.

Al-Thaʿālibī, Abū Manṣūr ʿAbd al-Malik (350–429/961–1038), *Kitāb Thimār al-Qulūb fī al-Muḍāf wal-Mansūb*, Cairo, 1908.

———, *Laṭāʾif al-Maʿārif*, ed. Ibrāhīm al-Abyārī and Ḥasan K. al-Ṣayrafī, Cairo, 1960; English tr. by C.E. Bosworth, *The Book of Curious and Entertaining Information*, Edinburgh, 1968.

———, *al-Tamthīl wal-Muḥāḍara*, ed. ʿAbd al-Fattāḥ Muḥammad Ḥulw, Riyad, 1983.

Al-Tujībī, al-Qāsim b. Yūsuf al-Sabtī (d.730/1329), *Mustafād al-Riḥla wal-Ightirāb*, ed. ʿAbd al-Ḥafīẓ Manṣūr, Tunis, 1975.

Al-Udfuwī, Kamāl al-Dīn Abū al-Faḍl Jaʿfar al-Shāfiʿī (d. 748/1347), *al-Ṭāliʿ al-Saʿīd al-Jāmiʿ li-Asmāʾ al-Fuḍalāʾ wal-Ruwāt*, Cairo, 1914.

Al-ʿUmarī, Shihāb al-Dīn Aḥmad Ibn Faḍl Allāh (700–749/1301–1349), *Masālik al-Abṣār fī Mamālik al-Amṣār: Mamālik Miṣr wal-Shām wal-Ḥijāz wal-Yaman*, ed. Ayman Fuʾād Sayyid, Cairo, 1985; *Masālik al-Abṣār fī Mamālik al-Amṣār: Qabāʾil al-ʿArab fī al-Qarnayn al-Sābiʿ wal-Thāmin al-Hijrīyayn*, ed. D. Krawulsky, Beirut, 1985; *Masālik al-Abṣār fī Mamālik al-Amṣār: Dawlat al-Mamālīk al-Ūlā*, ed. D. Krawulsky, Beirut, 1986.

———, *al-Taʿrīf bil-Muṣṭalaḥ al-Sharīf*, ed. Muḥammad Ḥusayn Shams al-Dīn, Beirut, 1988; ed. Samīr al-Durūbī, al-Karak, 1992.

Usāma b. Munqidh, Muʾayyad al-Dawla Abū al-Muẓaffar al-Shayzarī (488–584/1095–1188), *Kitāb al-Iʿtibār*, ed. P.K. Hitti, Princeton, 1930; English tr. by P.K. Hitti, *Memoirs of an Arab-Syrian Gentleman*, New York, 1929; repr., Beirut, 1964.

Al-Yaʿqūbī, Ibn Wāḍiḥ Aḥmad b. Abī Yaʿqūb (d. 284/897), *Kitāb al-Buldān*, BGA, VII, ed. M.J. de Goeje, Leiden, 1892; repr., Leiden, 1967.

———, *Taʾrīkh al-Yaʿqūbī*, ed. M. Th. Houtsma, 2 vols., Beirut, 1960.

Yāqūt, Shihāb al-Dīn Abū ʿAbd Allāh al-Ḥamawī al-Rūmī (d. 626/1229), *Kitāb Irshād al-Arīb ilā Maʿrifat al-Adīb*, ed. D.S. Margoliouth, 7 vols., London, 1923–31.

———, *Kitāb al-Mushtarak*, ed. F. Wüstenfeld, Göttingen, 1846.

———, *Muʿjam al-Buldān*, 5 vols., Beirut, 1955–57.

Al-Yūnīnī, Quṭb al-Dīn Mūsā (d. 726/1326), *Dhayl Mirʾāt al-Zamān*, 4 vols., Hyderabad, 1954–61.

Al-Yūsufī, Mūsā b. Muḥammad (d. 759/1358), *Nuzhat al-Nāẓir fī Sīrat al-Malik al-Nāṣir*, ed. Aḥmad Ḥuṭayṭ, Beirut, 1986.

Al-Ẓāhirī, Zayn al-Dīn ʿAbd al-Bāsiṭ b. Khalīl al-Ḥanafī (844–920/1440–1514), *Nayl al-Amal fī Dhayl al-Duwal*, ed. ʿUmar ʿAbd al-Salām Tadmurī, 9 vols., Saida and Beirut, 2002.

Secondary Works

ʿAbd Allāh, Ṣafī A. Muḥammad, *Mudun Miṣr al-Ṣināʿīya fī al-ʿAṣr al-Islāmī*, Cairo, 2000.

ʿAbd al-Bāqī, Muḥammad Fuʾād, *al-Muʿjam al-Mufahris li-Alfāẓ al-Qurʾān al-Karīm*, Beirut, n. d.

ʿAbd al-Mawlā, Muḥammad Aḥmad, *al-ʿAyyārūn wal-Shuṭṭār al-Baghādida fī al-Taʾrīkh al-ʿAbbāsī*, Alexandria, 1990.

ʿAbd al-Raḥmān, ʿĀṣim M., *Marākiz al-Ṣināʿa fī Miṣr al-Islāmīya*, Cairo, 1989.

ʿAbdul Jabbar M., "Agricultural and Irrigation Labourers in Social and Economic Life of ʿIrāq during the Umayyad and ʿAbbasid Caliphates," *IC*, 47 (1973), pp. 15–31.

Abu-Lughod, Janet L., *Cairo: 1001 Years of the City Victorious*, Princeton, 1971.
———, *Before European Hegemony: The World System AD 1250–1350*, Oxford, 1989; Japanese tr. by Tsugitaka Sato and others, *Yoroppa haken izen*, 2 vols., Tokyo, 2001.
Abū Sadīra, Sayyid T. al-Sayyid, *al-Ḥiraf wal-Ṣināʿāt fī Miṣr al-Islāmīya*, Cairo, 1991.
Academy of Arabic Language ed., *Modern Dictionary of Chemical and Pharmaceutical Terms*, Cairo, 2004.
Agius, Dionisius A., *Classic Ships of Islam: From Mesopotamia to the Indian Ocean*, Leiden and Boston, 2008.
Aḥmad, Aḥmad ʿAbd al-Rāziq, *al-Badhl wal-Barṭala: Zaman Salāṭīn al-Mamālīk*, Cairo, 1979.
Aḥmad, ʿAzīz, *A History of Islamic Sicily*, Edinburgh, 1975.
Ahsan, Muhammad M., *Social Life under the Abbasids*, London and New York, 1979.
Al-ʿAlī, Ṣāliḥ Aḥmad, *al-Tanẓīmāt al-Ijtimāʿīya wal-Iqtiṣādīya fī al-Baṣra fī al-Qarn al-Awwal al-Hijrī*, Beirut, 1969.
———, *Baghdād Madīnat al-Salām: al-Jānib al-Gharbī*, 2 vols., Baghdad, 1985.
Allouche, A., *Mamluk Economics: A Study and Translation of Al-Maqrīzī's Ighātha*, Salt Lake City, 1994.
Amīn, Muḥammad Muḥammad, *al-Awqāf wal-Ḥayāt al-Ijtimāʿīya fī Miṣr 648–923/1250–1517*, Cairo, 1980.
———, "Manshūr bi-Manḥ Iqṭāʿ min ʿAṣr al-Sulṭān al-Ghawrī," *Ḥawlīyāt Islāmīya*, 19 (1983), 1–23.
Amitai-Preiss, Reuven, *Mongols and Mamluks: The Mamluk-Ilkhānid War, 1260–1281*, Cambridge, 1995.
———, "The Remaking of the Military Elite of Mamluk Egypt by Al-Nāṣir Muḥammad b. Qalāwūn," *SI*, 72 (1990), 145–163.
Amitai-Preiss, Reuven and David O. Morgan ed., *The Mongol Empire and its Legacy*, Leiden, Boston, and Köln, 2000.
Al-ʿArīnī, al-Sayyid al-Bāz, *al-Iqṭāʿ al-Ḥarbī bi-Miṣr Zaman Salāṭīn al-Mamālīk*, Cairo, 1966.
———, *al-Mamālīk*, Beirut, 1979.
Arnold, Thomas W., *The Caliphate*, Oxford, 1924; repr. London, 1965.
Al-Ashqar, Muḥammad ʿAbd al-Ghanī, *Tujjār al-Tawābil fī Miṣr fī al-ʿAṣr al-Mamlūkī*, Cairo, 1999.
Ashtor, Eliyahu, *Histoire des prix et des salaires dans l'Orient médiéval*, Paris, 1969.
———, *A Social and Economic History of the Near East in the Middle Ages*, Berkeley and Los Angeles, 1976.
———, *Levant Trade in the Later Middle Ages*, Princeton, 1983.
———, *Technology, Industry and Trade: The Levant versus Europe, 1250–1500*, Variorum reprints, London, 1992.
———, "The Kārimī Merchants," *Journal of the Royal Asiatic Society*, 1956, 45–56.

———, "L'administration urbaine en Syrie médiévale," *Rivista degli Studi Orientali*, 31 (1956), 73–128.

———, "Un mouvement migratoire au haut moyen âge: Migrations de l'Irak vers les pays méditerranéens," *Annales: ESC*, 27 (1972), 185–214.

———, "Levantine Sugar Industry in the Late Middle Ages: A Case of Technological Decline," Abraham L. Udovitch ed., *The Islamic Middle East, 700–1900*, Princeton, 1981, 91–132.

ʿĀshūr, Saʿīd ʿAbd al-Fattāḥ, *al-Mujtamaʿ al-Miṣrī fī ʿAṣr Salāṭīn al-Mamālīk*, Cairo, 1962.

———, *al-ʿAṣr al-Mamālīkī fī Miṣr wal-Shām*, Cairo, 1965.

———, *al-Ḥarakat al-Ṣalībīya: Ṣafḥat Mushriqa min Taʾrīkh al-Jihād al-ʿArabī fī al-ʿUṣūr al-Wusṭā*, 2 vols., Cairo, 4th ed., 1982.

Atiya, A. S., *The Crusade: Historiography and Bibliography*, Bloomington, 1962; repr. Westport, 1976.

———, *A History of Eastern Christianity*, London, 1968.

———, "A Mamlūk 'Magna Carta'," George N. Atiyeh and Ibrahim M. Oweiss ed., *Arab Civilization: Challenges and Responses, Studies in Honor of Constantine K. Zurayk*, Albany, N.Y., 1988, 128–139.

Atiyeh, George N. and Ibrahim M. Oweiss ed., *Arab Civilization: Challenges and Responses, Studies in Honor of Constantine K. Zurayk*, Albany, N.Y., 1988.

Attié, B. A., "Les manuscripts agricoles arabes de la Bibliothèque Nationale de Paris," *Hespéris Tamuda*, 10 (1969), 241–261.

Ayalon, David, *L'ésclavage du Mamelouk*, Jerusalem, 1951.

———, *Gunpowder and Firearms in the Mamluk Kingdom: A Challenge to a Medieval Society*, London, 1956; 2nd ed., Totowa, N.J., 1978.

———, *Studies on the Mamlūks of Egypt (1250–1517)*, Variorum reprints, London, 1977.

———, *The Mamlūk Military Society*, Variorum reprints, London, 1979.

———, *Outsiders in the lands of Islam: Mamluks, Mongols and Eunuchs*, Variorum reprints, London, 1988.

———, *Islam and the Abode of War: Military Slaves and Islamic Adversaries*, Variorum reprints, London, 1994.

———, *Eunuchs, Caliphs and Sultans: A Study of Power Relationships*, Jerusalem, 1999.

———, "Studies on the Transfer of the ʿAbbāsid Caliphate from Baġdād to Cairo," *Arabica*, 7 (1950), 41–59.

———, "The Wafidiya in the Mamluk Kingdom," *IC*, 25 (1951), 89–104.

———, "Studies on the Structure of the Mamluk Army I-III, " *BSOAS*, 15 (1953), 203–228, 449–476; 16 (1954), 57–90.

———, "Notes on the *Furūsīya* Exercises and Games in the Mamluk Sultanate," U. Heyd ed., *Studies in Islamic History and Civilization*, Jerusalem, 1961, 31–62.

———, "The System of Payment in Mamluk Military Society," *Studies on the Mamlūks of Egypt (1250–1517)*, Variorum reprints, London, 1977, 37–65, 257–296.

———, "From Ayyubids to Mamluks," *REI*, 49 (1981), 43–58.
———, "Some Remarks on the Economic Decline of the Mamlūk Sultanate," *Jerusalem Studies in Arabic and Islam*, 16 (1993), 108–124.
Bacharach, Jere L. ed., *Fustat Finds: Beads, Coins, Medical Instruments, Textiles, and Other Artifacts from the Awad Collection*, Cairo, 2002.
———, "The Dinar Versus the Ducat," *IJMES*, 4 (1973), 77–96.
———, "Circassian Monetary Policy: Copper," *JESHO*, 19 (1976), 32–47.
———, "African Military Slaves in the Medieval Middle East: The Case of Iraq (869–955) and Egypt (868–1171)," *IJMES*, 13 (1981), 471–495.
Baer, Gabriel, *A History of Landownership in Modern Egypt 1800–1950*, London, New York, and Toronto, 1962.
———, *Studies in the Social History of Modern Egypt*, Chicago and London, 1969.
Baġdād: publié à l'occasion du mille deux centième anniversaire de la fondation, Arabica, volume special, 1962.
Bakhīṭ, Muḥammad ʿAdnān, *Mamlakat al-Karak fī al-ʿAhd al-Mamlūkī*, Amman, 1976.
———, *The Ottoman Province of Damascus in the Sixteenth Century*, Beirut, 1982.
Balog, P., *The Coinage of the Mamluk Sultans of Egypt and Syria*, New York, 1964.
Al-Baqlī, Muḥammad Qindīl, *al-Taʿrīf bi-Muṣṭalaḥāt Ṣubḥ al-Aʿshā*, Cairo, 1984.
Barthold, W., *Turkestan down to the Mongol Invasion*, Fourth Edition, Philadelphia, 1977.
Behens-Abouseif, Doris, *Fatḥ Allāh and Abū Zakariyya: Physicians under the Mamluks*, Cairo, 1987.
Behrens-Abouseif, Doris ed., *The Cairo Heritage; Essays in Honor of Laila Ali Ibrahim*, Cairo and New York, 2000.
Béllahsen, F. and D. Rouche, *Cuisine tunisienne*, Barcelona, 2003.
Ben Abdallah, Habib, *De l'iqta' étatique à l'iqta' militaire: Transition économique et changements sociaux à Baghdad, 247–447 de l'Hégire/861–1055 ap. J.*, Uppsala, 1986.
Berthier, Paul, *Les anciennes sucreries du Maroc et leur réseaux hydrauliques*, 2 vols., Rabat, 1966.
Bianquis, Thierry, *Damas et la Syrie sous la domination fatimide (359–468/969–1076)*, 2 vols., Damascus, 1986–89.
Bibliography of Islamic and Middle Eastern Studies in Japan 1868–1988, Compiled and Published by The Centre for East Asian Cultural Studies for UNESCO, The Toyo Bunko, 2 vols., Tokyo, 1992. As for the subsequent information after 1989, see http://www.james1985.org.
Bloom, Jonathan M., *Paper before Print: The History and Impact of Paper in the Islamic World*, New Haven and London, 2001.
Blume, Helmut, *Geography of Sugar Cane*, Berlin, 1985.
Borsch, Stuart J., *The Black Death in Egypt and England: A Comparative Study*, Cairo, 2005.

Bosworth, Clifford. E., *Medieval Arabic Culture and Administration*, Variorum reprints, London, 1982.

———, *The New Islamic Dynasties: A Chronological and Genealogical Manual*, Edinburgh, 1996.

Bosworth, Clifford. E., Ch. Issawi, R. Savory, and Abraham L. Udovitch ed., *The Islamic World from Classical to Modern Times: Essays in Honor of Bernard Lewis*, Princeton, 1989.

Brockelmann, Carl, *Geschichte der Arabischen Litteratur*, 5 vols., Leiden, 1937–49.

Browne, E. G., *Arabian Medicine*, Cambridge, 1921; repr. 1962.

Bulliet, Richard W., *The Camel and the Wheel*, Cambridge, Mass., 1975.

———, *Conversion to Islam in the Medieval Period*, Cambridge, Mass., 1979.

———, *Cotton, Climate, and Camels in Early Islamic Iran*, New York, 2009.

Busse, H., *Chalif und Großkönig–Die Buyiden im Iraq*, Wiesbaden, 1969.

———, "Iran under the Būyids," *The Cambridge History of Iran*, vol. 4, Cambridge, 1975, 250–304.

Cahen, Cl., *La Syrie du Nord à l'époque des Croisades et la principauté franque d'Antioche*, Paris, 1940.

———, *Pre-Ottoman Turkey*, Translated from the French by J. Jones-Williams, London, 1968.

———, *Makhzūmiyyāt*, Leiden, 1977.

———, *Les peuples musulmans dans l'histoire médiévale*, Damascus, 1977.

———, "Le service de l'irrigation en Iraq au début du XIe siècle," *BEO*, 13 (1949–50), 117–143.

———, "Documents relatifs à quelques techniques Iraqienne au début du onzième siècle," *Ars Islamica*, 15–16 (1951), 23–28.

———, "Quelques problèmes économiques et fiscaux de l'Irāq buyide d'après un traité de mathématiques," *Annales de l'Institut d'Études Orientales (Alger)*, 10 (1952), 326–363.

———, "L'évolution de l'iqṭāʿ du IXe au XIIIe siècle," *Annales:ESC*, 8 (1953), 25–52.

———, "Le régime des impôts dans le Fayyūm ayyūbide," *Arabica*, 3 (1956), 8–30.

———, "Mouvements populaires et autonomisme urbain dans l'Asie musulman du moyen âge I-III," *Arabica*, 5 (1958), 225–250; 6 (1959), 25–56, 233–265.

———, "Un traité financier inédit d'époque fatimide-ayyubide," *JESHO*, 5 (1962), 139–159.

———, "Al-Makhzūmī et Ibn Mammātī sur l'agriculture égyptienne médiévale," *AI*, 11 (1972), 141–151.

———, "Aperçu sur les impôts du sol en Syrie au moyen âge," *JESHO*, 18 (1975), 233–244.

———, "Monetary Circulation in Egypt at the Time of the Crusades and the Reform of al-Kāmil," Abraham L. Udovitch ed., *The Islamic Middle East, 700–1900*, Princeton, 1981, 315–333.

Campbell, Donald, *Arabian Medicine and its Influence on the Middle Ages*, 2 vols., London, 1926; repr. Amsterdam, 1974.

Canard, M., "Le riz dans le Orient aux première siècles de l'Islam," *Arabica*, 6 (1959), 113–131.

Centre national de la recherche scientifique ed., *Sucre, sucreries et douceurs en Méditerranée*, Paris, 1991.

Chamberlain, Michael, *Knowledge and Social Practice in Medieval Damascus, 1190–1350*, Cambridge, 1994.

Chapoutot-Remadi, M., "Agriculture dans l'empire mamluk au moyen âge d'après al-Nuwayrī," *Les Cahiers de Tunisie*, 22 (1974), 23–45.

———, "Une grande crise à la fin du XIIIe siècle en Égypte," *JESHO*, 26 (1983), 217–245.

Chipman, Leigh, *The World of Pharmacy and Pharmacists in Mamlūk Cairo*, Leiden and Boston, 2010.

Ciggaar, K. and H. Teule ed., *East and West in the Crusader States: Context-Contacts-Confrontations*, III, *Orientalia Lovaniensia Analecta 125*, Leuven and Dudley, MA., 2003.

Cohen, Mark R., *Jewish Self-Government in Medieval Egypt: The Origins of the Office of Head of the Jews, ca. 1065–1126*, Princeton, 1980.

Colloque internationale sur l'histoire du Caire (27 Mars-5 Avril 1969), Cairo, 1969.

Conermann, Stephan and Anja Pistor-Hatam ed., *Die Mamlūken: Studien zu ihrer Geschichte und Kultur. Zum Gedenken an Ulrich Haarmann (1942–1999)*, Asien und Africa, Band 7, Schenefeld, 2003.

Contadini, Anna ed., *Arab Painting: Text and Image in Illustrated Arabic Manuscripts*, Leiden and Boston, 2010.

Cuno, Kenneth M., *The Pasha's Peasants: Land, Society, and Economy in Lower Egypt, 1740–1858*, Cambridge, 1992.

Daniels, Christian, *Science and Civilization in China* (Joseph Needham). Vol. 6, Biology and Biological Technology, part III, *Agro-Industries: Sugarcane Technology*, Cambridge, 1996.

———, "The Adoption and Transfer of New Sugarmaking Technology within South China during the Late Ming – Early Qing Period (Minmatsu Shinsho ni okeru shin seito gijutsu taikei no saiyo oyobi kokunai iten, in Japanese)," *Shujitsu Joshi Daigaku Shigaku Ronshu*, 3 (1988), 77–156.

Darrag, Aḥmad, *L'Égypte sous le règne de Barsbāy*, Damascus, 1961

Deerr, Noel, *The History of Sugar*, 2 vols., London, 1949–50.

Denoix, Sylvie, *Décrire le Caire: Fusṭāṭ-Miṣr d'après Ibn Duqmāq et Maqrīzī*, Cairo, 1992.

D'Hulster, K. and J. van Steenbergen ed., *Continuity and Change in the Realms of Islam: Studies in Honour of Professor Urbain Vermeulen*, *Orientalia Lovaniensia Analecta 171*, Leuven, Paris and Dudley, MA., 2008.

El-Doğhim, Mahmoud El-Saied, *Fihris al-Makhṭūṭāt al-ʿArabīya wal-Turkīya wal-Fārisīya fī al-Maktabat al-Sulaymānīya*, 3 vols. Istanbul, 2010.

Dols, Michael W., *The Black Death in the Middle East*, Princeton, 1977.

Dozy, R., *Dictionnaire détaillé des noms des vêtements chez les Arabes*, Amsterdam, 1845; repr. Beirut, n. d.

———, *Supplément aux dictionnaires arabes*, 3rd ed., 2 vols., Paris, 1967.

Durand-Guédy, David, *Iranian Elites and Turkish Rulers: A History of Iṣfahān in the Saljūq Period*, London and New York, 2010.

Al-Dūrī, ʿAbd al-ʿAzīz, *Muqaddima fī al-Taʾrīkh al-Iqtiṣādī al-ʿArabī*, Beirut, 1969.

———, *Taʾrīkh al-ʿIrāq al-Iqtiṣādī fī al-Qarn al-Rābiʿ al-Hijrī*, Baghdad, 1948; 2nd ed., Beirut, 1974.

———, *The Rise of Historical Writing among the Arabs*, English tr. by Lawrence I. Conrad, Princeton, 1983.

———, "The Origins of Iqṭāʿ in Islam," *al-Abḥāth*, 22 (1969), 3–22.

———, "Nashʾat al-Iqṭāʿ fī al-Mujtamaʿāt al-Islāmīya," *Majallat al-Majmaʿ al-ʿIlmī al-ʿIrāqī*, 20 (1970), 3–24.

Edwards, Jill ed., *Historians in Cairo: Essays in Honor of George Scanlon*, Cairo and New York, 2002.

Ehrenkreutz, Andrew S., *Saladin*, Albany, N.Y., 1972.

———, *Monetary Change and Economic History in the Medieval Muslim World*, Variorum reprints, London, 1992.

———, "Contribution to the Knowledge of the Fiscal Administration of Egypt in the Middle Ages," *BSOAS*, 16 (1954), 502–514.

———, "The Crisis of Dīnār in the Egypt of Saladin," *JAOS*, 76 (1956), 178–184.

Elham, S. H., *Kitbuġā und Lāǧīn: Studien zur Mamluken-Geschichte nach Baibars al-Manṣūrī und an-Nuwairī*, Freiburg, 1977.

Ellenblum, Ronnie, *Frankish Rural Settlement in the Latin Kingdom of Jerusalem*, Cambridge, 1998.

Ernest, H., *Die mamlukischen Sultansurkunden des Sinai-Klosters*, Wiesbaden, 1960.

Ettinghausen, R., *Arab Painting*, Cleveland, 1962.

Fahd, B. M., *al-ʿĀmma bi-Baghdād fī al-Qarn al-Khāmis al-Hijrī*, Baghdad, 1967.

Fahd, T., "Conduite d'une exploitation agricole d'après L'Agriculture Nabatéenne," *SI*, 32 (1970), 109–128.

Fākhūrī, Maḥmūd and Ṣalāḥ al-Dīn Khawwā, *Mawsūʿat Waḥadāt al-Qiyās al-ʿArabīya wal-Islāmīya wa-mā Yuʿādilhā bil-Maqādīr al-Ḥadītha*, Beirut, 2002.

Fischel, W. J., *Ibn Khaldūn in Egypt: His Public Functions and His Historical Research (1382–1406)*, Berkeley and Los Angeles, 1967.

———, "Über die Gruppe der Kārimī-Kaufleute," *Analecta Orientalia*, 14 (1937), 67–82.

———, "The Spice Trade in Mamluk Egypt," *JESHO*, 1 (1958), 157–174.

Frantz-Murphy, G., *The Agrarian Administration of Egypt from the Arabs to the Ottomans*, Cairo, 1986.

Gacek, Adam, *The Arabic Manuscript Tradition: A Glossary of Technical Terms and Bibliography*, Leiden, Boston, and Köln, 2001.

Garcin, J. C., *Un centre musulman de la Haute-Égypte médiévale: Qūṣ*, Cairo, 1976.
———, *Espaces, pouvoirs et idéologies de l'Égypte médiévale*, Variorum reprints, London, 1987.
———, "Note sur les rapports entre bédouins et fellahs à l'époque mamluke," *AI*, 14 (1978), 147–163.
Ghabin, Ahmad, *Ḥisba, Arts and Craft in Islam*, Wiesbaden, 2009.
Ghawānima, Yūsuf Ḥasan, *Dimashq fī ʿAṣr Dawlat al-Mamālīk al-Thāniya*, Beirut, 2005.
Gibb, Hamilton A. R., *The Damascus Chronicle of the Crusades, extracted and translated from the Chronicle of Ibn al-Qalānisī*, London, 1932; repr. London, 1967.
———, *Studies on the Civilization of Islam*, London, 1962.
———, *The Life of Saladin from the Works of ʿImād ad-Dīn and Bahāʾ ad-Dīn*, Oxford, 1973.
Gilli-Elewy, Hend, *Bagdad nach dem Sturz des Kalifats: Die Geschichte einer Provinz unter ilkhānischer Herrschaft (656–735/1258–1335)*, Berlin, 2000.
Goitein, S. D., *A Mediterranean Society*, 6 vols., Berkeley and Los Angeles, 1967–93.
———, *Letters of Medieval Jewish Traders*, Princeton, 1973.
———, "The Documents of the Cairo Geniza as a Source for Mediterranean Social History," *JAOS*, 80 (1960), 91–100.
———, "The Beginning of the Kārim Merchants and the Nature of their Organization," *Studies in Islamic History and Institutions*, Leiden, 1966.
Graf, G., *Die Epitome der Universalchronik Ibn ad-Dwādārīs im Verhältnis zur Langfassung*, Berlin, 1990.
Grehan, James, *Everyday Life and Consumer Culture in 18th-Century Damascus*, Seattle and London, 2007.
Grunebaum, G.E. von, *Muhammadan Festivals*, London, 1951.
Guo, Li, *Commerce, Culture, and Community in a Red Sea Port in the Thirteenth Century: The Arabic Documents from Quseir*, Leiden and Boston, 2004.
Haarmann, Ulrich, *Quellenstudien zur frühen Mamlukenzeit*, Freiburg, 1970.
———, "The Sons of Mamluks as Fief-holders in Late Medieval Period," T. Khalidi ed., *Land Tenure and Social Transformation in the Middle East*, Beirut, 1984, 141–168.
———, "Arabic in Speech, Turkish in Lineage: Mamluks and their Sons in the Intellectual Life of Fourteenth-Century Egypt and Syria," *Journal of Semitic Studies*, 33 (1988), 81–114.
Al-Ḥajjī, Ḥayāt Nāṣir, *The Internal Affairs in Egypt During the Third Reign of Sultan al-Nāṣir Muḥammad b. Qalāwūn, 709–741/1309–1341*, Kuwait, 1978.
———, *Aḥwāl al-ʿĀmma fī Ḥukm al-Mamālīk, 678–784/1279–1382: Dirāsa fī al-Jawānib al-Siyāsīya wal-Iqtiṣādīya wal-Ijtimāʿīya*, Kuwait, 1994.
———, "Baʿḍ al-Abʿād al-Iqtiṣādīya li-Salṭanat al-Mamālīk," *Ḥawliyāt al-Ādāb wal-ʿUlūm al-Ijtimāʿīya*, 23 (2002–03), al-Risāla 189, 7–117.

Halm, H., *Ägypten nach den mamlukischen Lehensregistern*, 2 vols., Wiesbaden, 1979–82.

Ḥamārneh, Ṣāliḥ, "Zirāʿat Qaṣab al-Sukkar wa-Ṣināʿatuh ʿinda al-ʿArab al-Muslimīn," *Annual of the Department of Antiquities*, Amman, 22 (1977–78), 12–19.

Hamarneh, Sami Kh., *The Physician, Therapist and Surgeon Ibn al-Quff*, Cairo, 1974.

Haneda, Masashi and Toru Miura ed., *Islamic Urban Studies: Historical Review and Perspectives*, London and New York, 1994.

Hanna, Nelly, *An Urban History of Būlāq in the Mamluk and Ottoman Periods*, Cairo, 1983.

———, *Making Big Money in 1600: The Life and Times of Ismaʿil Abu Taqiyya, Egyptian Merchant*, New York, 1998.

———, "Coffee and Coffee Merchants in Cairo 1580–1630," M. Tuchscherer ed., *Le commerce du café avant l'ère des plantations coloniales*, Cairo, 2001, 91–101.

Hanna, Nelly and Raouf Abbas ed., *Society and Economy in Egypt and the Eastern Mediterranean 1600–1900*, Cairo and New York, 2005.

Harīdī, Aḥmad A., *Fihrist Khiṭaṭ Miṣr*, 3 vols., Cairo, 1983–84.

Hasebe, Fumihiko, "Abnormal Weather, Famine, Epidemics, and Population Decrease in Fourteenth-Century Egypt (14 seiki Egypt no ijo kisho, kikin, ekibyo, jinko gensho, in Japanese)," *Rekishi ni okeru shizen* (Nature in History). Reflections on World History 1, Tokyo, 1989, 57–82.

Hasebe, Fumihiko ed., *Poor Relief in the Medieval Mediterranean Cities* (*Chusei kan Chichukai-ken toshi no kyuhin*, in Japanese), Tokyo, 2004.

Hashimoto, Hitoshi and Akikazu Takada ed., *Science of Sugar* (*Sato no Kagaku*, in Japanese), Tokyo, 2006.

Al-Hassan, Ahmad Y. and Donald R. Hill, *Islamic Technology: An Illustrated History*, Cambridge, New York, New Rochelle, Melbourne and Sydney, 1986.

Hattox, Ralph S., *Coffee and Coffeehouses: The Origins of a Social Beverage in the Medieval Near East*, Seattle and London, 1985.

Havemann, A., *Riʾāsa und Qaḍāʾ*, Freiburg, 1975.

Hillenbrand, Carole, *The Crusades: Islamic Perspectives*, Edinburgh, 1999.

Hinz, W., *Islamische Masse und Gewichte*, Leiden, 1955; English tr. by M.I. Marcinkowski, *Measures and Weights in the Islamic World*, Kuala Lumpur, 2003.

Holt, Peter M., *Egypt and the Fertile Crescent 1516–1922*, London, 1966.

———, *The Memoirs of a Syrian Prince Abū'l-Fidāʾ, Sultan of Ḥamāh (672–732/1273–1331)*, Wiesbaden, 1983.

———, *The Age of the Crusades: The Near East from the Eleventh Century to 1517*, London, 1986.

———, *Early Mamluk Diplomacy (1260–1290): Treaties of Baybars and Qalāwūn with Christian Rulers*, Leiden, 1995.

———, "The Position and Power of the Mamlūk Sultan," *BSOAS*, 38 (1975), 237–249.

Holt, Peter M. ed., *Political and Social Change in Modern Egypt*, London, 1968.

———, *The Eastern Mediterranean Lands in the Period of the Crusades*, Warminster, 1977.

Horii, Yutaka, "The Mamūk Sultan Qānṣūh al-Ghawrī (1501–16) and the Venetians in Alexandria," *Orient*, 38 (2003), 178–199.

Humphreys, R. S., *From Saladin to the Mongols: The Ayyubids of Damascus 1193–1260*, Albany, N.Y., 1977.

———, *Islamic History: A Framework for Inquiry*, Princeton, 1991; Revised ed., London, 1995.

———, "The Emergence of the Mamluk Army," *SI*, 45 (1977), 67–99.

Hunsberger, Alice C., *Nasir Khusraw, The Ruby of Badakhshan: A Portrait of the Persian Poet, Traveller and Philosopher*, London, 2000.

Igarashi, Daisuke, "The Establishment and Development of al-Dīwān al-Mufrad: Its Background and Implications," *Mamlūk Studies Review*, 10–1 (2006), 117–140.

Inalcik, Halil, *The Ottoman Empire: The Classical Age 1300–1600*, English tr. by N. Itzkowitz and C. Imber, London, 1973.

———, *The Middle East and the Balkans under the Ottoman Empire: Essays on Economy and Society*, Bloomington, 1993.

———, *Essays in Ottoman History*, Istanbul, 1998.

Inalcik, Halil and Donald Quataert ed., *An Economic and Social History of the Ottoman Empire 1300–1914*, Cambridge, 1994.

ʿInān, Muḥammad ʿAbd Allāh, *Miṣr al-Islāmīya wa-Taʾrīkh al-Khiṭaṭ al-Miṣrīya*, Cairo, 1969.

Index Islamicus: 1906–1980, Compiled by J.D. Pearson, 7 vols., Cambridge and London, 1958–83; *1981–1985*, Compiled by G.J. Roper, 2 vols., London, 1991.

International Sugar Organization, *Sugar Year Book*, 2009

Irwin, R., *The Middle East in the Middle Ages: The Early Mamluk Sultanate 1250–1382*, London, 1986.

———, "Iqṭāʿ and the End of the Crusader States," P.M. Holt ed., *The Eastern Mediterranean Lands in the Period of the Crusades*, Warminster, 1977, 62–77.

Ito, Hiroshi ed., *A Cultural History of Sugar: Japanese and Sugar* (*Sato no bunkashi: Nihonjin to sato*, in Japanese), Tokyo, 2008.

Jamāl al-Dīn, A. M., *al-Nuwayrī wa-Kitābuh Nihāyat al-Arab fī Funūn al-Adab*, Cairo, 1984.

Johansen, B., *The Islamic Law on Land Tax and Rent*, London, 1988.

Al-Juʿaydī, Shalabī Ibrāhīm I., *al-Azamāt wal-Awbiʾa fī Miṣr fī ʿAṣr al-Mamālīk al-Jarākisa*, Alexandria, 2002.

Kabir, M., *The Buwayhid Dynasty of Baghdad*, Calcutta, 1964.

Kamal, Hassan, *Encyclopaedia of Islamic Medicine*, Cairo, 1975.

Kawakita, Minoru, *A World History of Sugar* (*Sato no sekaishi*, in Japanese), Tokyo, 1996.

Kennedy, Hugh, *The Prophet and the Age of the Caliphates: The Islamic Near East from the Sixth to the Eleventh Century*, London and New York, 1986.

———, *Al-Ṭabarī: A Medieval Muslim Historian and His Work*, Princeton, 2008.

Kennedy, Hugh ed., *The Historiography of Islamic Egypt (c. 950–1800)*, Leiden, Boston, and Köln, 2001.

Khalidi, Tarif ed., *Land Tenure and Social Transformation in the Middle East*, Beirut, 1984.

Khan, M. S., *Studies in Miskawayh's Contemporary History (340–369 AH)*, Ann Arbor, 1980.

———, "The Effects of the *Iqṭāʿ* (land-grant) System under the Buwayhids," *IC*, 58 (1984), 289–305.

Khowaiter, Abdul-Aziz, *al-Malik al-Ẓāhir Baybars*, Riyad, 1976.

———, *Baibars The First: His Endeavours and Achievements*, London, 1978.

Kikuchi, Tadayoshi, "*Muḥtasib* in Cairo during the Mamluk Dynasty: An Analysis of their Personal History (Mamluk-cho jidai Cairo no *muḥtasib*: shusshin kaiso to keireki wo chushin ni, in Japanese)," *The Toyo Gakuho*, 64–1/2 (1983), 131–176.

Kinshichi, Norio, *Henry the Navigator* (*Enrike kokai oji*, in Japanese), Tokyo, 2004.

Klausner, C. L., *The Seljuk Vezirate: A Study of Civil Administration 1055–1194*, Cambridge, Mass., 1973.

Kobayashi, Akio, *Coffeehouses: Urban Life in Eighteenth Century London* (*Kofi hausu: Toshi no seikatsushi 18 seiki no London*, in Japanese), Tokyo, 1984.

Kortantamer, S., *Ägypten und Syrien zwischen 1317 und 1341 in der Chronik des Mufaḍḍal b. Abī l-Faḍāʾil*, Freiburg, 1978.

Kubiak, Wladyslaw B., *al-Fustat: Its Foundation and Early Urban Development*, Cairo, 1987.

Labib, Subhi Y., *Handelsgeschichte Ägyptens im Spätmittelalter (1171–1517)*, Wiesbaden, 1965.

———, "Egyptian Commercial Policy in the Middle Ages," M.A. Cook ed., *Studies in the Economic History of the Middle East*, London, 1970, 63–77.

Lambton, Ann K. S., *Landlord and Peasant in Persia*, London, 1953.

———, *State and Government in Medieval Islam*, Oxford, 1981.

———, *Continuity and Change in Medieval Persia*, Albany, N.Y., 1988.

———, "Two Safavid Soyūrghāls," *BSOAS*, 14 (1952), 44–54.

———, "Reflections on the IQṬĀʿ," G. Maqdisi ed., *Arabic and Islamic Studies in Honor of Hamilton A.R. Gibb*, Leiden, 1965, 358–376.

———, "Reflections on the Role of Agriculture in Medieval Persia," Abraham L. Udovitch ed., *The Islamic Middle East, 700–1900*, Princeton, 1981, 283–312.

Lane, Edward W., *An Account of the Manners and Customs of the Modern Egyptians*, London, 1836; repr. from the definitive fifth edition of 1860, Cairo, 2003.

———, *Arabic-English Lexicon*, 8 vols., London, 1863–93; repr. New York, 1955–56.

Lane-Poole, Stanley, *Saladin and the Fall of the Kingdom of Jerusalem*, London, 1898; repr. Beirut, 1964.

Lapidus, Ira M., *Muslim Cities in the Later Middle Ages*, Cambridge, Mass., 1967.

———, *A History of Islamic Societies*, Cambridge, 1988.

———, "The Grain Economy of Mamlūk Egypt," *JESHO*, 12 (1969), 1–15.

———, "Muslim Urban Society in Mamlūk Syria," A.H. Hourani and S.M. Stern ed., *The Islamic City*, Oxford, 1970, 195–205.

Lassner, Jacob, *The Topography of Baghdad in the Early Middle Ages*, Detroit, 1970.

———, *The Middle East Remembered: Forged Identities, Competing Narratives, Contested Spaces*, Ann Arbor, 2000.

Laufer, Berthold, *Sino-Iranica: Chinese Contributions to the History of Civilization in Ancient Iran*, Chicago, 1919; repr. Taipei, 1973.

Le Strange, G., *Palestine under the Moslems*, London, 1890; repr. Beirut, 1965.

———, *Baghdad during the Abbasid Caliphate*, Oxford, 1900; repr. New York, 1972.

———, *The Lands of the Eastern Caliphate*, London, 1905; repr. London, 1966.

Lev, Efraim and Zohar Amar, *Practical Materia Medica of the Medieval Eastern Mediterranean according to the Cairo Genizah*, Leiden and Boston, 2008.

Lev, Yaacov, *State and Society in Fatimid Egypt*, Leiden and New York, 1991.

Lev, Yaacov ed., *War and Society in the Eastern Mediterranean, 7th-15th Centuries*, Leiden, New York, and Köln, 1997.

Levanoni, Amaria, *A Turning Point in Mamluk History: The Third Reign of al-Nāṣir Muḥammad Ibn Qalāwūn 1310–1341*, Leiden, 1995.

———, "The al-Nashw Episode: A Case Study of 'Moral Economy,'" *Mamlūk Studies Review*, 9–1 (2005), 207–220.

Levey, M., *Early Arabic Pharmacology*, Leiden, 1973.

Levey, Reuben, *A Baghdad Chronicle*, Cambridge, 1929; repr. Philadelphia, 1977.

Lewis, Bernard, *Race and Slavery in the Middle East*, New York, 1973.

———, "Sources for the Economic History of the Middle East," M.A. Cook ed., *Studies in the Economic History of the Middle East*, London, 1970, 78–92.

———, "Ottoman Land Tenure and Taxation in Syria," *SI*, 50 (1979), 109–124.

Lewis, Bernard and Peter M. Holt ed., *Historians of the Middle East*, London, 1962.

Lippmann, Edmund O. von, *Geschichte des Zuckers*, Leipzig, 1890.

Little, Donald P., *An Introduction to Mamluk Historiography*, Wiesbaden, 1970.

———, *A Catalogue of the Islamic Documents from al-Ḥaram aš-Šarīf in Jerusalem*, Beirut, 1984.

———, *History and Historiography of the Mamlūks*, Variorum reprints, London, 1986.

———, "Coptic Converts to Islam during the Baḥrī Mamluk Period," M. Gervers and R.J. Bikhazi ed., *Conversion and Continuity: Indigenous Christian Communities in Islamic Lands, Eighth to Eighteenth Centuries*, Toronto, 1990, 263–288.

———, "Notes on the early *naẓar al-khāṣṣ*," Thomas Philipp and Urlich Haarmann ed., *The Mamluks in Egyptian Politics and Society*, Cambridge, 1998, pp. 235–253.

Lyons, Malcolm C. and D.E.P. Jackson, *Saladin: The Politics of the Holy War*, Cambridge, 1982.

MacKenzie, Neil D., *Ayyubid Cairo: A Topographical Study*, Cairo, 1992.

Maejima, Shinji, *Some Aspects of the Cultural Exchange between East and West* (*Tozai bunka koryu no shoso*, in Japanese), Tokyo, 1971.

Mahdi, Muhsin, *The Thousand and One Nights*, Leiden, 1995.

Mājid, ʿAbd al-Munʿim, *Nuẓum Dawlat Salāṭīn al-Mamālīk wa-Rusūmhum fī Miṣr*, 2 vols., Cairo, 1964–67.

Makdisi, Saree and Felicity Nussbaum ed., *The Arabian Nights in Historical Context: Between East and West*, Oxford, 2008.

Martel-Thoumian, Bernadette, *Les civils et l'administration dans l'état militaire Mamlūk* (*IX*e*/XV* e *siècle*), Damascus, 1992.

Marzolph, Ulrich and Richard van Leeuwen, *The Arabian Nights Encyclopedia*, 2 vols., Santa Barbara, 2004.

Matsuura, Toyotoshi, *Wind and Earthenware: An Account of Sugar* (*Kaze to Kame: Sato no Hanashi*, in Japanese), Fukuoka, 1987.

Mazuel, Jean, *Le sucre en Égypte: étude de géographie historique et économique*, Cairo, 1937.

Mazumdar, Sucheta, *Sugar and Society in China; Peasants, Technology, and the World Market*, Cambridge, Mass., 1998.

Meloy, John L., *Imperial Power and Maritime Trade: Mecca and Cairo in the Later Middle Ages*, Chicago, 2010.

———, "Imperial Strategy and Political Exigency: The Red Sea Spice Trade and the Mamluk Sultanate in the Fifteenth Century," *JAOS*, 123 (2003), 1–19.

Melville, Charles, "'The Year of the Elephant': Mamluk-Mongol Rivalry in the Hejaz in the Reign of Abū Saʿīd (1317–1335)," *Studia Iranica*, 21 (1992), 197–214.

Mez, Adam, *Die Renaissance des Islams*, Heidelberg, 1922; repr. Hildesheim, 1968.

Michel, Nicolas, "Devoirs fiscaux et droits fonciers: la condition des fellahs égyptiens (13e-16e siècles)," *JESHO*, 43 (2000), 521–578.

———, "Villages désertés, terres en friche et reconstruction rural en Égypte au début de l'époque ottoman," *AI*, 36 (2002), 197–251.

Mintz, Sidney W., *Sweetness and Power: The Place of Sugar in Modern History*, New York, 1985; Japanese tr. Minoru Kawakita and Koichi Wada, *Amasa to kenryoku: Sato ga kataru kindaishi*, Tokyo, 1988.

Miura, Toru, "The Ṣāliḥīyah Quarter in the Suburbs of Damascus: Its Formation, Structure, and Transformation in the Ayyūbid and Mamlūk Periods," *BEO*, 47 (1995), 129–181.

———, "Administrative Networks in the Mamluk Period," Tsugitaka Sato ed., *Islamic Urbanism in Human History: Political Power and Social Networks*, London, 1997, 39–76.

Miura, Toru and John E. Philips ed., *Slave Elites in the Middle East and Africa*, London, 2000.

Modarresi, H., *Kharāj in Islamic Law*, London, 1983.

Montgomery, James E. ed., *'Abbasid Studies: Occasional Papers of the School of 'Abbasid Studies, Cambridge 6–10 July 2002, Orientalia Lovaniensia Analecta 135*, Leuven, Paris, and Dudley, MA., 2004.

Morimoto, Kosei, *The Fiscal Administration of Egypt in the Early Islamic Period*, Kyoto, 1981.

———, "What Ibn Khaldūn Saw: The Judiciary of Mamluk Egypt," *Mamlūk Studies Review*, 6 (2002), 109–131.

Mortel, R. (Mūrtīl, R.), *al-Aḥwāl al-Siyāsīya wal-Iqtiṣādīya bi-Makka fī al-'Aṣr al-Mamlūkī*, Riyad, 1985.

———, "Taxation in the Amirate of Mecca during the Medieval Period," *BSOAS*, 58 (1995), 1–16.

Mottahedeh, Roy P., *Loyalty and Leadership in an Early Islamic Society*, Princeton, 1980.

Müller-Wodarg, D., "Die Landwirtschaft Ägyptens in der frühen 'Abbāsidenzeit," *Der Islam*, 31 (1954), 174–227; 32 (1956), 14–78, 141–167; 33 (1957), 107–114.

Muṣṭafā, Māhir Aḥmad, *Ṣa'īd Miṣr fī 'Ahd al-Mamālīk al-Jarākisa (784–922 AH /1382–1517 AD)*, Cairo, 2004.

Al-Nadawī, 'Abd al-Ḥalīm, *Minhaj al-Nuwayrī fī Kitābih Nihāyat al-Arab fī Funūn al-Adab*, Damascus, 1987.

Naga, Shohachiro, *A History of Black Sugar as Seen from the Source Materials in Okinawa and Amami* (*Okinawa-Amami no Bunken kara mita Kurozato no Rekishi*, in Japanese), Naha, 2003

Al-Najjār, Muḥammad Rajab, *Ḥikāyāt al-Shuṭṭār wal-'Ayyārīn fī al-Turāth al-'Arabī*, Kuwait, 1981.

Nāṣir, 'Āmir Najīb M., *al-Ḥayāt al-Iqtiṣādīya fī Miṣr fī al-'Aṣr al-Mamlūkī*, Amman, 2003.

Northrup, Linda S., *From Slave to Sultan: The Career of al-Manṣūr Qalāwūn and the Consolidation of Mamluk Rule in Egypt and Syria (678–689 AH. /1279–1290 AD)*, Stuttgart, 1998.

Ohtoshi, Tetsuya, "The Manners, Customs, and Mentality of Pilgrims to the Egyptian City of the Dead: 1100–1500 AD," *Orient*, 29 (1993), 19–44.

Ohtsuka, Kazuo ed., *Food Culture in the World* (*Sekai no shokubunka*, in Japanese) , vol. 10, *Arab*, Tokyo, 2007.

Ouerfelli, Mohamed, *Le sucre: production, commercialisation et usages dans la Méditerranée médiévale*, Leiden and Boston, 2008.

Pedersen, Johannes, *The Arabic Book*, English tr. by G. French, Princeton, 1984.

Pellat, Ch., *Cinq calendriers égyptiens*, Cairo, 1986.

———, "Le calendrier agricole de Qalqašandī," *AI*, 15 (1979), 165–185.

Perry, Charles, "A Thousand and One 'Fritters': The Food of the Arabian Nights," M. Rodinson, A.J. Arberry, and Ch. Perry, *Medieval Arab Cookery*, Trowbridge, 2006, 487–496.

Peters, F. E., *The Hajj: The Muslim Pilgrimage to Mecca and the Holy Places*. Princeton, 1994.

Petersen, A., "Continuity and Renewal: The Medieval Hajj Route through Syria and Jordan," K. D'Hulster and J. van Steenbergen ed., *Continuity and Change in the Realms of Islam: Studies in Honour of Professor Urbain Vermeulen, Orientalia Lovaniensia Analecta, 171*, Leuven, Paris, and Dudley, MA., 2008, 495–505.

Petry, Carl F., *The Civilian Elite of Cairo in the Later Middle Ages*, Princeton, 1981.

———, *Twilight of Majesty: The Reigns of the Mamlūk Sultans al-Ashraf Qāytbāy and Qānṣūh al-Ghawrī in Egypt*, Seattle and London, 1993.

———, *Protectors or Praetorians?: The Last Mamlūk Sultans and Egypt's Waning as a Great Power*, Albany, N.Y., 1994.

Petry, Carl ed., *The Cambridge History of Egypt*, vol. 1, *Islamic Egypt, 640–1517*, Cambridge, 1998.

Philipp, Thomas and Ulrich Haarmann ed., *The Mamluks in Egyptian Politics and Society*, Cambridge, 1998.

Pipes, D., *Slave Soldiers and Islam: The Genesis of a Military System*, New Haven and London, 1981.

Poliak, A. N., *Feudalism in Egypt, Syria, Palestine and the Lebanon, 1250–1900*, London, 1939.

———, "Les révoltes populaires en Égypte à l'époque des Mamelouks," *REI*, 8 (1934), 251–271.

Popovic, A., *La révolte des esclaves en Iraq au IIIe/IXe siècle*, Paris, 1976.

Popper, W., *The Cairo Nilometer*, Berkeley and Los Angeles, 1951.

———, *Egypt and Syria under the Circassian Sultans 1382–1468 AD: Systematic Notes to Ibn Taghrī Birdī's Chronicle of Egypt*, 2 vols., Berkeley and Los Angeles, 1955–57.

Pormann, Peter E. and Emilie Savage-Smith, *Medieval Islamic Medicine*, Washington, D.C., 2007.

Powell, J. M., *Muslims under Latin Rule 1100–1300*, Princeton, 1990.

Powers, David S., *Law, Society, and Culture in the Maghrib, 1300–1500*, Cambridge, 2002.

Qāsim, Qāsim ʿAbduh, *Ahl al-Dhimma fī Miṣr al-ʿUṣūr al-Wusṭā*, 2nd ed., Cairo, 1979.

Rabbat, Nasser O., *The Citadel of Cairo: A New Interpretation of Royal Mamluk Architecture*, Leiden, New York, and Köln, 1995.

———, "Al-Maqrizi's Khitat, an Egyptian *Lieu de Mémoire*," Doris Behrens-Abouseif ed., *The Cairo Heritage*, Cairo, 2000, 17–30.

Rabie, Hassanein, *The Financial System of Egypt AH 564–741/AD 1169–1341*, London, 1972.

———, "Some Technical Aspects of Agriculture in Medieval Egypt," Abraham L. Udovitch ed., *The Islamic Middle East, 700–1900*, Princeton, 1981, 59–90.

Rafeq, Abdul-Karim, *The Province of Damascus 1723–1783*, Beirut, 1966.

———, *Buḥūth fī al-Taʾrīkh al-Iqtiṣādī wal-Ijtimāʿī li-Bilād al-Shām*, Damascus, 1985.

———, "The Socioeconomic and Political Implications of the Introduction of Coffee into Syria. 16th-18th Centuries," M. Tuchscherer ed., *Le commerce du café avant l'ère des plantations coloniales*, Cairo, 2001, 127–142.

Rāġib, Yūsuf, *Marchands d'étoffes du Fayyoum au IIIe/IXe siècle d'après leurs archives* (*actes et lettres*), 3 vols., Cairo, 1982–92.

Ramzī, Muḥammad, *al-Qāmūs al-Jughrāfī lil-Bilād al-Miṣrīya*, 6 vols., Cairo, 1953–68.

Raymond, André, *Artisans et commerçants au Caire au XIIIe siècle*, 2 vols., Damascus, 1973–74.

———, *Le Caire*, Paris, 1993.

———, "La population du Caire, de Maqrīzī à la Description de l'Égypte," *BEO*, 37 (1975), 201–215.

Raymond, A. and G. Wiet, *Les marchés du Caire: Traduction annotée du texte de Maqrīzī*, Cairo, 1979.

Richards, D.S. ed., *Islamic Civilisation 950–1150*, Oxford, 1973.

Rivlin, Helen A., *The Agricultural Policy of Muḥammad ʿAlī in Egypt*, Cambridge, Mass., 1961.

Rodinson, Maxime, A.J. Arberry, and Ch. Perry ed., *Medieval Arab Cookery*, Trowbridge, 2006.

Rosenthal, Franz, *A History of Muslim Historiography*, 2nd revised edition, Leiden, 1968.

———, *The Herb: Hashish versus Medieval Muslim Society*, Leiden, 1971.

Sabari, S., *Mouvements populaires à Baghdad à l'époque ʿAbbaside*, Paris, 1981.

Sabra, Adam, *Poverty and Charity in Medieval Islam: Mamluk Egypt, 1250–1517*, Cambridge, 2000.

Saleh, A., "Les migration bédouines en Égypte au moyen âge," *Annali* (Istituto Orientale di Napoli), 41 (1981), 1–33.

El-Sāmarrāie, Ḥusām Q., *Agriculture in Iraq during the 3rd Century AH*, Beirut, 1972.

Sanders, Paula, *Ritual, Politics, and the City in Fatimid Cairo*, Albany, N.Y., 1994.

Sato, Tsugitaka, *Mamlūks: Muslim Rulers from the Non-Islamic World* (*Mamurūku: Ikyo no sekai kara kita Isuramu no sihaishatachi*, in Japanese), Tokyo, 1991

———, *State and Rural Society in Medieval Islam: Sultans, Muqtaʿs and Fallahun*, Leiden, 1997.

———, *State and Kingship in Islam* (*Isurāmu no kokka to oken*, in Japanese), Tokyo, 2004.

———, *Sugar in the Social Life of Medieval Islam* (*Sato no Isurāmu seikatsushi*, in Japanese), Tokyo, 2008.

———, "Irrigation in Rural Egypt from the 12th to the 14th Centuries," *Orient*, 8 (1972), 81–92.

———, "The Evolution of the Iqṭāʿ System under the Mamluks: An Analysis of al-Rawk al-Ḥusāmī and al-Rawk al-Nāṣirī," *Memoirs of the Research Department of The Toyo Bunko*, 37 (1979), 99–131.

———, "The Iqṭāʿ System of Iraq under the Buwayhids," *Orient*, 18 (1982), 83–105.

———, "The Proposers and Supervisors of *al-Rawk al-Nāṣirī* in Mamluk Egypt," *Mamlūk Studies Review*, 2 (1998), 73–92.

———, "Sugar in the Economic Life of Mamluk Egypt," *Mamlūk Studies Review*, 8–2 (2004), 87–107.

———, "Slave Traders and Kārimī Merchants during the Mamluk Period: A Comparative Study," *Mamlūk Studies Review*, 10–1 (2006), 141–156.

———, "Fiscal Administration in Syria during the Reign of Sultan al-Nāṣir Muḥammad," *Mamlūk Studies Review*, 11–1 (2007), 19–37.

———, "The Origin and Expansion of Sugar Production in the Islamic World," *Bulletin of the Graduate Division of Letters, Arts and Sciences of Waseda University*, 54 (2009), 5–20.

Sato, Tsugitaka ed., *Islamic Urbanism in Human History: Political Power and Social Networks*, London, 1997.

Sauvaget, J., *Alep: Essai sur le développement d'une grande ville syrienne, des origines au milieu du XIXe siècle*, Paris, 1941.

———, *La poste aux chevaux dans l'empire des Mamelouks*, Paris, 1941.

———, *Introduction à l'histoire de l'Orient musulman*, Paris, 1961; English ed. based on the 2nd edition as recast by Cl. Cahen, *Introduction to the History of the Muslim East*, Berkley and Los Angeles, 1965.

———, "Sur un papyrus arabe de la Bibliothèque Égyptienne," *Annales de l'Institut d'Études Orintales* (Alger), 7 (1948), 29–38.

———, "Noms et surnoms des Mamelouks," *Journal Asiatique*, 238 (1950), 31–58.

Schacht, J., *An Introduction to Islamic Law*, Oxford, 1964.

Schafer, Edward H., *The Golden Peaches of Samarqand: A Study of T'ang Exotics*, Berkeley, Los Angeles, and London, 1963.

Schimmel, Annemarie, *Islamic Names*, Edinburgh, 1989.

Schwarz, P., "Die Zuckerpressen von Ahwāz," *Der Islam*, 6 (1916), 269–279.

Serjeant, R. B., *Islamic Textiles: Material for a History up to the Mongol Conquest*, Beirut, 1972.

Setton, K.M. ed., *A History of the Crusades*, 6 vols., Madison, Milwaukee, and London, 1969–89.

Sezgin, Fuat, *Geschichte des Arabischen Schrifttums*, 13 vols., Leiden, 1967–2007.

Sharon, M. ed., *Studies in Islamic History and Civilization in Honor of Professor David Ayalon*, Jerusalem and Leiden, 1986.

Shatzmiller, Maya ed., *Crusaders and Muslims in Twelfth-Century Syria*, Leiden, New York, and Köln, 1993.

Shaw, Stanford J., *The Financial and Administrative Organization of Ottoman Egypt 1517–1798*, Princeton, 1958.

Shimada, Johei, *State and Society in Islam* (*Isuramu no kokka to shakai*, in Japanese), Tokyo, 1977.

———, *Studies on the Early Islamic States* (*Shoki isurāmu kokka no kenkyu*, in Japanese), Tokyo, 1996.

Shimizu, Kosuke, "*Irshād al-Zirāʿa:* The Crop Cultivation Manual (*Irshād al-Zirāʿa* ni okeru sakumotsu saibaiho kakuron, in Japanese) 1–2," *Shien*, 133 (1996), 55–73; 134 (1997), 1–19.

Shoshan, Boaz, *Popular Culture in Medieval Cairo*, Cambridge, 1993.

Smith, G. R., *The Ayyūbids and Early Rasūlids in the Yemen (567–694/1173–1295)*, London, 1978.

Smith, S. D., "The Early Diffusion of Coffee Drinking in England," M. Tuchscherer ed., *Le commerce du café avant l'ère des plantations coloniales*, Cairo, 2001, 245–268.

Sobernheim, M., "Das Zuckermonopol unter Sultan Barsbāi", *Zeitschrift für Assyriologie*, 27 (1912), 75–84.

Steenbergen, Jo van, *Order Out of Chaos: Patronage, Conflict and Mamluk Socio-Political Culture, 1341–1382*, Leiden and Boston, 2006.

———, "*Taqwīm al-Buldān al-Miṣrīya* (C.U.L. MS. Qq.65). Identifying a Late Medieval Cadastral Survey of Egypt," U. Vermeulen and J. van Steenbergen ed., *Egypt and Syria in the Fatimid, Ayyubid and Mamluk Eras*, IV, Leuven and Dudley, MA., 2005, 475–489.

Stern, S.M. ed., *Documents from Islamic Chanceries*, S.M. Stern and R. Walzer ed., *Oriental Studies*, vol. 3, Oxford, 1965.

Surūr, Muḥammad Jamāl al-Dīn, *Dawlat Banī Qalāwūn fī Miṣr: al-Ḥālat al-Siyāsīya wal-Iqtiṣādīya fī ʿAhdihā bi-Wajh Khāṣṣ*, Cairo, 1947.

Suzuki, Kikuko, "On the Importance of the Arab Cookery Books in Medieval Islamic Period (Chusei Arabu ryorisho no keito to tokucho nitsuite, in Japanese)," *Oriento*, 37–2 (1994), 88–107.

Tadmurī, ʿUmar ʿAbd al-Salām, *Taʾrīkh Ṭarābulus al-Siyāsī wal-Ḥaḍārī ʿabra al-ʿUṣūr*, 2 vols., Tripoli, 1978–81.

Tai, Kokuki, *The Evolution of Sugar Production in China* (*Chūgoku Kansho-togyo no tenkai*, in Japanese), Tokyo, 1967.

Takayama, Hiroshi, *The Administration of the Norman Kingdom of Sicily*, Leiden, New York, and Köln, 1993.

Taqizadeh, S. H., "Various Eras and Calendars Used in the Countries of Islam," *BSOAS*, 9 (1937–39), 903–922; 10 (1940–42), 107–132.

Thorau, P., *Sultan Baibars I von Ägypten*, Wiesbaden, 1987; English tr. by P.M. Holt, *The Lions of Egypt: Sultan Baybars I & the Near East in the Thirteenth Century*, London and New York, 1987.

Tsunoyama, Sakae, *A World History of Tea* (*Cha no sekaishi*, in Japanese), Tokyo, 1980.

Tuchscherer, M. ed., *Le commerce du café avant l'ère des plantations coloniales*, Cairo, 2001.

Tucker, William, "Natural Disasters and the Peasantry in Mamlūk Egypt," *JESHO*, 24 (1981), 215–224.

———, "Environmental Hazards, Natural Disasters, Economic Loss, and Mortality in Mamluk Syria," *Mamlūk Studies Review*, 3 (1999), 109–128.

Ṭurkhān, Ibrāhīm ʿAlī, *al-Nuẓum al-Iqṭāʿīya fī al-Sharq al-Awsaṭ fī al-ʿUṣūr al-Wusṭā*, Cairo, 1963.

Udovitch, Abraham L., *Partnership and Profit in Medieval Islam*, Princeton, 1970.

———, "England to Egypt, 1350–1500: Long-term Trends and Long-distance Trade, IV. Egypt," M.A. Cook ed., *Studies in the Economic History of the Middle East*, London, 1970, 115–128.

———, "Technology, Land Tenure, and Rural Society: Aspects of Continuity in the Agricultural History of the Pre-Modern Middle East," id. ed., *The Islamic Middle East, 700–1900: Studies in Economic and Social History*, Princeton, 1981, 11–26.

———, "Merchants and Amīrs: Government and Trade in Eleventh Century Egypt," *Asian and African Studies (Haifa)*, 22 (1988), 53–72.

Udovitch, Abraham L. ed., *The Islamic Middle East, 700–1900: Studies in Economic and Social History*, Princeton, 1981.

Ullmann, Manfred, *Islamic Medicine*, Edinburgh, 1978.

Varisco, D. M., *Medieval Agriculture and Islamic Science: The Almanac of a Yemeni Sultan*, Seattle, 1994.

Vermeulen, U., "Some Remarks on a Rescript of an-Nāṣir Muḥammad b. Qalāʾūn on the Abolition of Taxes and the Nuṣayris (Mamlaka of Tripoli, 717/1317)," *Orientalia Lovaniensia Periodica*, 1 (1970), 195–201.

Vermeulen, U., D. de Swet, etc. ed., *Egypt and Syria in the Fatimid, Ayyubid and Mamluk Eras*, I-III, Leuven, 1995–2001.

Waines, David, *In a Caliph's Kitchen: Medieval Arabic Cooking for the Modern Gourmet*, London, 1989.

Waley, Muhammad Isa ed., *Islamic Codicology: An Introduction to the Study of Manuscripts in Arabic Script*, London, 2005.

Walker, Bethany J., "The Role of Agriculture in Mamluk-Jordanian Power Relations," *BEO*, Numéro Supplément 57 (2008), 79–99.

Watson, Andrew M., *Agricultural Innovation in the Early Islamic World*, Cambridge, London, and New York, 1983.

Willcocks, W., *Egyptian Irrigation*, London, 1889.

Winter, Michael and Amalia Levanoni ed., *The Mamluks in Egyptian and Syrian Politics and Society*, Leiden and Boston, 2004.

Yajima, Hikoichi, *The Formation of the Islamic World and the International Commerce: With Special Reference to Changes of the International Commercial Networks* (*Isuramu sekai no seiritsu to kokusai shogyo: kokusai shogyo network no hendo wo chushin ni*, in Japanese), Tokyo, 1991.

———, *A History as Seen from the Sea* (*Kaiiki kara mita rekishi*, in Japanese), Nagoya, 2006.

———, "The International Trade Routes connecting the Nile Valley Basin with the Red Sea Coast: On the Qūṣ–ʿAydhāb Route based on al-Tujībī's *al-Riḥlah* (Nile gawa keikoku to Kokai wo musubu kokusai route: tokuni Qus–ʿAydhab route wo megutte, in Japanese)," *Isuramu Sekai* (*The Islamic World*), 25–26 (1986), 1–25.

———, "On the Date of Decline of ʿAydhāb, an International Port of Trade on the Red Sea," *Journal of East-West Maritime Relations*, 1 (1989), 167–197.

Yanagihashi, Hiroyuki, *A History of the Early Islamic Law of Property: Reconstructing the Legal Development, 7th-9th Centuries*, Leiden and Boston, 2004.

Young, M.J. L., J.D. Latham, and R.B. Serjeant ed., *Religion, Learning and Science in the ʿAbbasid Period*, Cambridge, 1990.

Yusuf, M. D., *Economic Survey of Syria during the Tenth and Eleventh Centuries*, Berlin, 1985.

Zaouali, Lilia, *Medieval Cuisine of the Islamic World*, English tr. by M.B. DeBevoise, Berkeley and Los Angeles, 2007.

Ziadeh, N. A., *Urban Life in Syria under the Early Mamlūks*, Beirut, 1953; repr. Westport, Conn., 1970.

———, *Damascus under the Mamlūks*, Norman, 1964.

Ziyāda, Muḥammad Muṣṭafā etc., *Dirāsāt ʿan al-Maqrīzī*, Cairo, 1971.

Index

www.ingramcontent.com/pod-product-compliance
Ingram Content Group UK Ltd.
Pitfield, Milton Keynes, MK11 3LW, UK
UKHW022224051026
15624UKWH00002B/334

9 789004 277526